Working With Interpreters and Translators

A Guide for Speech-Language Pathologists and Audiologists

Henriette W. Langdon, EdD, FASHA, CCC-SLP
Terry Irvine Saenz, PhD, CCC-SLP

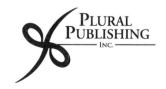

PLURAL
PUBLISHING
INC.

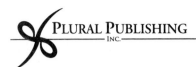

PLURAL PUBLISHING
INC.

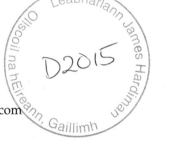

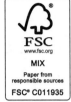

5521 Ruffin Road
San Diego, CA 92123

e-mail: info@pluralpublishing.com
Website: http://www.pluralpublishing.com

Copyright © by Plural Publishing, Inc. 2016

Typeset in 11/14 Palatino by Flanagan's Publishing Services, Inc.
Printed in the United States of America by McNaughton & Gunn, Inc.

Cover image courtesy of Kevin Starr.

Library of Congress Cataloging-in-Publication Data

Langdon, Henriette W., author.
  Working with interpreters and translators : a guide for speech-language pathologists and audiologists / Henriette W. Langdon, Terry I. Saenz.
      p. ; cm.
  Includes bibliographical references and index.
  ISBN 978-1-59756-611-7 (alk. paper)—ISBN 1-59756-611-X (alk. paper)
  I. Saenz, Terry I. (Terry Irvine), author. II. Title.
  [DNLM: 1. Interprofessional Relations. 2. Speech-Language Pathology—methods. 3. Translating. 4. Audiology—methods. 5. Cultural Diversity. 6. Multilingualism. WL 340.2]
  RC423
  616.85'5—dc23
                                                    2015019519

Contents

List of Videos

Henriette W. Langdon and Maxine B. Langdon Starr

Video Clip 1. Expectations of Interpreters and Translators Who Collaborate With Interpreters and Translators
 A Quick Background of the Profession
 Types of Interpreting
 Types of Translation
 Expectations

Video Clip 2. Interpretation in Action: Interviews and Conferences
 Contents
 Following the BID Process
 Briefing (Demonstration)
 Interaction for Interviews (Demonstration)
 Interaction for Conferences (Demonstration)
 Debriefing (Demonstration)

Video Clip 3. The Role of the Interpreter/Translator in Hearing Assessments
 General Statement
 A Typical Day in the Life of a Hearing Aid Dispenser
 Assessment Conducted by a Hearing Aid Dispenser
 Demonstration of Typical Hearing Aids
 The Sound-Proof Booth[1]

Video Clip 4. The BID Process in SLP Assessments: When There Are Normed Tests in the Language (e.g., Spanish)
 Change of Roles
 Obtaining and Analyzing a Language Sample
 When There Are Normed Tests in the Language (Spanish)
 What to Be Aware of When Using a Normed Test
 Scenario With an 8-Year-Old
 Responding to Selected Subtests of the CELF-4 (Spanish)
 Debriefing the Assessment Process

---

[1]This video addresses the dilemmas in working with a hearing aid dispenser instead of an audiologist. It was carried out to offer an additional perspective of situations where the assistance of an interpreter might be needed when a client's proficiency is limited in English.

Foreword

I am not a speech-language pathologist (SLP), an audiologist, an interpreter/translator (I/T), a psychologist, counselor, linguist, teacher, or a school/hospital administrator. So, why would I be interested in writing the foreword to a guide on collaborating with interpreters and translators with practitioners whose fields, speech-pathology and audiology, are tangentially related to mine? For all the titles and qualifications I may not seem to have, I nevertheless consider that I possess some background and experience to offer comments on this very important topic of collaborating with I/Ts.

We all are well aware that we live in a world that is increasingly culturally and linguistically diverse, a phenomenon that we are experiencing not only in the United States but throughout the entire globe. Despite a greater number of bilingual specialists available in different fields, there continues to be a vast discrepancy between supply and demand for services for clients whose English is limited and who have very diverse linguistic backgrounds. Even if you are considered a bilingual specialist, you may need to know how to collaborate effectively with an I/T when you are not proficient in your client's language, and an assessment is needed to evaluate his or her skills in an equitable, ethical, and legally appropriate manner.

I am a bilingual licensed marriage and family therapist (LMFT), and I have been working as a mental health specialist (MHS) for almost 3 years. My services are contracted to a large school district,

and I work with many bilingual primarily Spanish-speaking students. My job requires that I participate in individual education plan (IEP) meetings, collaborate with general education and subject-matter teachers, school administrators and staff, parents, and I/Ts to plan and evaluate students' progress. My major charge is to assist these students with their social and emotional goals so that they have a fair chance to succeed academically, vocationally, and personally.

As the only child of an ambitious and hardworking SLP who also happens to be my accomplished mother, I have been exposed to many of the roles taken in the profession. During most of my upbringing, she was eager to conduct every test on the planet known to SLPs in the languages of French, English, and Spanish to try out the test or collect some norms (yes, I'm trilingual). I can attest to being thrown into the client chair more times than most children are ever asked to do. More important, I enjoyed trying my best to impress my mother and her eager SLP graduate students with my intelligence and linguistic skills. Aside from this, however, I decided along the way of being used as a testing "guinea pig" that my mother had already saturated the SLP field, and so I chose the field of psychology instead. My choice to ultimately become a therapist was not that simple, as many therapists and helping professionals say the field chose them as much as they chose their vocation.

Similarly to any lengthy test used in speech-language pathology, which typically comprises multiple parts with many sections, the individual who is asked to take this test is also multifaceted. There are some characteristics of that individual that cannot be measured by a standardized test. Human beings have strengths and weaknesses that are unique to their own personal character and may not be measured by their responses to a given set of test items. Upon entering my field, I believed that my strengths were observation and language expression. Also, we need to consider that we only have a limited number of tests in a few languages for monolingual speakers and an even fewer number for bilingual speakers of Spanish-English or other frequently spoken languages like Chinese-English or French-Spanish. The fact is that, overall, the fields of speech and language pathology and audiology lack materials to equitably assess the numerous languages and combinations of two languages that may come across during our daily work. Therefore, other measures that may be attained through careful observation need to be considered. Many of the conclusions we might reach need to be carefully interpreted taking into account the background, growth and development, experiences, the culture, and the specific structures and uses of the languages of the client we are with, to say the least. My own early development illustrates some of these aspects.

Early on during my infancy, I frustrated my mother extensively because I was silent for over 2 years. I did not utter a complete or "true" word as a baby. She tells me almost every year around my birthday of how much I made her worry that I was going to be a mute child. However, in hindsight, I have given her an explanation saying that I was not mute but rather observing the world around me. I was acting like an absorbent sponge, immersing myself in all the sights, smells, sounds, tastes, and touches available within my reach. I was listening and watching. I have always been somewhat intuitive, as I can guess what a person is thinking simply by observation. Naturally, these personality traits have assisted me a great deal as a mental health professional. I also imagine they are advantageous to SLPs and also especially to I/Ts.

There is a well-known saying that I grew up with and continue saying, which is, "There is no 'I' in 'TEAM.'" I have always been part of a professional team when I work in the schools, with other disciplines, or among my colleagues in supervision, trainings or collaborating on difficult cases. Even when I was growing up, I was competing on a sports team (figure skating drill team, cheerleading), performing concerts as part of the school orchestra, or providing the soundtrack for the school plays. I could not have accomplished these personal or professional feats alone, but yet I always had a distinct role to play. In IEP meetings, I am the prime commentator on the student's emotional or behavioral goals and presentation. In sporting events, I was the support and the base so that our flyer could hit a back-tuck basket toss. In the orchestra, I have played the roles of concert chair and also background percussionist. In both aspects, I had to do my part and play my role, so that the student, the team or the patient/client/consumer benefited but also so that I had felt that I had made an impact or a difference. Who is going to be the one to advocate for these children, clients, students, parents, or those without the ability to communicate? Of course, the SLPs, teachers, administrators, psychologists, mental health professionals, school and hospital personnel, and graduate students reading this book should already have the answer: US. Not only just YOU can make a difference, but also working as a team, the effects become united and have a resounding effect on everyone as a whole.

I would imagine this book is not only for those who work with I/Ts in various settings but also so that the I/T can have a voice, an importance, a distinction, and an identity of his or her own. We who provide human services do not carry on this work for our own personal benefit (although, of course, being paid for what one loves to do is an added bonus). Everyone who is on a team has his or her own distinct role, even if it is just to sit back and observe (as I know from my own experience). We must begin to take the role of the I/T more seriously and definitively. Let us give I/Ts their own voice and recognition, just as the SLP helps give the gifts of language and communication to those who could not otherwise facilitate those skills independently. Without the I/Ts' unique skills that allow us to bridge the needed communication with our clients and their families, we would be unable to serve many individuals who seek our services.

I hope this book will inspire those of us who make a difference every day in people's lives to also acknowledge and recognize the unique skills and strengths the I/T brings and to be better prepared and trained to work and interact with these professionals going forward.

With gratitude, admiration, and respect for all the work I/Ts, SLPs, audiologists, mental health professionals, administrators of all sorts, and staff do to better the lives of everyone around them.

—Maxine B. Langdon Starr,
PhD, LMFT

Contributor

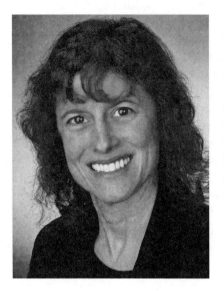

Teresa L. Wolf, MS, CCC-SLP, is a clinical professor in speech-language pathology at the University of Memphis. She holds the Certificate of Clinical Competence from the American Speech-Language-Hearing Association. Her areas of clinical interest include voice, articulation, and working with culturally and linguistically diverse populations. She has presented nationwide on the topic of working with interpreters and has been a coauthor on several journal publications. She is currently the coprincipal investigator on a grant funded by the U.S. Department of Education, which focuses on training graduate students to work with interpreters in the field of speech-language pathology.

Acknowledgments

I have always enjoyed reading or composing this section because a book, a guide, or any created work cannot be completed without the help and support of others.

First, I find it necessary to provide the readers a short history that precedes the birth of this second edition on collaborating with interpreters and translators in speech-language pathology and audiology. The conception of this new edition was not easy, and I realize my story mirrors that of many other authors. But, I needed to share with readers how seemingly unrelated events can ultimately converge to create a positive ending. Thinking Publications, under the leadership of its founder and editor Nancy McKinley, produced the two guides on speech-language pathologists and audiologists collaborating with interpreters and translators in 2002. As of 2010, the company that bought out Thinking Publications, after Nancy's passing in 2005, decided to no longer reprint the guides. It had been my intent to rewrite the guides, and I tried to negotiate a contract with another editing company, but it resulted in an unsuccessful endeavor. Toward the end of 2010, Carl, my husband, was diagnosed with lung cancer, and he passed in the spring of 2012. Due to this unfortunate event, my project to write a second edition was pushed to the side. Then one day, in the fall of 2013, I received a copy of an e-mail written by Dr. Linda Jarmulowicz, Associate Professor and Associate Dean in the School of Communicative Sciences and Disorders at the University of Memphis in Tennessee, addressed to one of the editors of the company that terminated the printing of the guides asking for additional copies, and she was told they were out of print. Linda had used the two publications to train her students on working with interpreters and translators in speech-language pathology and audiology through a grant that she had written with this volume's guest author, Clinical Professor Teresa L. Wolf. This e-mail provided me with the necessary incentive to contact Plural Publishers. By then, I had had the pleasure to meet Valerie Johns, Senior Editor, at the Spring California Speech-Language-Hearing Association Convention, who had encouraged me to write a proposal. But, I had not taken any action until I received the magical e-mail. Therefore, my first thank you goes to Linda for giving me the incentive to embark on this project, and the second thank you is for Teresa, who graciously accepted my invitation to write Chapter 7 on training issues, adding on her first-hand experience and expertise in training graduate students to work effectively with interpreters and translators.

My third thank you goes to my coauthor, Dr. Terry Irvine Saenz, who agreed to navigate with me on this venture after my former writing partner, Dr. Lilly Cheng, decided she needed to put her effort into her multiple new projects. Terry, who had been my writing partner in the past, was once again an excellent collaborator. Terry wrote Chapters 3 and 4, which include entirely new material and the latest literature to support her information. Terry would like to acknowledge the input she received from Dr. HyeKyeung Seung for a draft of Chapter 3. In addition to writing her two chapters, Terry offered invaluable support and patience by reading at least two drafts of the four chapters I rewrote, including Chapter 7, written by Teresa. Also, her help in reading the entire manuscript once it came to us in the typesetting edition was invaluable. Her attention to detail is immeasurable! Altogether, my writing partners proved to be the most punctual and reliable team I have ever had.

Terry, Teresa, and I wish to thank Valerie Johns, Executive Editor, and Kalie Koscielak, Project Editor, in facilitating the distribution and feedback from our reviewers and for coordinating the editing and final product, and Megan Carter and Alya Hameed for their assistance in the copyediting phase of the project. We also very grateful for the feedback from our reviewers, Dr. Elisabeth Wiig, Nancy Castilleja, and Kristin McNeil. Their comments assisted all of us in producing a clearer text. A few other anonymous reviewers took the time to read and comment on earlier drafts of the manuscript, and we greatly appreciate their feedback as well.

Direct input through e-mails and phone conversations from several audiologists and/or specialists in deaf and hard-of-hearing individuals was extremely helpful in securing that the material would be as accurate and up-to-date as possible in the area of working with interpreters and translators in audiology covered in Chapters 5 and 6. I want to extend my thanks to Dr. Sandy Bowen, Susan Clark, Dr. Mitzarie A. Carlo Colón, Evelyn Merritt, and Dr. Christine Yoshinaga-Itano who took time to answer multiple questions and offer their own insights on this issue. Special thanks to my colleague, Dr. June McCullough, who was willing to discuss some of the dilemmas of working with a language interpreter/translator in audiology and provided me with very

needed comments on some sections of Chapters 5 and 6. Dr. Lu-Feng Shi, professor of audiology at Long Island University, kindly suggested some feedback and further references. Last but not least, I wish to thank my old friend and colleague, Dr. Lilly Cheng, who agreed to give away some of her time to write the Epilogue.

I also wish to thank Dr. Katarzyna Węsierska, Professor from the University of Silesia in Katowice, Poland, for encouraging her doctoral student, Katarzyna Gaweł, to undertake a dissertation topic on collaborating with interpreters and translators in Poland. Last but not least, my great appreciation also goes to Dr. Barbara Morrill who has offered me encouragement and support during the completion of this project, and Dr. Gloria Weddington for her continued support of my work.

The zeal to try my best and continue to learn has been instilled by two exceptional individuals who both have served as my mentors, and I want to thank them both for being excellent models: Dr. Paula Menyuk and Dr. Elisabeth Wiig, both Emerita Professors from Boston University, where I received my doctorate degree.

And, finally, the book could not have been completed without the help of Maxine Langdon Starr, who is directly related to me, as she is my daughter. Maxine reviewed the entire manuscript and wrote the Foreword. She also helped me design, produce, and edit the video clips that are part of this guide. We spent many hours together planning and editing each tape. We are most grateful to those who were brave and accepted to take on various roles in these tapes. Another person I wish to thank is Kevin Starr, Maxine's husband, who kindly let her go when I needed her to complete work on this project and offered his artistic talent by giving his input on the cover of the book.

Last, Spottie Dottie, a little white dog with brown and black spots on her ears and a few others spread around her body, played a very important role. During the course of writing this guide, she spent her time lying next to me or on my lap. And, she also offered me some of the unconditional love and tenderness that I have needed following the loss of my husband Carl. Thank you Spottie Dottie!

In memory of Nancy McKinley, MS, CCC-SLP Founder and CEO of Thinking Publications, who believed in my ideas and work and who edited as well as published the first edition of the guide on Collaborating With Interpreters and Translators and the Interpreters and Translators in Communication Disorders: A Practitioner's Manual, both in 2002.

—Henriette W. Langdon

I dedicate this book to my daughter, Sara Elizabeth Saenz; my parents, Dr. Robert Philip and Jacqueline Lee Irvine; and my siblings, Holly Anne Irvine, Karen Irvine Tait, and Robert Scott Irvine. I am grateful beyond words for their support over the years.

—Terry Irvine Saenz

Part I

A Guide for the Speech-Language Pathologist and Audiologist

Working with Interpreters and Translators: A Guide for Speech-Language Pathologists and Audiologists Part I is a revision of two original publications, *Collaborating With Interpreters and Translators: A Guide for Communication Disorders Professionals* (Langdon & Cheng, 2002) and *Interpreters and Translators in Communication Disorders: A Practitioner's Handbook* (Langdon, 2002), originally published by Thinking Publications (Eau Claire, WI). A revision seemed necessary of this important process because everyone is well aware that demographics in the United States are continually growing and changing. A recent report by Bager (2013) indicates that 17.9% of American households reported they spoke another language than English in 2000, and as of 2011, that percentage increased to 20.8%. At the same time, the number of English-language learners or ELL has grown significantly in most states in the nation. In some states such as California, close to 25% of students enrolled in the public schools are ELL. Although the reader may encounter variations from study to study, a recent

document available through the National Center on Statistics (2014) reported that "the percentage of public school students in the United States who were English-language learners was higher in the school year 2011–12 (9.1 percent, or an estimated 4.4 million students) than in 2002–03 (8.7 percent, or an estimated 4.1 million students)." These statistics have implications not only for education and health but also for the provision of specialized services in allied health professions such as speech-language pathology and audiology. Additionally, federal and state laws mandate that all individuals be assessed in an equitable manner by utilizing these individuals' preferred language or modality of communication. Even though efforts have been put forth to train bilingual professionals to provide services in a variety of languages, the demand most often exceeds the supply of these professionals. And, in the past 10 to 15 years, there are more certified bilingual personnel in the fields of speech-language pathology and audiology, but demands for such professionals continue to exceed their supply. This is a dilemma that exists not only in the United States but also over the entire globe as more people immigrate to various countries for political reasons or in search of a better life.

Thirty years ago, in 1985, I was fortunate to attend one of the most rewarding meetings at the American Speech-Language-Hearing Association (ASHA) that I can recall in my long career of 40 years in speech-language pathology. The primary goal of that meeting, headed by Dr. Lorraine Cole, then director of ASHA's Multicultural Affairs office, was on how we, as a profession, can best serve the growing diverse population in our nation., An entire publication of *ASHA* followed that highlighted important points discussed in that meeting, including some position papers. A reference to this document is made in Chapter 1 (ASHA, 1985). One of the intents was to delineate best practices in assessing and serving multilingual and multicultural populations in our field with the message that in case there is no access to a bilingual speech-language pathologist or audiologist who can provide services in our client's language, the second best approach is to work with a trained interpreter/translator. During the past 30 years that have elapsed since then, I have had a chance to collaborate with colleagues in drafting a manual and the two books mentioned at the beginning of this introduction, as well as training speech-language pathologists (SLPs), audiologists, psychologists, teachers, and special education personnel, including individuals assigned to be interpreters on how to best collaborate with interpreters and translators when assessing ELL students and communicating with their families. Most of my work has been conducted in specifically serving the pediatric population in the public school or clinic settings but not excluding the medical setting, and this is the focus of this guide. Therefore, the focus of this

guide is on the younger population (ages infancy through 22 years of age), with which all of the authors of this guide are most familiar. However, many of the strategies described can be applied in serving the adult population as well. The book is written for SLPs, audiologists, general and special educators, psychologists, administrators, students, and, very importantly, personnel who act as interpreters/translators. We hope the content will serve as a foundation to perform a job that ultimately will benefit the student and his or her family. Although there is virtually no research on best practices to follow in this process, the content may perhaps serve as a platform for future research in documenting preferred approaches and strategies. The information presented is extracted from practices used in various fields where interpreting and translation are necessary, such as international conferences, legal settings, and medical and community settings, including interpreting for the deaf and hard-of-hearing population. Additionally, the content is supported by a review of the most current relevant literature, observations, personal experiences, and practice in training various professionals and students over the years by the authors in using many of the strategies described in this guide as well as direct feedback from those who have direct experience with the process.

The guide includes a Foreword written by Maxine B. Langdon Starr and 10 different chapters written by one of the two authors of this guide, Henriette W. Langdon or Terry Irvine Saenz, and our invited guest author, Teresa L. Wolf. An Epilogue written by Lilly Cheng can be found at the end of the guide. Each chapter in Part I includes a list of topics to be reviewed, content, some follow-up activities, and references. This new version includes a great deal of new information even though some sections of the first volumes still remain. For example, the chapter on demographics (Chapter 1) has been updated and expanded, and there is much more material on cultural aspects that are covered as well as the specific roles played by the interpreter in this process (Chapters 3 and 4). The chapter on assessment has been expanded and includes more detailed information for each of the two disciplines, speech-language pathology and audiology (Chapter 6). Chapter 7 covers material that has been adapted in training interpreters and translators in a speech-pathology and audiology university department.

DESCRIPTION OF PART I CHAPTERS

Chapter 1, "Bridging Linguistic Diversity" (Henriette W. Langdon), includes a brief historical perspective of the process of interpretation and translation, and it discusses the need for interpreters and translators in the fields of speech-language pathology and audiology based on mandated federal and state laws while presenting statistics pertaining to languages spoken in the world and some of their characteristics. Additionally, current data on the top 10 most frequently languages spoken in the world, including the ones that are most frequently spoken by English-language learners (ELL) in the United States, are reported. Finally, interpreting and translating methods used in various contexts such as international conferences, medical settings, and court proceedings are described.

Chapter 2, "Communication Issues in a Multilingual Society" (Henriette W. Langdon), serves as a review for the experienced SLP or audiologist but may be helpful to the practicing student and interpreter/translator (I/T). The content includes a description of verbal and nonverbal aspects of interpretation and a brief discussion of the difference between language and dialect.

Verbal aspects of communication such as phonology, suprasegmentals, grammar, semantics, and pragmatics, as well as the use of gestures, facial expressions, and emotions with ramifications for speech and language and audiological evaluations, are described next. A discussion follows on phenomena that occur when two languages are in contact, that is, early awareness of two languages, code-switching, and language loss. A description of specific skills to achieve successful written translations follows. Identifying how both verbal and nonverbal patterns of communication affect the interpretation process is discussed at the end of the chapter.

Chapter 3, "Cultural Elements" (Terry Irvine Saenz), includes topics on definitions of specific terms such as *culture* and *acculturation* as well as descriptions of *disability, handicap, illness,* and *pain* from a multicultural perspective. The issue of confidentiality is discussed next with a review of cross-cultural beliefs about different causes of disabilities that may be broadly categorized as *visible* or *invisible.* Access and exposure to resources by multicultural populations are described as well as the varying role family members play as decision makers for services. The impact of the consumer's degree of formal education and experiences on acceptance of specialized services is addressed as well. Finally, the crucial role played by the I/T as a *cultural broker* in this process is discussed.

Chapter 4, "Interpreting and Translating in Speech-Language Pathology and Audiology" (Terry Irvine Saenz), provides a review of the ASHA Code of Ethics for SLPs and audiologists with application to their collaborating with I/Ts. Issues such as recruiting I/Ts, the necessary preparation of I/Ts by SLPs or audiologists, and these professionals' need for updating their knowledge about the process are discussed. Other topics included are ways to evaluate I/Ts' performance as well as their bilingual skills and the multiple functions provided by the I/Ts, of serving as message converter, message clarifier, cultural clarifier, and patient (client) advocate. A description of a proposed Code of Ethics for I/Ts working in our fields and their important roles in the process are part of this chapter.

Chapter 5, "Three Important Steps: Briefing, Interaction, Debriefing (BID Process)" (Henriette W. Langdon), outlines the BID process for various scenarios such as interviews, conferences, assessments, and interventions and the roles and collaboration protocols that need to be maintained between the SLP or audiologist and the I/T to ensure that the process is running smoothly. The end of the chapter outlines a path to enable the creation of a formal certification for I/Ts collaborating with SLPs and audiologists that was written in conjunction with guest writer Teresa L. Wolf.

Chapter 6, "Assessing Bilingual/Culturally/Linguistically Diverse Children" (Henriette W. Langdon), addresses issues such as when services of a trained I/T should be requested to evaluate an ELL student. It covers a review of tests in languages other than English; preassessment considerations; the RIOT, a suggested procedure for assessment; and what to do when there are tests in the first language

of the student and what alternatives to take when such tests are not available. Separate sections of the chapter include unique dilemmas that surface during assessments, and offer possible solutions for each of the two disciplines of speech-language pathology and audiology.

Chapter 7, "Enhancing Professional Development Programs and the Future of Interpreters" (Teresa L. Wolf), describes the challenges facing I/Ts working with communication disorders professionals and offers a professional development program designed specifically for interpreters/translators working with speech-language pathologists and audiologists while providing checklists, which may be duplicated for training purposes as well for use by consumers to evaluate the effectiveness of the interpreting/translating service. It also suggests activities that may help build the future for interpreters in speech-language pathology and audiology.

An Epilogue at the end of the guide, written by Li-Rong Lilly Cheng, summarizes the importance and future of this alternative process to equitably assess and work with our nation's culturally and linguistically diverse population.

REFERENCES

American Speech-Language-Hearing Association (1985). *Clinical management of communicatively handicapped minority populations. ASHA, 7*(6), 29–32.

Bager, C. (August, 2013). Where 60 million people in the United States don't speak English at home. Washington, DC: CityLab. Retrieved March 20, 2015, from file://localhost/Users/henriettelangdon/Desktop/BOOK%20 I%3FT%20/Where%2060%20Million%20 People%20in%20the%20U.S.%20Don't%20 Speak%20English%20at%20H

Langdon, H. W. (2002). *Interpreters and translators in communication disorders: A practitioner's handbook.* Eau Claire, WI: Thinking Publications.

Langdon, H. W., & Cheng, L.-R. L. (2002). *Collaborating with interpreters and translators: A guide for communication disorders professionals.* Eau Claire, WI: Thinking Publications.

National Center for Education Statistics. (2015). English language learners. In *The condition of education 2014* (NCES 2014-083). Washington, DC: U.S. Department of Education.

Chapter 1

Bridging Linguistic Diversity

Henriette W. Langdon

CHAPTER GOALS

- Provide a brief historical perspective of the process of interpretation and translation
- Discuss the need for interpreters and translators in the fields of speech-language pathology and audiology based on mandated federal and state laws
- Present statistics pertaining to languages spoken in the world and some of their characteristics
- Provide current data on the top 10 languages most frequently spoken languages in the world, in the United States, and those speakers' proficiency in English
- Describe the various methods used in interpreting and translating and various specialties in the field to include conference, medical, and court interpreting

I don't have any memories about living in a monolingual world. From early infancy when my first words and sentences developed, I switched from Spanish to Polish without being conscious of it. Specific persons and situations made this switch a natural and effortless process. Then at age 5, I was introduced to French by attending a full-immersion school program. In the beginning, I recall listening to the teacher speak to the whole class, singing songs, repeating what she said, then suddenly, "it all sank in," and French was miraculously integrated into my linguistic repertoire. From that moment on, the development of the three languages seemed to continue, with each one following its own track like a train arrival or departure at the time and location needed. In upper elementary school, we were introduced to English, but its acquisition proceeded at a slower pace due to the lack of opportunities to use the language with peers or adults even though Mexico, where I grew up, bordered the United States. When I moved to America to start my graduate studies, I remember needing to make more effort to express myself and having to rehearse internally what I wanted to say in English by using one of the three other languages. However, this period lasted only a few months, and after that, I was able to pave my fourth language track. Since those days, I have traveled on four different "tracks" continuously, and

I have been able to communicate with a number of people coming from different corners of the world where one of the four languages I knew were spoken.

I had never encountered a situation where I had to negotiate my communication with the help of someone who could interpret for me. Quite the contrary, I was the one who facilitated the interaction between my clients who were primarily Spanish speaking and teachers or other professionals who spoke English. I performed this task without any specific training, relying only on my knowledge of English and Spanish as well as my intuition to secure that the parties were communicating effectively. I must admit that as the interpreter, I felt empowered by the fact that I was the only one in the group who had the knowledge and skills in two languages, which enabled me to perform this job. But when it was my turn to be in an interaction where I had to rely on an interpreter to communicate with a child (Vietnamese), I was left at the mercy of that interpreter. It was an uncomfortable experience; I felt as if a screen separated me from the child I was assessing. On another occasion, I participated in a conference in Holland and I had to rely on an interpreter to understand the various lectures delivered in Dutch. It was exhausting to watch and listen to the speakers while at the same time trying to pay attention to the interpreter's translation into English. I found myself traveling on two tracks that were moving simultaneously at different speeds. Perhaps if I were in a booth where I could only concentrate on the translation, it would have been easier. As a matter of fact, working with deaf students with the assistance of a sign language interpreter was a much easier process because I did not try to understand the sign language but watched the student and heard the interpreter instead.

My interest in the area of interpreters and translators as applied in our field of speech-language pathology and audiology began 25 years ago, when I was asked to write a manual on training interpreters and special educators (which included speech-language pathologists). After completing the manual with input from some colleagues (Langdon, with Siegel, Halog and Sánchez-Boyce, 1994), we all traveled extensively in California and to some other states to offer training to both interpreters/translators and special educators. Subsequently, I became involved more deeply in this topic because of my personal multilingual and multicultural background and because I firmly believe that bilingual individuals need to be assessed in their preferred languages if needed, in addition to English when appropriate. Otherwise, the client's entire linguistic abilities are not evaluated fairly. The client might be more dominant in one language than the other in different domains. For example, the client may be able to express certain ideas in the first language (L1) but may be able to read and write with greater ease in the second language (L2). Assessing only one language is almost like assessing vision in only one eye or hearing in only one ear.

There are many challenges in carrying out an equitable speech-language or audiological assessment on a client whose language is limited in English and living in the United States. This guide centers on collaborating with an interpreter and/or translator to provide speech-language or audiology services when the professional is not fluent in the client's language and is a significant revision of two previous volumes (Langdon, 2002; Langdon & Cheng, 2002). Although the content relates to situations that occur in the United States, it can be applied to any country where service providers and clients do not share the same language and need services from an interpreter/translator (I/T). As early as 1985, the American Speech-Language-Hearing Association (ASHA) provided guidelines on the utilization of services from interpreters and translators in case there were no bilingual certified speech-language pathologists (SLPs) or audiologists in the client's language. Among some guidelines, some important statements were made that include the following:

> If the use of interpreters or translators is the only alternative, the speech-language pathologist or audiologist should:
>
> 1. Provide extensive training to the assistant on the purposes, procedures and goals of the tests and therapy methods. The assistant also should be taught to avoid the use of gestures, vocal intonation, and other cues that could inadvertently alert the individual to the response during test administration.
> 2. Pre-plan for an individual's services to insure the assistant's understanding of specific clinical procedures to be used.
> 3. Use the same assistant(s) with a given minority language client rather than using assistants on a random basis.
> 4. Use patient observation or other nonlinguistic measures as supplements to the translated measures, such as (1) child's interaction with parents, (2) child's interaction with peers, (3) pragmatic analysis.

It is recommended that the speech-language pathologist and audiologist state in their written evaluation that a translator was used and the validity of the results may be affected. (p. 31)

Since those remarks, more awareness about the need to assess bilingual clients in their languages has occurred in the two fields of speech-language pathology and audiology because it is required by law, and there has been a steady increase of language minority populations represented in the school setting. For example, a comprehensive report carried out by Uro and Barrio (2013) from responses by 46 major school districts nationwide indicated that there were 38 different languages among the five most frequently spoken languages in those districts. Many school districts have addressed this issue by making interpreting and translation services available. Specifically, in the New York public school system alone, students attending the schools may speak one of as many as 200 different languages. The New York City Department of Education website advertises that it offers free translation services in several languages including Arabic, Bengali. Chinese, French, Haitian Creole, Korean, Russian, Spanish, and Urdu. The department indicates that there are on-site interpretation services in 80 languages and over-the-phone interpretation services in 200 languages (New York City Department of Education, 2014).

However, many challenges remain and will be elaborated upon in the various chapters of the guide that include the adequate training of bilingual individuals to assist in our specific and specialized fields of speech-language pathology and audiology and the training of our own professionals (SLPs and audiologists) to collaborate with an I/T. Even when an individual is a certified medical interpreter, it does not necessarily signify that she or he is familiar with procedures and terminology that are used in speech-language pathology or audiology. Furthermore, the greatest need for adequately trained I/Ts is evident in the public schools, where there is an increasingly greater number of students who speak a variety of languages other than English. In those settings, the experience and training of I/Ts are highly variable, affecting quality of services. It is further affected by the professionals' lack of training in collaboration with those I/Ts as well. (This issue is further explored in Chapter 6 of this guide.) It is not uncommon to hear that "anyone who speaks another language is called upon to assist in a conference, assessment, or individual education plan (IEP) meeting." At times, a clerical staff member who may know the language, a neighbor, or even a relative may be called at the last minute to perform the job. Additional elaboration on preferred selection and training of I/Ts who work with SLPs and audiologists will be discussed throughout the guide. Although most of the content may be more applicable to the preschool through high school population, it can be easily implemented when working with older bilingual populations. Many more resources exist for students and their families who may not be proficient in English through websites as applied to the school setting, but it does not mean that the day-by-day delivery of services is of the highest quality. One of the issues is that the I/T working in the school setting is not required to have any particular training. Most of the training occurs on the job over time. It is hoped that in the near future, those individuals working as interpreters and translators in the public school setting will be adequately trained and certified just like those same professionals who work in the medical, court, and international arenas. This topic is addressed at greater length in Chapter 7.

HISTORICAL PERSPECTIVES ON INTERPRETING AND TRANSLATING

Interpretation and *translation* are complementary terms that may be used differentially depending on the context. For the purposes of this guide, *interpretation* means transmitting the same oral information from one language to another, and *translation* means the same, but using written information. In this guide, there will be more reference to the interpreting term, as it occurs more frequently in the fields of speech-language pathology and audiology. Although the differentiation of the two terms clarifies the process, it is sometimes difficult to separate interpretation from translation, as the two terms may be used interchangeably.

Since ancient times, people who spoke different languages had to rely on the assistance of someone who could bridge the communication barrier between the two languages. There are reports of ancient Egypt (3000 BC) indicating even then languages had a word for *interpreter*. During Roman and Greek times, the services of interpreters were utilized to bridge the communication between the various conquered nations and their conquerors. During medieval times, interpreters were hired to interpret in monasteries, where monks who spoke different languages attended religious events and participated in various councils and business and diplomatic meetings. When Christopher Columbus landed in the New World, he had to rely on Indians who were able to learn Spanish and served as interpreters. Hernán Cortés, the Spanish conquistador, relied on an Indian woman named "La Malinche" (who eventually became his mistress) to interpret between

Nahuatl and Mayan, her two native languages, and Spanish (Díaz del Castillo, 1963). Some people credit her for the success with which the Spaniards conquered the Aztecs. In this case, the role of interpreter transcended its regular function of bridging the communication between two parties who did not share a common language to one of traitor toward one's own people. Similarly, Roberts (1997) reports that early French settlers in Canada saw the need for interpreters and sent two native Iroquois speakers to France to be trained, and thus interpreters' roles expanded beyond serving as a bridge between parties that did not share a common language. Roberts states, "French resident-interpreters adopted the Indian lifestyle and acted not only as linguistic intermediaries, but also as commercial agents, diplomats and guides" (p. 7). A lengthier discussion on the responsibilities and function of interpreters follows in subsequent chapters, primarily in Chapter 4.

Until the end of the 18th century, whenever two European countries were at war, the official peace treaties were negotiated and written in Latin and later on in French (even when Great Britain and France were involved, as during the Treatise of Paris of 1783). However, with the involvement of the United States following World War I, it became necessary to conduct negotiations in English, hence the need for trained English-French interpreters. Initially, military personnel acted as interpreters (Gerver & Sinaiko, 1977). The increased participation of the United States in military affairs and the greater need for communication between various nations to enhance diplomatic, scientific, and commercial exchanges between nations served as bases for the creation of world language interpreting and trans-lation centers of the world (Institute of Geneva in Switzerland; Georgetown University; Monterey Language Institute). A greater demand for interpreters and translators in assisting second-language learners in the community grew from various federal and state laws to protect the rights of citizens such as Title VI of the 1964 Civil Rights Act, reviewed by Chen, Youdelman, and Brooks (2007). Specific applications to the fields of speech-language pathology and audiology are discussed in the next section.

NEED FOR TRAINED INTERPRETERS AND TRANSLATORS IN THE FIELD OF COMMUNICATIVE DISORDERS

Both federal and state laws that require that clients who are not proficient in English be assessed fairly by using their first and second languages grew from PL-94-142, which was originally drafted in 1975 to protect the rights of children with disabilities. Among several provisions, the law specifies that the child's assessment must be conducted by a multidisciplinary team in all areas of suspected disability using tests that are not racially, culturally, or linguistically biased. The Individual Disabilities Education Act (IDEA, 2004) (which is a revision of PL-94-142) and subsequent amendments spell out specific federal legislative guidelines for the identification, assessment, and intervention for children with educational needs. In the case of English-language learner (ELL) students, "In making a determination of eligibility a child shall not be determined to be a child with a disability if the determinant factor for such determination is limited English proficiency" (P.L. 108-446 §614(b)(5)(C)). The statute also requires that "Local Educational Agencies or LEAs ensure that assessments and other evaluation materials are provided and administered in the language and form most likely to yield accurate information unless it is not feasible to so provide or administer" (P.L. 108-446 §614(b)(3)(A)(ii)). With so many diverse languages and the movement of various linguistic groups within the United States and around the globe, there is an increasing need for individuals who can help bridge the linguistic barrier between individuals who cannot communicate in the same language. Therefore, it is evident that the supply for I/Ts who can collaborate with SLPs and audiologists is a necessity when professionals are not sufficiently fluent in the language of the client and/or the client's family. Thirty years ago, ASHA (1985) drafted a position on this topic: "Interpreters or translators could be used with minority language speakers when the following circumstances exist: (a) when the certified speech-language pathologist or audiologist on the staff does not meet the needed competencies to provide services to limited-English proficient speakers; (b) when an individual who needs services speaks a language which is uncommon for that local area; and (c) when there are no trained professionals readily available with proficiency in that language that would permit the use of one of the previously described alternative strategies" (p. 31). A more recent ASHA (2004) position statement, entitled *Knowledge and Skills Needed by Speech-Language Pathologists and Audiologists to Provide Culturally and Linguistically Appropriate Services* [Knowledge and Skills], includes the importance of clinicians knowing how to work effectively with an I/T.

In the past, ASHA published a directory of certified SLPs and audiologists who self-nominated themselves as being able to provide clinical services in other languages than English. A recent report by ASHA (2012) indicated that only 7,039 or 5% of the total of 150,000 members met ASHA's definition of bilingual service provider; 6,282 were ASHA-certified SLPs, and 574 were ASHA-certified audiologists. The remainder included members with dual certification. More than 50% of bilingual ASHA-certified members were Spanish-speaking providers (57%) (3,790 were ASHA-certified SLPs, and 186 were certified audiologists).

An ASHA professional issues reference, entitled *Bilingual Service Delivery* (ASHA, n.d.), provides step-by-step procedures to assess ELL students, including all the ethical principles and considerations that need to be taken into consideration and references on how to most successfully collaborate with interpreters (http://www.asha.org/PRPSpecific Topic.aspx?folderid=8589935225&section =Key_Issues).

From the combined experiences of the two editors of this guide, which amount to about 75 years, we have witnessed that, traditionally, interpreters working in the schools have had varying experiences and have not had much training other than that offered by the clinicians they collaborate with. Their role as an important part of the team is not recognized, and their impact is most often not respected. In several cases, an SLP/assistant (SLP/A) may serve as an I/T under the supervision of an SLP. For details, the reader is referred to the Speech-Language Pathology Scope of Practice document (2013; http://www.asha.org/policy/SP2013-00337/#r1). Nevertheless, there are no developed guidelines to determine the level of linguistic and performance necessary for an SLP/A to take on the role of an I/T. The objective of this guide is to offer both the communication disorders professional (SLP or audiologist) and the I/T an outline of best practices known in other fields where interpreters and translators services are utilized, such as medicine, courts, international conferences, and with the deaf population, as well as to offer ideas on training those individuals. Evidence-based practice research in this area is almost nonexistent and should be addressed by researchers in the future.

LANGUAGE STATISTICS

World Languages

The 17th edition of Ethnologue (2013) lists 7,106 languages spoken by 6.7 billion people. Of those languages, five distinct categories include (1) 652 *Institutional*, (2) 1534 *Developing*, (3) 1502 *Vigorous*, (4) 1401 *In Trouble*, and (5) 906 *Dying*. Each category includes a specific numbering system: (1) Institutional (0–4), (2) Developing (5), (3) Vigorous (6a), (4) In Trouble (6b–7), and (5) Dying (8a-8b). The various languages are classified according to two criteria: (1) overall status from developing to endangered and (2) grade on the expanded graded intergenerational disruption scale, which has 13 different gradations (Lewis & Simons, 2010). Specifically, (1) an *institutional* language is one that is used in various institutions such as government agencies, places of worship, courts, and schools (scale 1–4); (2) a *developing* language is one where "the language is in vigorous use, with literature in a standardized form being used by some though this is not yet widespread

or sustainable" (scale of 5); (3) a *vigorous* language is "one which is used for face-to-face communication" (scale of 6a); (4) a language *in trouble* (scale of 6b–7) is one that may be used for face-to-face communication but there is a decreasing number of speakers of that language; and (5) a *dying* language is one that is spoken by only the grandparent generation (8a,8b) (Lewis & Simons, 2010). Specific definitions can be found on the Ethnologue website (http://www.ethnologue.com/about/language-status). A listing of the total populations and different types of languages for each of the five continents can be found in Table 1–1.

The statistics reported below indicate that there is no correlation between size of population and number of different languages. For example, the Americas and Africa have similar population sizes, yet twice as many different languages are spoken in Africa (2,145) compared to the Americas (1,000). Also, relatively few languages (284) are spoken in Europe with a population of 728 million, compared to the Pacific with only a population of about 33 million and over 1,000 languages. The percentages of languages that are in trouble and dying are equally disproportionate in comparison to the total number of languages spoken on any given continent. Table 1–2 reports these percentages.

The continent with the most languages that are in the *In Trouble* or *Dying* categories are the Americas (64.6%), whereas in Africa, this number is only 16.1%. On average, one third of the world's languages are *In Trouble* or *Dying*, which is significant. A pessimistic perspective is that as many as 50% of languages will die within the next 100 years unless drastic measures are taken to preserve them. Baker (2011) comments that figures are often relative and change from

Table 1–1. Percentage of Languages by Status in Each Continent

Continent	Population Size	Number of Languages	Status
Africa	938,190,060	2,145	Institutional: 11% Developing: 23% Vigorous: 50% In Trouble: 10% Dying: 6%
Americas	900,743,578	1,000	Institutional: 5% Developing: 22% Vigorous: 12% In Trouble: 29% Dying: 32%
Asia	4,114,950,000	2,304	Institutional: 10% Developing: 16% Vigorous: 36% In Trouble: 30% Dying: 8%
Europe	728,090,620	284	Institutional: 29% Developing: 21% Vigorous: 17% In Trouble: 16% Dying: 17%
Pacific	33,684,149	1,311	Institutional: 7% Developing: 28% Vigorous: 31% In Trouble: 18% Dying: 16%

Source: Adapted from Ethnologue (2013). Retrieved December 17, 2014, from http://www.ethnologue.com

study to study, but there is no question that many languages are nearly extinct. According to Lewis (2009), as many as 516 languages are nearly extinct, with the largest proportion being in South America (170) and in the Pacific (210). For the most part, languages survive as a result of their prestige; their position vis-à-vis the dominant culture, depending on whether the speakers feel proud of using the language and there are speakers of that language; and, last but not least, if the language has a script, that is, a writing system. Thus, the survival of a language in a given soci-

Table 1–2. *Percentages of Languages in Trouble and Dying in Each Continent*

Continent	Total Number of Languages	Total Number of Languages in Trouble and Dying	Combined Percentage
Worldwide	7,105	2,389	33.6
Americas	1,000	646	64.6
Africa	2,145	346	16.1
Asia	2,304	863	37.4
Europe	284	93	32.7
Pacific	1,311	438	33.2

Source: Adapted from Ethnologue (2013). *Languages of the world.* Retrieved September 15, 2014, from http://www.ethnologue.com

ety is bound to some of these factors as populations migrate from various corners of the globe to others.

Top 10 Most Frequently Spoken Languages in the World

Table 1–3 lists the top 10 languages spoken in the world, including the number of speakers as of 2013 (Ethnologue, 2013), the percent of the population that speaks the particular language, and the regions and areas where the language is spoken most frequently.

As could be expected, the most widely spoken language in the world is *Chinese,* used by as many as one fourth or 25% of the total global population, which includes several varieties of the language, many of which are mutually unintelligible in that speakers of the same language family name may not be able to communicate with one another. Chinese is followed by *Spanish, English, Hindi, Arabic, Portuguese, Bengali, Russian, Japanese,* and *Javanese* (in decreasing order), which are spoken by

5% or less by the global population. In sum, about 52% of the total population speaks the first 10 of the most frequently spoken languages, whereas the other 48% speak one or more of the remaining 7,100 languages! This is quite significant and emphasizes the fact that we will always need to rely on interpreting and translation services to communicate with others.

In addition to estimating the number of speakers of a given language, languages have been classified according to *families,* meaning that they have "common ancestors" with subsequent species similar to a phylogenetic tree. This information, which can be found in Ethnologue (2013), indicates that there are 136 language families, including 6 of which are each spoken by at least 5% of the population. For details, the reader is referred to http://www.ethnologue.com/statistics/family. Table 1–4 lists the six major families, the number of languages, and the percent of the total world population who speak those languages.

When considering language *families* instead of *single* languages, a total of

Table 1–3. *Top 10 Languages Spoken in the World*

Language	Approximate Number of Speakers	Percent Based on 7.2 Billion Global Population[a]	Locations Where the Language Is Official
1. Chinese (Mandarin) and Varieties	1,917,000,000	25	China and Singapore
2. Spanish	406,000,000	5.5	Central and South America, Spain
3. English	335,000,000	4.2	Australia, some Caribbean islands, Great Britain, Guyana, Hong Kong, some countries of Africa, United States, and others[b]
4. Hindi	260,000,000	3.6	India and Fiji
5. Arabic	223,000,000	3.1	North Africa and other African countries, Egypt, United Emirates, Israel, Jordan, Lebanon, and Libya[c]
6. Portuguese	202,000,000	2.6	Angola, Brazil, Cape Verde, East Timor, Guinea-Bissau, Macau, Mozambique, Portugal, and Sao Tomé e Principe (Off Guinea)
7. Bengali	193,000,000	2.5	Bangladesh, India
8. Russian	162,000,000	2.2	Part of Georgia (Abkhazia), Belarus, Kasakhstan, Kyyrgyztan, Russia, Transnistria (part of Moldovia)
9. Japanese	122,000,000	1.6	Japan, Palau
10. Javanese	84,300,000	1.1	Indonesia (Java)

[a]Calculated by Langdon (2014).
[b]Main countries.
[c]Takes into account several varieties of Arabic.

Source: Adapted from Ethnologue (2013). Retrieved July 12, 2014, from http://www.ethnologue.com

85% of the world population speaks 65% of the existing languages. This means that a small percentage of the world's population (15%) speaks one third of all other languages (35%). Thus, there are many languages that are spoken by very few people. The opposite is also true; for example, Indo-European languages (437) are spoken by half of the world's population.

Languages may also be classified into *typological systems* that are based on

Table 1–4. *Major Language Families of the World*

Family Name	Number of Languages	Percent of Living Languages	Percent of World Speakers
Afro-Asiatic	367	5.16	5.95
Austronesian	1,222	17.20	5.50
Indo-European	437	6.15	46.46
Niger-Congo	1,526	21.47	6.92
Sino-Tibetian	455	6.40	20.14
Trans–New Guinea	460	6.70	00.6
Totals	4.483	63.09	85.03

Source: Adapted from Ethnologue (2013). *Languages of the world.* Retrieved September 15, 2014, from http://www.ethnologue.com

their sentence or morphological structure. In *sentence structure*, three main categories are considered: (1) *subject-verb-object* (SVO), (2) *subject-object-verb* (SOV), and (3) *verb-subject-object* (VSO). Examples of SVO languages include English, French, Italian, Romanian, Polish, and Russian. Some of these languages may also have the SOV structure in some of their forms like Spanish, French, Polish, and Russian. German, Dutch, and Japanese have the subject-object-verb (SOV) structure, while Welsh, Arabic, Classical Hebrew, Mayan, Tagalog, and Tongan are considered VSO languages. Based on *morphological* structure, four groups of languages have been identified: (1) *isolating* (e.g., Chinese), those languages including words that are invariable and do not use inflections (i.e., prefixes and suffixes), and word order determines the meaning of what is said; (2) *fusional or inflecting* (e.g., English, German), languages where word inflections add meaning to what is said; (3) *agglutinative* (e.g., Japanese), languages using combinations of inflections to a word to denote different categories, such as person, number, tense, voice, and mood; and (4) *polysynthetic* (e.g., many Native American languages), languages, not among the most common spoken, that combine individual word elements into a composite word that would be expressed as a phrase or sentence in most other languages.

Today, more than ever before, many countries with a majority language, such as French and German, report a greater diversity of languages spoken among their residents because of immigrants who speak Turkish, Kurdish, Russian, Arabic, Italian, Polish, and other languages. For example, in addition to French, Spanish, Italian, Portuguese, Maghrebic Arabic (spoken in Northern Arabic countries), Dutch, and English are spoken in France. Additionally, some countries have more than one official language: Belgium has three official languages, Dutch, French, and German; Bolivia has Spanish and Quechua; Canada has English and French;

Cyprus has Greek and Turkish; Finland has Finnish and Swedish; Haiti recognizes both French and Creole as official languages; New Zealand has English and Maori; and Paraguay has Spanish and Guaraní (Central Intelligence Agency, n.d.; https://www.cia.gov/library/publications/the-world-factbook/fields/2098.html).

Languages Spoken in the United States

According to data provided by Shin and Kominski (2010) from the U.S. Census Bureau, 55.4 million people, or 20% ages 5 and older, reported speaking another language than English at home, and of those, 24.5 million indicated they did not speak English "very well" or "at all." Table 1–5 presents the rank order of speakers of English as a second language who don't speak the language "well" or "not at all" according to the 10 most frequently languages spoken languages in the United States.

Shin and Kominski (2010) report that larger numbers of 18- to 40-year-olds who speak another language than English at home speak Spanish, and also a larger proportion of older persons speaking this language who are 65 years and older report not speaking English "very

Table 1–5. *Rank Order of Speakers of English as a Second Language "Who Don't Speak the Language Well" or "Not at All" According to the 10 Most Frequently Spoken Languages in the United States*

First Language Spoken in Order of Number	Number	Percent	Percentage Change From 1980–2007	Percentage Speaking English "Not Well" or "At All"	Rank
Total	55,444,485	100	140.4	25.6	
Spanish	34,547,077	62.3	210.0	29.1	3
Chinese	2,464,579	4.5	290.7	29.9	2
Tagalog	1,480,429	2.7	212.2	7.1	9
French	1,355,805	2.5	28.0	7.2	8
Vietnamese	1,207,004	2.2	510.9	31.7	1
German	1,104,354	2.0	−30.9	4.7	10
Korean	1,062,337	1.9	299.0	28.9	4
Russian	851,174	1.5	391.4	24.9	5
Italian	798,801	1.4	−50.6	11	7
Portuguese or P. Creole	687,128	1.2	95.3	21.3	6

Source: Adapted from Shin and Kominski (2010).

well." For the most part, those individuals who were "foreign born" are less likely to speak English very well, especially within the Spanish-speaking group. Also, the percentage of Spanish speakers nationwide significantly exceeds those of speakers of other languages (62.3%), followed by 4.5% Chinese speakers and Tagalog (2.7%). The other languages are spoken by fewer than 2.5% of people with a succession of mostly Indo-European languages and Asian languages for the rest of the languages listed. Overall, the number of speakers in other languages than Spanish has increased significantly from 1,980 to 2,007, including Vietnamese, Korean, and Tagalog as well as Russian. Among those speakers, the rank order of those who don't speak English "very well" or "at all" fluctuates between 31.7% (Vietnamese) and 4.7% (German). The first five groups that fall into the category of those who don't have a good command of English include the Vietnamese, Chinese, Spanish, Korean, and Russian. Therefore, it is important to keep those statistics in mind when assessing the languages in which more I/Ts might be needed. Naturally, the needs will vary from region to region and community to community and, very importantly, individual differences must always be considered as well.

Information on English language proficiency of school-age children has important implications for education and, therefore, assessment and intervention. Batalova and McHugh (2010a) report that during the 2007 to 2008 year, there were 49.9 million pre-kindergarten to Grade 12 students enrolled in U.S. public schools. Of those students, 5.3 million, or 10.7%, were English-language learners. The number of pre-K–12 English-language learners (ELL) has steadily increased in the past 40 years since the passage of the Bilingual Act of 1968. In the last decade alone from 1997–1998 to 2007–2008, the number of ELL students has increased from 3.5 million to 5.3 million or 53.2%, whereas the general student population has only increased 8.5% from 46.0 to 49.9 million.

The states with the largest numbers of ELL students are California (1.5 million), Texas (701,799), Florida (234,934), New York (213,000), Illinois (175,454), and Arizona (166,572) (Batalova & McHugh, 2010a). As can be noted, 11 states have experienced an increase of 200% in the influx of ELL students in the past 20 years (between 1997–1998 and 2007–2008), and those states are located primarily in the Southeast United States. A detailed report on various statistics regarding the public school population including ELL students may be found in the report written by Aud et al. (2012). Figure 1–1 lists the 10 top languages spoken by those ELL students.

The most frequently spoken language by ELL students is Spanish (73.1%), followed by significantly fewer numbers who speak Chinese (3.8%) or Vietnamese (2.9%). The frequency of these languages mirrors the number of less proficient speakers of English whose first language is one of those three. Spanish is the top language spoken by ELL students in most states with the exception of six states: Hawaii, North and South Dakota, Montana, Vermont, and Maine.

The five most common languages spoken by ELL students for several states can be found in Batalova and McHugh (2010b). Figure 1–2 illustrates the states with the fastest growing numbers of ELL students, and Table 1–6 lists the five top languages spoken by ELL students in selected states.

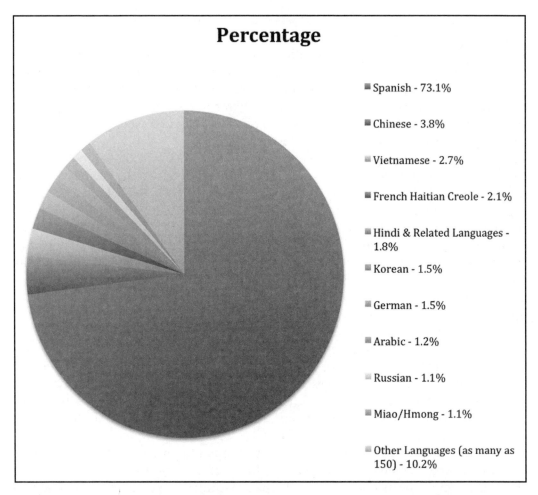

Percentage

- Spanish - 73.1%
- Chinese - 3.8%
- Vietnamese - 2.7%
- French Haitian Creole - 2.1%
- Hindi & Related Languages - 1.8%
- Korean - 1.5%
- German - 1.5%
- Arabic - 1.2%
- Russian - 1.1%
- Miao/Hmong - 1.1%
- Other Languages (as many as 150) - 10.2%

Figure 1–1. Top 10 languages spoken by ELL students in the United States. Adapted from Batalova and McHugh (2010b).

Thus, even though we have data on the most frequently spoken languages in the United States, there are variations from state to state and even region or community within a state. However, the information presented above indicates that English is not the only language spoken in the United States, and there are growing numbers of speakers of other languages, including ELL, who speak a variety of different languages and have insufficient command of the language. There are not enough bilingual professionals in the fields of speech pathology and audiology, and for that matter any professional field, who can provide services in all the languages represented in the United States or any country of the world. Thus, there is the pressing need to collaborate with a well-trained interpreter and translator.

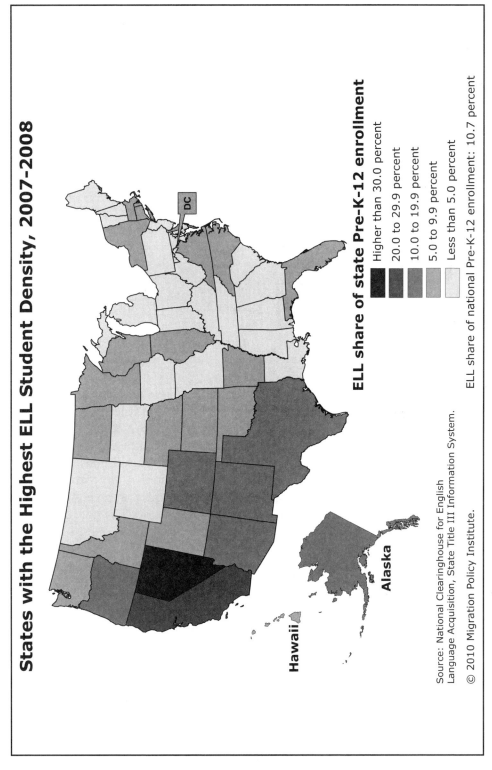

Figure 1–2. States and districts with the highest number and share of English-language learners. Originally published by the Migration Policy Institute, an independent, nonpartisan think tank dedicated to the study of movement of people worldwide. Reprinted with permission.

Table 1–6. Examples of the Five Top Languages Spoken in Selected States

State	Language 1	Language 2	Language 3	Language 4	Language 5
California	Spanish	Vietnamese	Chinese	Tagalog	Hmong
Arizona	Spanish	Navajo	Vietnamese	Arabic	Somali
Vermont	Bosnian	Cushitic[a]	Spanish	Vietnamese	Chinese
Minnesota	Spanish	Hmong	Somali	Vietnamese	Russian
Utah	Spanish	Navajo	Vietnamese	Tonga	Samoan

[a]Cushitic family of African languages spoken in the Northeast.

Source: Batalova and McHugh (2010b).

INTERPRETING AND TRANSLATING METHODS

There are two basic methods of interpreting: *consecutive* and *simultaneous*. In *consecutive interpreting*, the message is transmitted into the second language (L2) once it is spoken in the first language (L1). This results in a short lag time between when the message is heard in L1 and then needs to be conveyed in L2. The *consecutive* method is the one used in most contexts such as court/legal or medical interpreting. This method enables a more personal contact between members who cannot communicate in the same language and who, therefore, need an I/T. This is the suggested method to be implemented during the SLP or audiologist and I/T collaboration process.

In *simultaneous interpreting*, there is no time lag between when a message is conveyed in L1 and transmitted in L2. This is the method used during international conferences. "Simultaneous interpretation is like driving a car that has a steering wheel but no breaks and no reverse" (Pyotr Avaliani, former chief of the Russian Interpretation Service) (Language Outreach by the United Nations, n.d.). It can be implemented in other contexts when there might be many participants and/or a great deal of material to share. In some instances, the I/T may *whisper* the message to the person who needs the message interpreted, but this is not the preferred method because the others present cannot easily follow the flow of the interaction. It may be used in conferences where many professionals are sharing information on a given child. However, this author has not found it to be effective because no one in the team may hear the verbal exchange between the interpreter and the parent/family member. Often, participants may detect a possible miscommunication if the verbal output may be too short or too long and may "read" the interpreter's or the parent's facial expression with ease.

There are two basic methods of translation: *prepared or sight*. In a *prepared translation*, a letter, document, or IEP is completed ahead of time. In a *sight translation*, the information is translated (orally) into L2 as it is read in L1.

SPECIALIZATIONS IN THE FIELD OF INTERPRETING AND TRANSLATING

A list of accredited institutions in the world and United States can be found in the American Translators Association (ATA; http://www.atanet.org/certification/eligibility_approved.php#us). Each institution lists the specific specialization programs offered such as legal/court (the terms seem to be used interchangeably), medical, and/or international conference as well as the languages offered, but some of the listings include interpreting training for the deaf within those fields, which is not the focus of this book. Other institutions offer certificates in translation only.

A few examples of specific specialization programs in the United States and languages are listed in Table 1–7.

Conference Interpreting

As was previously mentioned, *conference interpreting* was instituted as a field of specialization following World War I and became very important during the Nuremberg trials at the conclusion of World War II. This type of interpreting is oral and simultaneous. It is practiced at international meetings, gatherings between heads of state, and various summits and professional seminars as well as when heads of state or government get together. For further information, the reader may

Table 1–7. Selected List of Institutions, Specializations, and Languages Offered in Training Interpreting/Translating in the United States

Institution	Specialization	Languages
Hunter College in NY	Court and Medical	Spanish-English
Monterey Institute of International Studies in CA	Conference	Chinese, French, German, Japanese, Korean, Russian, and Spanish
New York University	Court and Medical	Spanish-English and Chinese-English
Montclair State University in NJ	Court, Medical, and Government	Spanish-English
Georgetown University in DC	Conference	English, French, Spanish, Portuguese, German, Japanese and Passive Italian
University of California, Los Angeles (UCLA) in CA	Legal	Spanish-English
University of Arizona in Tucson (AZ)	Legal/Court	Spanish-English and Navajo-English

Source: American Translators Association (2015).

access an illustration on YouTube: *A Day in the Life of an Interpreter* (http://www.youtube.com/watch?v=aut2Wy-sSoU).

Medical Interpreting

It is important to ensure that medical procedures are followed adequately. The You-Tube segment, entitled *The Road for Certification for Medical Interpreters*, illustrates these procedures (http://www.youtube.com/watch?v=7zvlQNVof7U). Patients who seek medical care in various health settings such as clinics, hospitals, and private practices can find guidelines on adequate provision of interpreting services by referring to the report written by Youdelman and Perkins (2005). The document describes various ways to serve patients utilizing services from bilingual personnel who have been specifically trained to work in the medical field. These services are required by law as specified in various pieces of legislation, which include among others (a) National Standards for Culturally and Linguistically Appropriate Services for Health Care from the U.S. Department of Health and Human Services Office of Minority Health (http://www.minorityhealth.hhs.gov/omh/browse.aspx? lvl=2&lvlid=53), (b) Title VI of the Civil Rights Act of 1964, and (c) Executive Order 13166, signed by the president in 2000, entitled *Improving Access to Services for Persons With Limited English Language Proficiency* (http://www.lep.gov/13166/eo13166.html). The website provides various other resources, which are also available in different languages, including for deaf interpreters. Additionally, each health agency must develop standards for the type of interpreting offered, such as face-to-face, tele-phone, or video. More discussion on this topic follows in Chapters 4 and 6.

Court/Legal Interpreting

Legal/court interpreters work in various settings that may include city, county, state, and federal courts. They may be involved in depositions, trials, hearings, and legal and arbitration cases and any other situation that requires legal procedures. As is the case for health care/medical interpreting, there are specific guidelines that individuals need to abide by if they wish to serve as I/Ts in the court/legal context. Specific training and certification are offered in this field (see examples in Table 1–7). NAJIT or National Association for Judiciary Interpreters and Translators is the major association, which has approximately 12,000 members nationwide. Members of this association work with various languages, including American Sign Language (ASL). Several documents include standards and procedures for court interpreters such as *28 USC § 1827—Interpreters in Courts of the United States* (http://www.law.cornell.edu/uscode/text/28/1827), with adaptations for each state, since laws vary from state to state. The reader may refer to the Internet to find those laws. References are listed at http://www.mass.gov/courts/ocis-standards-procedures.pdf (2009) for Massachusetts and http://www.courts.ca.gov/documents/CIP-Ethics-Manual.pdf (2013) for California.

Guidelines for I/Ts in allied health professions such as speech-language pathology, audiology, and occupational or physical therapy are absent. The SLP and the audiologist often work in two different settings, educational and medical.

Although there are guidelines and certification for medical interpreting, guidelines for interpreting on behalf of SLPs and audiologists in that setting are lacking. Similarly, there are no guidelines or certification requirements for I/Ts who work with SLPs and educational audiologists who work in the school setting.

The purpose of this guide is to bridge the gap that currently exists in providing guidelines for the SLPs and audiologists who collaborate with I/Ts in the educational setting. Some reference to the medical setting will be offered as well since SLPs and audiologists work in that environment. It is hoped that some formal guidelines will be eventually developed as well as a certification process to offer more credibility and respect to the I/T working in the educational/public school setting.

With the advent of technology, the interpreter-training process may become more effective and widely accessible. The use of various electronic platforms, including Skype or Chrome and many others, facilitates more contact between client, clinician, and I/T. Translations using computers are becoming more accessible today; however, a human element will always be needed to edit the information. Thus, trained bilingual and multilingual individuals will be in great demand to interpret and translate for all nations, as these nations become increasingly multilingual and need to interact globally.

SUMMARY

There is no question that the demographics of the United States are changing dramatically, as they are in the entire globe.

This fact has significant implications for adequate communication between individuals who might not speak the same language. Ideally, there should be equivalent representation of linguistic skills between clients and service providers, but this is an unrealistic goal. The need to bridge communication between individuals who do not speak the same language is a pressing issue in our world today. Therefore, professionals in all fields should know how to effectively collaborate with interpreters and translators, and those individuals should be adequately trained. Specific state and federal laws mandate that clients be assessed in their first/preferred language when seeking specialized services such as those provided in the fields of speech-language pathology and audiology. Throughout this chapter, we have described some main responsibilities of I/T specialties such as legal/court, medical, deaf, or international conferences, but there is clearly an absence of formal programs or official established protocols for those I/Ts who collaborate with SLPs or audiologists in either the educational or medical fields. One of the few programs that trains SLPs and audiologists to work collaboratively with I/Ts is the University of Memphis under the direction of Dr. Linda Jarmulovicz (PhD, CCC-SLP), Teresa Wolf (MS, CCC-SLP), and Dr. Jennifer Taylor (AudD, CCC-A). This team of professionals has created a program where students in both professions develop their skills in working with I/Ts. The I/Ts who have participated in this project have had experience working as I/Ts in the medical setting but were interested in collaborating more specifically with SLPs and audiologists working with prekindergarten to 12th-grade populations. Most of their caseloads have been with Spanish-speaking clients. The team has used one of the author's books to gather some preliminary ideas, which have evolved into specific strategies on how to best train SLPs and audiologists to work with I/Ts. Further ideas to develop a comprehensive program to train these professionals can be found in Chapters 6 and 7.

We have also reviewed the types and numbers of languages spoken in the world and found that there are several languages that are dying or are nearly extinct. There is no question that the world population has migrated considerably in the past half century and most likely will continue to migrate. It will always be necessary to have persons who can bridge the communication between individuals who do not share a common language. Therefore, there is a need for trained I/Ts in all sectors, including the allied health professions, which is the topic of this guidebook.

DISCUSSION ITEMS AND ACTIVITIES

1. What changes have occurred in the general field of interpreting/translation (consider various contexts) in the United States in the past 50 years?

2. What are the most commonly spoken languages in your community, and how are the ELL individuals assessed?

3. What are the resources available for those individuals?

4. Why is consecutive versus simultaneous interpreting preferred in most contexts with the exception of international conferences?

5. List three areas that were most surprising to you as you read the chapter. Discuss the reason for each one of the areas.

6. View the video *Qualified Health Interpreting* on YouTube (http://www.youtube.com/watch?v=Dzxq162N4jQ; retrieved January 5, 2014). Divide your participants into small groups of two to three individuals and write down at least 10 important points discussed in the video. Select a spokesperson in your group to share your 10 points with the all of the participants. Have the leader of the group write down the points brought about by each small group and tally the number of times a certain point has been brought about. Divide the points into the responsibilities of each team member (health care provider, patient, and I/T) as well as what seems to be best practice. What are some of the highlights? Why might they be important?

7. Role-play a scenario where you, as an SLP, have assessed a child who has a given disability (TBI–CP-autism). You are sharing your findings with the family through an interpreter. How would you deliver this information so that the interpreter can more easily interpret the definitions of the diagnoses?

REFERENCES

American Speech-Language-Hearing Association. (n.d.). *Bilingual service delivery*. Retrieved October 21, 2014, from http://www.asha.org/PRPSpecificTopic.aspx?folderid=8589935225&section=Overview
American Speech-Language-Hearing Association. (1985). Clinical management of commu-

nicatively handicapped minority populations. *ASHA, 7*(6), 29–32.

American Speech-Language-Hearing Association. (2004). *Knowledge and skills needed by speech-language pathologists and audiologists to provide culturally and linguistically appropriate services* [Knowledge and skills]. Retrieved from http://www.asha.org/policy

American Speech-Language-Hearing Association. (2012). *Demographic profile of ASHA members providing bilingual services.* Retrieved from http://www.asha.org/uploadedFiles/Demographic-Profile-Bilingual-Spanish-Service-Members.pdf

American Speech-Language-Hearing Association. (2013). *Speech-language pathology assistant scope of practice* [Scope of practice]. Retrieved from http://www.asha.org/policy

American Translators Association (ATA). (2015). *Certification Program.* Retrieved June 21, 2015, from http://www.atanet.org/certification/aboutcert_overview.php#1

American Translators Association. (2015). *List of approved interpreting and translating schools.* Retrieved from http://www.atanet.org/certification/eligibility_approved.php#us

Aud, S., Hussar, W., Johnson, F., Kena, G., Roth, E., Manning, E., Wang, X., & Zhang, J. (2012). *The condition of education 2012* (NCES 2012-045). Washington, DC: U.S. Department of Education, National Center for Education Statistics. http://nces.ed.gov/pubsearch

Baker, C. (2011). *Foundations of bilingual education and bilingualism.* Clevedon, UK: Multilingual Matters.

Batalova, J., & McHugh, M. (2010a). *Number and growth of students in US schools in need of English instruction.* Washington, DC: Migration Policy Institute.

Batalova, J., & McHugh, M. (2010b). *Top languages spoken by English language learners nationally and by state.* Washington, DC: Migration Policy Institute.

Central Intelligence Agency. (Ed.). (n.d.). *The world factbook.* Retrieved August 14, 2014, from https://www.cia.gov/library/publications/the-world-factbook/fields/2098.html

Chen, A. H., Youdelman, M. K., & Brooks, J. (2007). The legal framework for language access in healthcare settings: Title VI and beyond. *Journal of General Internal Medicine, 22*(Suppl. 2), 362–367. Retrieved November 4, 2014, from http://www.ncbi.nlm.nih.gov/pmc/articles/PMC2150609/

Civil Rights Act of 1964, Pub.L. 88-352, 78 Stat. 241 (1964).

Díaz del Castillo, B. (1963). *The conquest of New Spain* (J. M. Cohen, Trans.). Harmondsworth, England: Penguin Books. (Original work published 1632)

Ethnologue. (2013). *Languages of the world.* Dallas, TX: International Linguistics Center.

Gerver, D., & Sinaiko, H. W. (Eds.). (1977). *Language interpretation and communication.* New York, NY: Plenum Press.

Individuals with Disabilities Education Act of 2004, Pub. L. No. 108-446 (2004).

Judicial Council of California/Administrative Office of the Court. (Ed.). (2013). *Professional standards and ethics for California interpreters* (5th ed.). Retrieved October 22, 2014, from http://www.courts.ca.gov/documents/CIP-Ethics-Manual.pdf

Langdon, H. W. (2002). *Interpreters and translators in communication disorders: A practitioner's handbook.* Eau Claire, WI: Thinking Publications.

Langdon, H. W., & Cheng, L.-R. L. (2002). *Collaborating with interpreters and translators: A guide for communication disorders professionals.* Eau Claire, WI: Thinking Publications.

Langdon, H. W. (with Siegel, V., Halog, L., & Sánchez-Boyce, M.) (1994). *Interpreter/translator process in the educational setting.* Sacramento, CA: Resources in Special Education (RISE).

Language Outreach by the United Nations. (n.d.). *Conference interpreting in the United Nations.* New York, NY: Department for General Assembly and Conference Management, United Nations. Retrieved October 21, 2014, from http://www.unlanguage.org/Careers/Interpret/default.aspx

Lewis, M. P. (Ed.). (2009). *Ethnologue: Languages of the world* (16th ed.). Dallas, TX: SIL International.

Lewis, M. P., & Simons, G. F. (2010). Assessing endangerment: Expanding Fishman's GIDS. *Revue Roumaine de Linguistique, 55*(2), 103–120.

Limited English Proficiency (LEP): A Federal Interagency Website. (2011). *Improving access to services for persons with limited English language proficiency* (Executive order 13166). Retrieved October 22, 2014, from http://www.lep.gov/13166/eo13166.html

Monterey Institute of International Studies. (2008, January 31). *A day in the life of an interpreter.* Retrieved October 22, 2014, from http://www.youtube.com/watch?v=aut2Wy-sSoU

National Standards for Culturally and Linguistically Appropriate Services for Health Care from the U.S, Department of Health and Human Services Office of Minority Health. (2001). Retrieved from http://www.hablamosjuntos.org/signage/PDF/omh.pdf

New York City Department of Education. (2014). *Language access.* Retrieved October 20, 2014, from http://schools.nyc.gov/RulesPolicies/languagepolicy.htm

Roberts, R. (1997). Community interpreting today and tomorrow. In S. E. Carr, R. Roberts, A. DeFour, & D. Steyhn (Eds.), *The critical link: Interpreters in the community* (pp. 7–20). Philadelphia, PA: John Benjamins.

Shin, H. B., & Kominski, R. A. (2010). *Language use in the United States* (American Community Surveys Report ACS-12). Washington, DC: United States Census Bureau.

Standards and Procedures of the Office of Court Interpreter Services Massachusetts. (2009). Retrieved October 22, 2014, from: http://www.mass.gov/courts/ocis-standards-procedures.pdf

The Road for Certification in Medical Interpreting (CMI). (2010). Retrieved http://www.youtube.com/watch?v=7zvlQNVof7U

28 US Code Chapter 119 § 1827—interpreters in courts of the United States. Retrieved October 22, 2014, from http://www.law.cornell.edu/uscode/text/28/1827

Uro, B., & Barrio, A. (2013). *English language learners in American great city schools: Demographics, achievement, and staffing.* Washington, DC: Council of the American Great City Schools. Retrieved October 20, 2014, from http://www.cgcs.org/cms/lib/DC00001581/Centricity/Domain/87/ELL%20Survey%20Report%202013.pdf

Youdelman, M., & Perkins, J. (2005). *Providing language services in small health care provider setting.* Washington, DC: Commonwealth Fund. Retrieved October 22, 2014, from http://www.commonwealthfund.org/usr_doc/810_Youdelmanproviding_language_services.pdf? section=4039

Chapter 2

Communication Issues in a Multilingual Society

Henriette W. Langdon

CHAPTER GOALS

- Describe verbal and nonverbal aspects of interpretation
- Discuss the difference between language and dialect
- Describe verbal aspects of communication: phonology, suprasegmentals, grammar, semantics, and pragmatics with ramifications for speech-language and audiological evaluations
- Describe nonverbal aspects of communication such as gestures, facial expressions, and emotions
- Describe phenomena that occur when two languages are in contact, that is, early awareness of two languages, code-switching, and language loss
- Describe specific skills to achieve successful written translations
- Identify how both verbal and nonverbal patterns of communication affect the interpretation process

An interpreter/translator (I/T) must have specific skills and knowledge to perform an effective oral interpretation of verbal and/or written communication. The primary focus of this chapter is a discussion of the oral interpretation of verbal and written language with a briefer overview of translation (conveying a written translation from a written document).

A detailed oral language interpreter/translator's job description is available online (http://www.onetonline.org/) (Bureau of Labor Statistics, 2014). Among other skills and knowledge, the I/T must have strong verbal and nonverbal communication in both the English language and the target language (L1). Verbal communication includes "(1) Knowledge of the structure of the English language including the meaning and spelling of words, composition, and grammar and, (2) Knowledge of the structure and content of a foreign (non-English language) including pronunciation, meaning and spelling of words, composition, grammar and pronunciation." Additionally, "(3) the I/T must understand written sentences and paragraphs in work related documents and communicate effectively in writing as appropriate for the needs of the audiologist." Even though the term *non-verbal communication* as such is not mentioned in the job description of the I/T's oral language skills, certain components are listed, like interpreting gestures, facial expressions, and tone of voice in others and oneself to facilitate the communication of two individuals who do not share the same language. These components include "(1) giving full attention to what other people are saying, taking time to understand the points being made, asking questions as appropriate, and not interrupting at inappropriate times; (2) talking to others to convey information effectively; (3) the ability to listen to and understand ideas presented through spoken words; (4) the ability to communicate information and ideas in speaking so others can understand; (5) the ability to identify the speech of another person; and (6) the ability to speak clearly so others can understand you." These specific skills are included in O-NET Resource Center at http://www.onetonline.org/link/details/27-3091.00.

In line with the knowledge and skills of language required of an I/T, it is important to review the structure of language and its components in addition to variations that occur across languages. This information is familiar to all professionals working with clients who have speech, language, communication, and hearing problems but is presented here so that the professional can share it with the I/T or a student. The I/T, who may collaborate with the speech-language pathologist (SLP) or audiologist, might have received more formal training in the analysis of English and the target language. However, many individuals who take on the charge as I/Ts, especially in the public school setting, may not have received any formal training in the area of interpreting

and translating and the skills needed to be an effective professional. The information is especially important in the field of speech-language pathology and audiology, as the primary focus of these professions is the identification of speech and language disorders in the areas of oral language, hearing, processing, comprehension, and production, as well as various aspects commonly referred to as form (phonology, grammar, and syntax), content (semantics or word meanings), and use (pragmatics) (Bloom & Lahey, 1978), as well as written language (reading and writing) and phonological awareness.

The SLP's charge is to assess the level of the client's performance in each of the components of language that include articulation/phonology, morphology, syntax, and pragmatics. These components are marked differently in many languages; therefore, it important to be aware of some differences across languages. Given the scope of this guide, it is impossible to cite all possible variations across languages. The current author has compiled some information on language variations to offer the SLP or audiologist and the I/T as a reminder to avoid a misinterpretation in the analysis of a client's response. For example, certain languages make a differentiation between genders (French, Polish, Spanish, and Hebrew), whereas others do not (Chinese, Japanese, Vietnamese and many other Asian languages, and Turkish). Certain phonemes that exist in English may not exist in other languages. Idiomatic expressions are difficult to translate from one language because there may not be equivalent terms. A selected list of cross-linguistic references is presented in Table 2–1. Some key references include Campbell and King (2011) and McLeod and Goldstein (2012).

Table 2–1. References for Linguistic Characteristics of Various Languages

Languages Areas	Languages	Reference
Phonology, grammar, written system	100 different languages	Campbell and King (2011)
Phonology, grammar, written system, culture, proverbs, description of some features of the country where the language is spoken, practice phrases, and several other types of references	A great number of languages, listed in alphabetical order	Omniglot (The language encyclopedia) http://omniglot.com
Phonology, including information on research. Compiled from 44 different authors.	112 languages	McLeod and Goldstein (2012)

Source: Campbell and King (2011) and McLeod and Goldstein (2012).

Additionally, it important for all team members, including the SLP/audiologist and the I/T, to consider the phenomena that occur when two languages are in contact, such as awareness of each language, code-switching, and language loss. This information is important in analyzing the patterns of a client's languages to accurately determine if the client's language patterns reflect a difference or a disorder. A separate section of this chapter with the heading of phenomena that occur when two languages come in contact covers this aspect.

THE INTERPRETING AND TRANSLATING PROCESS IN SPEECH-LANGUAGE PATHOLOGY AND AUDIOLOGY

Specific preferred interpreting procedures will be described in greater detail in Chapters 4 and 5. This section covers verbal and nonverbal aspects of language that may impact the collaboration between

I/Ts and SLPs/audiologists. Accurate interpretation of meaning entails bridging together two different languages that do not share the same phonology, suprasegmentals, grammar, syntax, and/or pragmatic as well as nonverbal communication features such as gestures, facial expressions, eye contact, or voice volume.

Some schools of thought advocate that the role of interpreters should be limited to conveying meaning rather than assisting in bridging two cultures (Penney & Simmons, 1997). However, the interpreter is at the center of the turn-taking process (Englund Dimitrova, 1997). In addition, the interpreter is the one who ultimately negotiates the speaking time, indicating to each party that the message might be too long, complex, or unclear to convey in the other language. The dynamics of the process requires that the interpreter tend to both verbal and nonverbal communication signals. To be successful, the interpreter must understand the context of the interaction. For example, a different type of discourse takes place when an SLP asks questions regarding a child's language development, medical history, or social behavior compared to when a parent is given information about specific goals or programs that will assist the child, or when an audiologist describes the results of a hearing test, indicates the need for and use of a specific hearing aid, or recommends a cochlear implant.

Also, the SLP may need to rely on the I/T to administer specific tasks in L1 (first language/target language) and trust that it will be done accurately. Additionally, the I/T may be asked to serve as an assistant in interpreting data accurately. Therefore, the I/T should have a conscious knowledge of all components of language in both English and the target language. However, both the SLP and audiologist should be aware of the target language characteristics to decide whether the patterns observed in the client's speech in English reflect a language disorder or language difference. Furthermore, because the I/T is the only person on the assessment team who knows the client's first language, he or she will need to be skilled on how to obtain a language sample, transcribe it, and analyze its various components with the assistance of the SLP. This responsibility given to the I/T may sound controversial to some readers, but it is the best solution to obtain a more natural speaking sample from the client. How else would the SLP obtain a sample, other than requesting the parent or someone familiar with the client to record a conversation at home and have it analyzed by a speaker who is attuned to errors that may occur in the various components of language such as phonology, grammar, syntax, and pragmatics? Thus, the job of an I/T is not an easy one because he or she will have different roles depending on the situation (conference as opposed to assessment).

During a conference or assessment with an SLP or audiologist, the interpreter does not act as a machine that conveys word-by-word renditions; the emotion and tone of the original message must be maintained, even if it offensive or vulgar as stated by Nicholson and Martinsen (1997). Furthermore, when the I/T takes "the front seat" in interacting with a client during assessment, his or her responsiblities multiply.

Breakdowns in communication occur when the conversational participants make erroneous interpretations about each other's meaning and intent. Language is embedded in people's history and culture. Therefore, understanding the history, culture, and socialization patterns of a given group is crucial in securing cross-cultural communicative competence. True communicative competence in a second language requires an ability to integrate language, culture, history, social knowledge, and cognition. As Hall (1977) so aptly said, "All cultures have their own identity, language systems of nonverbal communication, material culture, history and *ways of doing things*" (p. 2). More on this topic is discussed in the next two chapters, but this author wanted to prepare the reader for the complexity of the charges that become the responsibility of the interpreter. The discussion regarding verbal and nonverbal aspects of language and their role in interpreting and translating begins with a review of the difference between language and dialect.

WHAT IS THE DIFFERENCE BETWEEN LANGUAGE AND DIALECT?

The difference between a language and a dialect is often unclear. When the difference lies in grammar, and rules are different from any other language, it is considered to be a language. If the distinction lies primarily in pronunciation and semantics (vocabulary), with possibly some grammatical differences, it is considered a regional dialect. Multiple languages and dialects may be spoken in any given region or country. Regional dialects of English, Spanish, and many other languages are easily identified as being one united language because other than differences in pronunciation and some vocabulary, these dialects are mutually intelligible. Speakers from Boston can communicate with speakers from Louisiana, and Spanish speakers from Argentina can easily communicate with speakers from Mexico or Cuba. Individuals who speak Puerto Rican Spanish, for example, use vocabulary words that are different from speakers of Mexican or Castilian Spanish and pronounce some sounds differently like the /s/ and /r/, but they can still understand each other because the dialects share the same grammatical rules. However, for many years, a great deal of debate and controversy has existed regarding whether African American Vernacular English or (AAVE) should be considered a dialect or a language, as it has its own grammatical rules, pronunciation, and vocabulary. A robust literature is available on this topic and cannot be reviewed fairly in this type of volume. AAVE shares many features with Creole English as well as various Western African languages. Implications for education are numerous, and professionals should be cautious in avoiding labeling children who speak AAVE as having speech and/or language problems. The reader may refer to sources such as Hudley and Mallinson (2011) and Wolfram and Schilling-Estes (2006), among many others. In essence, AAVE should be considered a variety of English such as American English, British English, or Australian English.

A difference in how words are pronounced is referred to as an *accent*. In other cases, even when dialects are mutually intelligible, they are considered as separate languages for political reasons. For example, Swedish, Danish, Norwegian, and Icelandic are mutually intelligible and could be considered dialects of the same language, but for political reasons, they are each considered different languages. The opposite can also occur. Different varieties or dialects of Chinese are mutually unintelligible, but they are thought to be the same language (Crystal, 1997). Languages and regional dialects vary in phonology, suprasegmental aspects, grammar, semantics, and pragmatics. Some broad characteristics of each parameter are described in the sections below.

VERBAL ASPECTS OF COMMUNICATION

Phonology and Suprasegmentals

Phonology includes the study of speech sounds in a language. Phonological differences (i.e., pronunciation) across languages and dialects account for languages' most noticeable characteristics. Phonological differences in dialects may manifest themselves through single phonemes that are pronounced differently across the same language. On the other hand, *suprasegmentals* refer to segments (usually a syllable) and includes stress, intonation, and tone. Stress is conveyed through pitch, loud-ness, and duration. For example, the word *loudness* has the stress in the first syllable (*loud*ness), whereas the stress is on the last syllable for the word *comprehend* (compre*hend*). In some languages like Spanish, changes in stress may alter the meaning of a word. Frequently, the difference is marked by a written accent on the vowel. For example, *to*mo means (*I take*, present tense) versus tom*ó* (*he, she, it took*, past tense), or *dó*mino (*domino*) versus domin*ó* (*he, she, it mastered*). Changes in meaning can occur in several Asian languages as well. For example, in Vietnamese, different tones on the same syllables affect the meaning of the syllable as in Vietnamese: *Bẫy nay bây bầy bẩy bẫy bây.* [IPA: [/ɓ̌ǐ̯/ /naɨ̯/ /ɓʌɨ̯/ /ɓʌ̀ɨ̯/ /ɓã̀ɨ̯/ /ɓ̌ʔɨ̯/ /ɓ̌ʔɨ̯/] ("All along you've set up the seven traps incorrectly!").

Words across languages may have similar common roots and are often referred to as *cognates* but are pronounced differently across languages. For example, the word *merchandise* is pronounced *merchandise* in English, *marchandise* in French, and *mercancía* in Spanish. But other words that appear to mean the same are different. For example, *embarazada* means *pregnant* in Spanish and not *embarrassed*, and *molestado* means *bothered* and not *molested*. *Biblioteca* in Spanish means *library*, whereas *librairie* in French means *bookstore*. *Cartoons* and *cartones* (*cartons* in Spanish), two nouns that share similar configurations, are two different words: *Cartoons* should be translated as *caricaturas*, but instead, this author has heard many use the word *cartones*, which is a borrowed word from the English word, *cartoons*. Therefore, the bilingual interpreter needs to be attuned to the particular variety of Spanish used for a given region or location. This example is applicable to any other language.

Intonation relates to the rising and falling pitch of an utterance. There is a difference between "John went home?" versus "John went home." Another classic example is, "I went to the *White House*" versus "I went to the *white* house," where the intonation is different. In Spanish, questions may have the affirmative structure (SV0) and raising intonation in oral speech and markings of ¿?. For example, "*Juan fue a la casa*" ("John went home") versus "¿*Juan fue a la casa*?" ("John went home?" or "Did John go home?").

The contrasts described above are very important for every individual working in assessing the pronunciation of a second-language learner or user of a dialectal variation of any language. A second-language learner or dialect speaker of any language may not pronounce a given phoneme or use the correct stress or intonation because of a language difference in contrast to a language disorder. For example, English has 12 vowels contrasted by only 5 vowels in Spanish, 16 vowels in French (some are nasalized), and 12 vowels in Polish (some of which are nasalized as well). Spanish speakers may have some difficulty pronouncing words like *pin* or *chick*. Also, they may have challenges pronouncing certain consonants in specific positions of words such as /ʃ/, /v/, /r/, /k/, /p/, and others. Different dialects exist in the mainland of the United States, which are reflected in the pronunciation of certain vowels and consonants like /r/, which is pronounced differently in Boston and California. The same is applicable to many other languages, which either do not have sounds in their repertoire or sounds that appear in only certain positions of words. Table 2–2 provides examples of some consonants that may be challenging for speakers of some languages. Very helpful resources in identifying difficulty in pronouncing consonants and vowels in English by speakers of other

Table 2–2. *Selected English Consonants That Are Challenging for Second-Language Learners*

Consonant	Spanish	Vietnamese	Hmong	Korean	Chinese	Arabic	Russian
/b/	3	3	1		2		
/tʃ/		1					
/d/		3			2		3
/g/	3	3	1		2	1	3
/j/	1	1	1				
/k/	2	2					2
/p/	2	2				1	2
/ʃ/	1	1		1			
/θ/		1		1		1	1
/d/	1	1			1	1	1
/v/	1	3		1	1	1	
/z/	1	1		1	1		
/r/	1			1		1	
/s/				1			
/l/	1					1	

Note. 1 = often a problem; 2 = may be a problem at the beginning of words; 3 = may be a problem at the end of words.

Source: Langdon (2008). Reprinted with permission from Cengage.

languages include Echevarría, Vogt, and Short (2012) as well as Swan and Smith (2001). A list of sounds and their development in various languages, including various dialects of English as well as diverse languages ranging from Dutch, Tagalog, Thai, Turkish, and even Maltese and Zapotec, can be found in McLeod (2007). Sound differences and audiological perception are important aspects of audiological assessments.

Abreu, Adriatico, and DePierro (2011) outline several testing challenges that audiologists face when assessing clients whose English is still developing. In addition to general communication barriers between clinicians, patients, and their families, the researchers reported that there is a lack of word discrimination tests and audiological processing materials such as calibrated lists of phonetically based words or spondees in different languages, which typically prevents the audiologist from completing a comprehensive evaluation of individuals who are not fluent or comfortable in English. This concern is discussed in greater detail in Chapter 6. Also, bilingual individuals may respond to discrimination tests differently in each one of their languages. For example, Shi and Sánchez (2010) found that bilingual children who had acquired English after the age of 10 responded better in Spanish even though they were fluent in English, and they recommend that children ages 7 to 10 be tested in both languages. In their research to obtain more accurate measures of speech reception thresholds (SRTs), Ramkissoon, Proctor, Lansing, and Bilger (2002) concluded that digit pairs are a good option to replace the usual spondee words. Therefore, when working with bilingual students, it is important to consider sound production and perception and their influence on the comprehension of language. Personal comments by audiologist and researcher, Dr. McCullough (personal communication, July 2014),[1] are as follows:

> I can't see that an interpreter will be much help in the audiological evaluation itself. First, there really aren't a lot of *calibrated* or *normed* word lists in other languages. Second, even if there were, an interpreter can't sit in front of an audiometer and pronounce test words and then score them. It just doesn't work that way. So really, if a child or an adult is not fluent or comfortable in English, it turns out that we just can't get information about their discrimination abilities unless the audiologist either (1) speaks the language and can administer/score materials in that language or (2) uses a picture-pointing system where test items are given in a patient's language and scored by the computer following a picture-pointing response, like my research.

Grammar

Grammar is the system of rules for combining words and word parts into sentences. Throughout history, languages have undergone continual change reflecting two levels of grammatical variation: (a) the formation of words from meaningful units of the language (morphology) and (b) combination of words into larger structures, such as phrases and sentences (syntax). Variations exist in word class, sentence structure, arrangements of structure, and word placement within phrases. Verbs, verb auxiliaries, negatives, inflectional suffixes in nouns, various forms of pronouns, articles, and adverbs all undergo variations over time. Also, tenses such as present, past, future, and mood such as indicative, imperative, conditional, and subjunctive undergo variations over time. Different languages may have different sentence structures (Chapter 1), as well as different voices (affirmative, negative, interrogative, and passive). In certain languages, there are two or three genders in nouns; in others, there is only one. In still others, the ending of the noun may vary depending on the position of the word in the sentence, as in Latin. For example, in Polish, the word *rose* has a different ending depending on the place of the word in the sentence: The morphological ending is different when the sentence reads as "I see the *rose*" as opposed to the "The *rose* is beautiful" or "I found a bee on the *rose*." Additionally, in some languages, certain word structures change depending on the person who is addressed, and some Asian languages have a great variety of forms

---

[1]Dr. June McCullough is a professor of audiology at San José State University, California, and has more than 30 years of clinical experience.

compared to others. In several European languages, a distinction is made between the *you* when referring to a familiar as compared to a respected person. In English, the same pronoun, *you*, is used for both forms. Another consideration is to keep in mind the formation of the plural form, the place of adjectives and pronouns within the noun phrase, and the place of auxiliaries.

With increasing access to the Internet, the SLP or audiologist may find basic information on the grammatical aspect of several languages and be better prepared for a session where the collaboration of an I/T might be needed. The professional may double-check the information obtained with the I/T. Some resources such as those listed in Table 2–1 might be very helpful. Grammatical rules in a speaker's native language may be misapplied to English and could be misinterpreted by the SLP or audiologist as part of a language development difficulty. For example, a grammatical feature that does not exist in the speaker's first language may be used when not expected in English. The I/T's feedback may be very helpful in identifying patterns of errors that may reflect the structure of the speaker's first language. However, the SLP will be the one who will need to direct the I/T's attention to the particular linguistic feature(s) that are questioned, such as the appropriate use of sounds in words, grammar, syntax, or use of language.

Semantics

Semantics is the study of word meanings. All words have recognized meanings. These meanings are not static but change over time. Some words change

their meanings completely and take on different cultural twists. Furthermore, the sociocultural events that are associated with the words, such as idioms and sayings, may not be readily transparent to all communicators. For example, in the United States, when someone asks if "he or she can buy somebody a drink," it usually means an alcoholic beverage, not milk or soda. In other cultures, nonalcoholic beverages would be included in the reference. Idioms and proverbs are very difficult to translate word by word because the meaning would be lost. Examples among several others include *all ears, basket case, call it a day, don't have a cow,* or *spill the beans*. When interpreted into other languages, idioms include completely different words and, in their back translation to the other language, lose their original meaning to some degree. For example, the French equivalent of the English proverb "It's Greek to me" is *"C'est du chinois"* ("It's Chinese to me"), "Give him an inch, and he will take a mile" becomes *"Le da la mano y se toma el pie"* in Spanish ("You give him a hand and he takes a foot"), and "Go jump in the lake" is translated as *"Vete por un tubo"* or "Go through a pipe." Several examples of idioms in various languages translated into English may be found on the website for Omiglot.com.

Originally, the study of semantics focused on vocabulary. However, because words undergo continual changes due to language use, it is difficult to separate words from their context. Words can take on a different meaning as a result of prosody, for example, "I want to buy the yellow *roses*" (difference between roses and other flowers) and "I want to buy the *yellow* roses" (difference between yellow and another color). Also, the setting in which a given sentence is used may change the meaning of a word as in "The door is open"; it may signal that either the door needs to be closed, or a person can come in. Some word changes may be introduced or used by specific segments of the population, like teens or young adults (*busted*, which used to mean, "to be broken," now means "needing to be fixed or repaired," "in trouble," or "ugly." *LOL* means "laugh out loud"). Other words change as a result of scientific progress, like technology and medicine, and still others from contact with other languages, like the influence of English on Spanish (*lonchear, to have lunch*, instead of *almorzar; parquear, to park*, instead of *estacionar; carpeta, rug*, instead of *tapete; troca, van*, instead of *camioneta*; or *retirarse, to retire*, instead of *jubilarse*), or the example given above about the translation of *cartoons* into Spanish.

Semantic variations are important considerations for I/Ts. When words or phrases are directly translated into their dictionary meanings, the intended meaning of the speaker may be lost. I/Ts must be aware of intonation and other cues for meaning. Speakers of languages that use vocabulary that may reflect dialectal variations need to make a conscious effort to be aware of the differences to avoid confusion. For example, the English word *grass* (like in a garden) may be referred to as *pasto* (Mexico, Argentina), *grama* (Guatemala, Puerto Rico), *césped* (Spain), or *sacate* (Mexican/Central-American Spanish). And, the word *kite* may be referred to as *papalote* (Mexico), *chiringa* (Puerto Rico), *volantín* (Chile), *barrilete* (Argentina), *cometa* (Colombia), or *pandorga* (Paraguay). A helpful resource where the reader might find the equivalents of various Spanish-speaking countries is Florián (2010).

Pragmatics

Pragmatics refers to the relationship between signs or linguistic expressions and their use in a sociolinguistic context. Content, social setting, connotation, inflection, and intonation play a role in the transmission of meaning in communication. Note that many of these items are subject to individual interpretation based on personal experience and cultural beliefs. Distinctions between literal and nonliteral meaning, nuance, and innuendo may be lost or misinterpreted in a cross-cultural setting where two communication partners perceive a situation differently. One of the essential roles of language is to establish and maintain social interaction. The social context and the relationship between participants are crucial to conversation. Several steps are involved in the communication process, including selection of a topic, initiation of speech, turn-taking, maintenance of the topic, and closure of the conversation. Pragmatics plays a role in the construction of narratives in bilinguals due to cultural and experiential variations.

Narratives Across Cultures

Narrative assessment can be a powerful tool for evaluating language use. A narrative is an organizer of human experiences consisting of a unique sequence of events containing the essence of the message and the speaker's communicative intent. The use of narratives demands a degree of cognitive and linguistic ability for its construction. A narrative is an account of various happenings from a range of various experiences common in all languages. However, the construction of narratives may vary across cultures and languages, and this must be taken into account. Researchers such as Bliss and McCabe (2008), Heath (1983), and Westby (1994) have studied the structure and significance of narratives in various cultures. Oral narratives seem to share a similar macrostructure and follow six steps: (a) *Abstract*: What is the story about? (b) *Orientation:* Who, when where, how? (c) *Complicating Action*: Then what happened? (d) *Evaluation*: How or why is this interesting? (e) *Result/Resolution*: What finally happened, the outcome? and (f) *Coda*: What is the ending, bringing the story back from the past to the present? Berman (2001), who studied narrative construction among various cultures and socioeconomic groups, found that children share similar cognitive, conceptual, and developmental abilities regarding narrative competence, as all cultures have some form of narratives. Westby (1994) reports that recounts or series of events may be rare among Mexican American, Chinese American, and African American working classes but frequent among mainstream and European American working classes. Essentially, stories are prevalent in all cultures except they have certain characteristic features. For example, among mainstream cultures, frequent story reading and imaginative accounts occur, while among Mexican Americans, the *"bruja"* (witch) stories are common as well as stories with historical figures, and the latter is also frequent among Chinese Americans. Bliss and McCabe (2011) outline the structures of narratives among African American, Mexican American, and Asian American children. These structures are listed in Table 2–3.

It is important to remember not to generalize; however, the authors' comments about children with possible language disorder problems can be applied to bilingual children from various backgrounds. That is, the listener will note that the narrative lacks topic maintenance, information, sequencing, referencing, and fluency. The narrative is presented in chunks, and the listener has difficulty following the story due to many disruptions reflecting "a reduced ability to plan, monitor, and/or revise utterances" (p. 218). This type of narrative is often referred to as a *"leapfrogging narrative."*

Table 2–3. Narrative Structures in Three Different Cultures

Culture	Description
African American	Topic associated-lengthy description of events is linked semantically rather than chronologically; ideas include emotional terms.
Mexican American	Broad topic maintenance that includes several characters in the scene; reference to characters is sometimes made, sometimes not.
Japanese American	Reference to not only the event described but to other similar events. Concise discourse and referents are frequently omitted to emphasize brevity. The authors indicate that conciseness has also been observed with children from Chinese and Korean American backgrounds.

Source: Adapted from Bliss and McCabe (2011).

Recounting stories with greater detail has been used as a tool to diagnose a possible language disorder in children from multicultural/multilingual backgrounds (Gillam, Peña, & Miller, 1999). The researchers found that students from such backgrounds who do not have a language disorder benefit from mediation sessions compared to those who have a true disorder. During those sessions, the students are explicitly taught how to differentiate relevant from irrelevant facts and how to express their ideas more clearly. Picture books such as *Frog, Where Are You?* (Mayer, 2003a), and *One Frog Too Many* (Mayer & Mayer, 2003b) are most helpful. These studies have been replicated on preschool African children with risks in language disorders as well as third-grade children from Canada-speaking Cree (Kramer, Mallet, Schneider, & Hayward, 2009). This technique could be very helpful in assessing a language disorder in languages other than Spanish where there are no tests with the collaboration and training of an I/T. More on this topic and its importance in assessment can be found in Chapter 6.

NONVERBAL ASPECTS OF COMMUNICATION

There is no question that in each communication act, nonverbal aspects such as facial expression, movement, posture, and voice play an important role in conveying a certain message. Knapp (1972) indicated that less than 33% of a message's social meaning is transmitted through words alone, whereas 65% of that social meaning is transmitted through nonverbal communication.

Gile (1995) states that "there are no formal sets of rules to provide a systematic list of the meanings of a culture's nonverbal code system. But, we cannot ignore that nonverbal messages can be used to accent, complement, contradict, regulate or contradict the verbal message" (p. 226). It is unrealistic to be able to offer a comprehensive review of nonverbal aspects of communication in a resource such as this one. Therefore, only a few aspects are reviewed here in greater detail: (a) gestures and (b) eye contact, emotions, and sense of time.

Gestures

Morris (1994) reported that as many as 3,000 possible gestures can be expressed using one's hands and fingers alone. Fontes (2008) comments that gestures have a purpose in aiding us to express ourselves. Even when we are on the phone and no one can see us, we use gestures because these gestures "help us think" (p. 83). However, interpretation of gestures may be misleading because they may mean different things in different countries. For example, shrugging in the United States means "I don't know," but among Latinos it may mean "I don't care" or "I don't wish to respond." Pointing is not polite among certain Asian groups, including those from India, Indonesia, or the Philippines. Asking someone to approach using a bent index finger as may be customary in the United States is considered very inappropriate in many parts of the world, as in China, Malaysia, Australia, and Indonesia. Fontes (2008) interprets the meaning of other gestures such as the one we do in the United States using the thumb and index in the shape of an *O* to signify *O.K.*, but it means *zero* in France and *money* in Japan, and making the *O* circle with the middle finger and index to indicate "go ahead" is considered obsene in many parts of the world.

During our interactions with others, we may note if our interviewees may change their facial expressions, cross and uncross their legs, and/or angle their torso. If this happens, Fontes (2008) advises stopping the interview to ask the person(s) about the particular gesture noticed to ensure that all is proceeding smoothly. One should also consider that different gestures for greeting and farewell are used across cultures such as hugging, kissing, and handshaking, and some of these gestures may be acceptable within genders or across genders depending on a specific group. In a professional encounter, shaking hands is a good form of greeting or farewell but not for some Muslim or Orthodox Jewish men. In those cases, a smile and a nod are acceptable substitutes. Age, gender, and personality differences must also be considered.

Therefore, while interacting with persons with diverse languages, cultures, and backgrounds, it is important to focus on the verbal interactions as well as non-verbal aspects to ensure that the interviewee is comfortable. The task of checking on the interviewee should lie not only with the I/T, who is more knowledgeable about verbal and nonverbal communication aspects, but also the SLP and/or audiologist as well as all team members.

Eye Contact, Emotions, and Sense of Time

Eye contact in the mainstream of the United States signifies that a person is attending to his or her communication parter. Grossman (1995) reports that North American listeners tend to gaze into the speaker's eyes, whereas African American listeners tend to look away, and in Japan, the gaze is directed toward the listener's neck (Burgoon, Buller, & Woodall, 1996). Lack of eye contact in Latino and Asian cultures signifies respect but may be interpreted to mean the opposite by European cultures. Fontes (2008) suggests lowering one's eyes or looking away while being observed to ease the interaction.

There is universality in the facial expressions of happiness, sadness, fear, surprise, anger, and disgust (Burgoon et al., 1996). But the specific manner in how these emotions are expressed does vary from culture to culture and may change depending on individual differences as well as each person's unique acculturation to prevalent cultural norms. Specifically, Ekman (1975) found that fear is indicated by a furrowed brow, raised eyebrows, wide-open eyes, creased or pinched base of the nose, taut cheeks, partially open mouth, and upturned upper lip. On the other hand, a smile is often interpreted differently cross-culturally, including embarrassment, friendliness, or a sign of possible tension (Lustig & Koester, 1999). For example, people from the mainstream in the United States lower their heads and use a lower tone of voice when expressing bad news. In some Asian countries as well as Japan, emotions are not openly displayed (Uba, 1994). The opposite may be experienced while interacting with Jews, Latinos, and African Americans. However, overall, many cultures accept that women display their emotions more openly compared to men.

Emotions are conveyed by facial expressions as well as through touch. In Latino and Slavic cultures, touch is more prevalent. When showing their feelings toward a person, many Polish and Slavic persons express it through verbal comments as well as hugs, kisses, and touch.

Likewise, when interacting with Latinos and especially Puerto Ricans, it is common to see conversants touching and grabbing each others' arms, hands, and shoulders. Persons from North America may appear "cold" because touch is not as frequently used in interactions with others (Fontes, 2008). Although it is not unusual for adults to pat children's heads as a sign of comfort or friendship, it is important to remain cautious when interacting with some children from Chinese, Filiipino, Indonesian, and even Central American or African American backgrounds, as the gesture is reserved for animals (Fontes, 2008).

In some countries of the Middle East and Africa, people greet each other with the left hand (which is used for toileting as well) while the right hand is used for eating and for purification before prayer. Still, observant Amish, conservative Christians, Muslims, and Orthodox Jews may not extend their hand to greet an interviewer of the opposite sex.

One other important aspect to consider in successful communication is the sense of time, as it is perceived very differently in many parts of the world. Many North American countries, especially Canada and the United States, as well as European countries, have a linear sense of time as we divide time from millennia into centuries, decades, years, months, weeks, days, hours, and minutes (Fontes, 2008). Many other cultures do not quite have a similar sense of time. For example, this author grew up in Mexico, where some activities did occur following the Western sense of time, while others did not. It required some understanding and adjustment on the part of those who were accustomed to a more predictable schedule. However, after her interaction with many Hispanic families who settled in the

United States, she has noticed a shift in these families' sense of timing and schedules. Over the years, many of these families have adjusted to being punctual for medical and professional appointments, but social appointments are conducted according to more lax schedules. For more extended information on the significance of several nonverbal aspects of communication, the reader is referred to two extensive resources (Fontes, 2008; Graves, 2014). More detailed information on nonverbal communication can be found in Chapters 3 and 4.

In conclusion, some of the greatest challenges in interpretation and translation include idiomatic expressions, the emotional connotations of words, and humor. Probably one of the last aspects of culture to be understood by a second-language learner is the emotional and even legalistic implications of a given word in a given situation. This aspect was exemplified in the dispute between the United States and China regarding the loss of a military plane in early 2001. The word *sorry* was translated into Chinese as *yihan*, which does not carry the connotation of guilt. Instead, *sorry* or *regret* should have been translated as *bao qan*, which renders the more apologetic tone that was expected by the Chinese (Smith, 2001).

Effective communication between two parties mediated by an interpreter is often difficult to achieve for several reasons, particularly those related to training issues. In some cases, interpreters have not received formal training, and in others, the training has been inconsistent. The philosophy of what constitutes effective interpreting in specific settings like education or health (with the exception of the medical setting) has not been defined. The lack of recognition for those interpreters working in educational/school settings is often mentioned (Carr, 1997). Another reason is the lack of consensus regarding the role of the interpreter as conveyer of meaning or mediator of communication. The interpreter must simultaneously balance two variables, verbal/linguistic and nonverbal, taking into consideration culture and context.

The next section is written as a reminder to both the SLP/audiologist that various phenomena may occur as a result of a client's contact with two languages, and this knowledge is considered important in evaluating a client's linguistic performance in order to be more effective when assessing a bilingual client.

PHENOMENA THAT OCCUR WHEN TWO LANGUAGES ARE IN CONTACT

Three phenomena are reviewed when two languages are in contact: (a) early awareness of two languages, (b) code-switching, and (c) language loss.

Early Awareness of Two Languages

Studies of children growing up in a bilingual environment document their awareness of two languages as early as 18 months; the child may be able to respond in the language in which she or he is addressed, or may even comment, "I speak like mommy" or "I speak like daddy" (Burling, 1973 [Garo and English]; Leopold, 1970 [German-English]; Vihman, 1981 [English-Estonian]). However, Vihman and McLaughlin (1982) indicate that the consciousness of being able to express the difference between two languages is

not apparent until age 4. This awareness depends on factors such as the level of language proficiency of the parents and caregivers as well as the language patterns used in the community. Nevertheless, the experience of the first writer is that even individuals with moderate to severe cognitive deficits can differentiate the two languages. Greenlee (1981) documents how adult individuals with severe cognitive disabilities switched to English when approached by Anglo persons who had learned Spanish as a second language and had an apparent non-native–like accent to ease the interaction. This fact indicates that even individuals who have severe cognitive impairments are aware of two languages when they are raised bilingually, and they can differentiate if the person can speak the language with ease. On the other hand, this author has found that some bilingual children who have language disorders are unable to differentiate between two languages, that is, they have difficulty identifying that *avión* is Spanish and *plane* is English. Yet, other students and individuals who can make this distinction may still have challenges in various comprehension and expression areas in both languages to varying degrees depending on their experience with and use of each language.

Code-Switching

Contrary to what may be believed, the majority of the world's population is bilingual (Baker & Jones, 1998). As Crystal (1997) stated, "Multilingualism is the natural way of life for hundreds of millions all over the world . . . it is obvious that an enormous amount of language contact must be taking place" (p. 362). Bilingual individuals often code-switch or code-mix (the two terms have been used interchangeably), a very common phenomenon, when they come in contact with other bilingual or even monolingual individuals. Paradis, Genesee, and Crago (2011) list various studies that document how young bilingual children use each of their languages and how they may switch to the other language depending on the context of the interaction. For example, they may use one or the other language more even with the parent who is not proficient in the other language they speak. When interacting with strangers, they switch to the strangers' language as much as possible, indicating they are aware of their preferred language. At times, children use a word in one language because they do not have that word available in the other language and/or there is not an equivalent word in the other language. In many instances, the code-mixing pattern is similar to the one used by adults. To summarize, Paradis et al. (2011) indicate that code-switching has a pragmatic effect, such as to emphasize what is being said, to quote what someone has said, to protest, and/or to narrate. Furthermore, the authors report that some of the children they observed used a given language more frequently to express emotions or to relate what had happened in a given situation. For example, they would switch to Spanish when speaking about school matters or when they would play with their friends during recess. Examples from Paradis et al. (2011) include *"Dame el spoon"* for ("Give me the spoon") or using the same word in the two languages to make an emphasis, as in *"Donne-moi le cheval, le cheval, the horse"* ("Give me the horse, the horse . . . ") (Genesee & Sauve, 2000) as well as intra-utterance code-switching, as in *"Alguién se murió en este cuarto, that he sleeps in"* ("Someone died in that room"

(Zentella, 1999, p. 119) and inter-utterance as in *"Pa, ¿me vas a comprar un jugo? It costs 25 cents"* ("Dad, are you going to buy me a juice?" [Zentella, 1999, p. 118]). The examples provided above do not violate the syntactic rules of any of the two languages. Thus, *"Elle est allée au mall"* ("She went to the mall") is an example of code-switching at the word level, but *"She est allée au mall"* would violate the rule between the subject pronoun and the verb. For specific rules of code-switching, the reader is referred to Milroy and Muysken (1995) and Myers-Scotton (1992).

Martin-Jones (1995) conducted several classroom observations where bilingual assistants were participating in the instructional process. She noted that each language was used for different purposes; English was used when the assistant was emphasizing some key concepts, but the native language was used to give directions. There was a difference between *curriculum talk* and *learner talk*. Furthermore, there may be situations when a child infuses the two languages within the same sentence or a given word. This author, who raised her daughter bilingually, finds herself switching to French when conveying a special feeling or opinions that convey emotions in her interactions instead of continuing the conversation in English. This behavior is far from unusual.

Until the past 20 years, code-switching was believed to result from an individual's inability to converse effectively in either of the two languages. Terms such as *Spanglish, Tex-Mex, Franglais, and Hinglish* were used to denote the alternation of two languages within discourse, and these terms were used in a derogatory manner. Currently, code-switching is considered to be a communication strategy used by proficient bilingual speakers. Reasons for code-switching include (a) emphasizing a given point, (b) relating something that was learned or occurred while using the alternate language, (c) accessing words in the alternate language when there are no equivalent words in the language of interaction (e.g., *quinceañera, bar* or *bat mitzvah*, which have cultural connotations, or words where an equivalent in another language is difficult to find, such as the English word *background* or the word *gemütlich* [*cozy* in German], *cul-de sac*), (d) expressing a specific feeling or emotion that is connected to the alternate language, (e) interjecting humor into the conversation, (f) excluding someone from the conversation, (g) adding authority, and (h) showing expertise (Grosjean, 1982, 2012; Myers-Scotton, 1992).

An additional example of code-switching, which is often referred to as *borrowing*, is when a child uses the prefix of one language and the ending of another within the same word, as described in the following situation. When a bilingual Spanish-Polish-speaking child said to his sister, "*Jéchame más*," using the root of Polish *jechać* meaning *to drive* and the suffix *me* for the Spanish imperative making the phrase "Drive me," the sister responded, "*Ya te jeché bastante*" ("I have driven you enough"), using the Polish verb *jechać* within a Spanish sentence. Other examples include "*está parqueando*" (from the root *park* and Spanish *ando*–progressive form), "*está mopeando*" (from the root *mop* and the Spanish progressive form *ando*). Or, "*Maman tu peux me taier (tie) mes chaussures?*" ("Mom, can you tie my shoes") (Grosjean, 2012, p. 59).

The following quote stresses the positive aspects of code-switching, "Mixing speech or speaking styles is common in everyday discourse, it makes discourse colorful, authentic, and varied. Bilingual children have the advantage of being able to use two languages to enrich their discourse" (Paradis et al., 2011, p. 99).

Language Loss

When a speaker is bilingual or multicultural, proficiency in the weaker language(s) may decline over time. Anderson (2004) differentiates *language loss* from *language attrition*. Language loss is a more rapid phenomenon compared to language attrition, which is generally considered a slower process. Several personal, social, cultural, and linguistic reasons may explain this phenomenon, specifically, a decreased number of speakers in a given geographical area caused by political and personal factors, distance from the country where the language is spoken, greater use of the majority language (which is necessary for employment), and possible belief that use of the language might not be needed for future social or vocational promotions. Other reasons for language attrition include when one spouse does not speak the same languages as the other spouse and no other relatives are living close by, or the individual's literacy in the first language is limited and/or written materials in that language are unavailable.

This author has equated the preservation of her languages to that of flowers and trees growing in a garden. "*Bilingualism and for that matter, multilingualism, is something one has to continually develop and take care of, just like flowers and trees in a garden, which need water and exposure to sun to grow and bloom.*" Specifically, this author grew up speaking two languages, Polish and Spanish, while being raised in Mexico City. When she enrolled in school, French became her language for academic learning. She began speaking more English once she moved to the United States to pursue her graduate education. A special effort was needed to preserve her three languages other than English. She is still fluent in both Spanish and French and reads the languages well even though she has resided over 45 years in the United States. She has been using her Spanish to work with Hispanic students and their families, and she has preserved her French language skills through reading and conversation with French speakers. Polish has been maintained through conversations with Polish-speaking relatives and some acquaintances as well as more recent frequent visits to Poland to present on her academic expertise in Polish. A conscious effort on her part has been needed to cultivate those three languages.

When assessing bilingual children, SLPs need to consider the frequency and proficiency of each language used by their students. For example, a child may not be able to read or write in Spanish or Russian, because he or she has not been exposed to the language in an academic setting, or the formal teaching has been sporadic or simply stopped at a certain point in the child's school career. The student may know a certain word in one language but not in the other language due to exposure/experience. Therefore, taking a detailed history of language use is important in determining if language loss or attrition might be a contributing factor in decreased performance in certain aspects of the student's first-language proficiency.

TRANSLATION SKILLS

The job description of an I/T lists the following knowledge and skills needed to be an effective translator: (a) knowledge of the English language and target language as mentioned earlier in this chapter, (b) understanding written sentences and paragraphs in work-related documents, (c) communicating effectively in writing as appropriate for the needs of the SLP or audiologist, (d) the ability to read and understand information and ideas presented in writing, and (e) the ability to communicate information and ideas in writing so others will understand (http://www.onetonline.org/link/summary/27-3091.00). Being bilingual and having good reading and writing skills in two languages does not make one an effective translator. Some specific skills are necessary, such as being familiar with the terms used in the given profession as well as the particular style for the profession.

Translating a legal document is a different task than translating a speech-language or audiological report. One of the main differences between interpreting and translating is that unless the task is to translate a written document verbally, there is no urgency to transfer the information from one language to the other immediately. One can take the time to read and think about the written material in the original language and compose the translation at any necessary pace. Some important ideas to keep in mind when translating include the following: (a) Read the entire text before beginning to translate; (b) do not translate each word, but focus on the meaning; (c) write a draft of the entire document; (d) take a break before going back to the text once again; (e) ask someone else to read the translation, especially if it is in a language that may not be your native language (it is possible that you are an English speaker who is very fluent in a second language, or the opposite), as it will depend on whether the translation is from L1 (target language) to L2 (English) or the opposite; and (f) check punctuation and spelling, including accents, because they may change the meaning of what is being said, for example, *tomo* versus *tomó* (in Spanish, "I take" vs. " I took"). Paper dictionaries were utilized in the past, but today there are many software products that are easily accessed that save time in finding equivalent terms in other languages. However, it is still very important to verify if the translation is accurate, including checking the spelling, grammar, and syntax. This is especially important for languages that are spoken in countries where services in speech-language pathology and audiology are not that frequent.

All readers of this guide should keep in mind that translating test items from English into another language should be avoided at all costs. This topic is further discussed in Chapter 6, which describes the process of assessment in speech-language pathology and audiology using services from an I/T.

VERBALLY/LINGUISTICALLY BASED APPLICATIONS TO THE INTERPRETING PROCESS

The verbal component of the interpretation process requires understanding, visualizing, and re-creating the message in the target language (Gile, 1995). Furthermore, specialized training may be required to translate to and from particular languages. Researchers who have focused on this issue have different opinions. Some feel that the process is universal, others that it is language specific. For example, interpreting from French to German may require different skills than interpreting from Japanese and English. Gile (1986)

reported that certain words in Japanese are pronounced identically but may have different meanings, so the challenge in interpreting Japanese is greater than it is for many other languages. He further noted that for a long time, researchers have neglected considering the specificity of languages and have masked the process with other than purely linguistic issues, such as attention and memory. It is time to analyze the linguistic aspect more carefully.

In typical discourse, "the number of grammatical structures that emerge (given a specific context, in this case, the process of assessment and the assessment itself) is finite and . . . what really varies is the lexicon" (Gile, 1995, p. 213). Content words, such as nouns, verbs, adjectives, and adverbs, are carriers of information and differ across languages in length and phonetic richness. Vocabulary shows essential differences because it reflects what is important in that language (Lustig & Koester, 1999). Specific linguistic features remind us about differences within members of a given group. For example, as stated earlier, in Spanish there are two types of *you*, and in many Asian languages, several different forms of *you* are used depending on who is addressed. Some languages may have very specific words to denote variations or subtleties for a concept. However, a talented interpreter can find a way to render the concept in an alternate language when there is no equivalent word for it. But, when unsure, the interpreter should check with the person who made a given comment or remark.

The process of interpreting is challenging because some structures are definitely more difficult to translate. For example, embedded sentences (e.g., "The specialist who told me that my son had autism was the one that was recommended by my physician when I belonged to Kaiser two years ago") can put a heavy demand on short-term memory skills. Furthermore, some languages do not have a term to translate *autism*, and the I/T may be the one person who will need to inform the professional about this fact.

When one of the parties has an accent in a given language that may interfere with smooth communication, or when a child or an adult has a speech-language impairment, the process of interpreting becomes even more challenging. A speaker's accent may unjustly convey a negative impression to native speakers of a given language. Unfortunately, the perception of accents varies from listener to listener: Some people may react neutrally, others negatively. The reality is that the moment one leaves one's place of residence, a listener who comes from another area may perceive an accent. Accents may be regional or foreign, and the burden of carrying on the conversation rests on the person whose accent is different. The ultimate success of the conversation rests on sociolinguistic variables. For example, French or Swedish accents may be perceived more positively in certain parts of the United States, compared to vernacular English or Spanish accents. This type of phenomenon is also true in Hawaii when considering Tagalog or Chinese accents. For more information on this topic, the reader is referred to Lippi-Greene (2004, 2012). Nevertheless, a client's perception of an interpreter may depend on the interpreter's accent, which may influence the trust in the process.

The interpreting process may also be complicated because of differences in the parties' educational levels; therefore, certain forms or words may need to be used with greater care. This author's experience is to be generally cautious in utilizing technical terms often referred to as professional jargon, such as *auditory processing, articulation, phonology, syntax, semantics, phonemic awareness, conductive hearing loss, discrimination*, and many others. A definition is preferred, and this practice is even recommended in cases where the SLP or audiologist interacts with members of the mainstream.

Interpretation is also complex because many words include two types of meaning. The denotative meaning carries the public, objective, and legal meaning of a given word. The connotative meaning carries more of the personal, emotionally charged private meaning (Lustig & Koester, 1999).

Other complicating matters in the interpreting process may be due to phenomena such as code-switching, language interference, and possible language loss. Specifically, interpreters may code-switch when the participants have at least receptive knowledge of the two languages. For example, the interpreter might repeat some of the information that was expressed by the SLP or a professional in the language of interaction instead of the client's or family's first language. Also, there may not be an equivalent for a given word in a given language, which interferes with smooth interpreting. In that case, a synonym or a definition for the word in the target language may be necessary, and this is the responsibility of the professional and not the interpreter. For example, if there is no equivalent for a given term like *autistic*, the SLP or audiologist will need to define the word.

Interference between two languages may also occur because of similarities between two words in the two languages (Gile, 1995). This might happen when words in two languages resemble each other in structure, like *embarazada* (Spanish, *pregnant*) for *embarrassed*, instead of using the Spanish equivalents, *apenada* or *con pena*.

At times, interpreters may not remember the translation of a word while performing an interpretation, and they may need to access a dictionary. Language loss is a common phenomenon for any bilingual individual, and everyone should keep in mind that living languages are changing. Therefore, there is a need for I/Ts to continue practicing their languages as much as possible. More on this topic is discussed in Chapter 4.

In summary, verbal and nonverbal means are part of the communication process. A native speaker of a given language can readily associate the verbal and nonverbal components of a language. However, this synchrony is unfamiliar to the party who does not know a given language. Part of the interpreter's role is to manage two languages that depend on two different verbal and nonverbal messages. The role of the interpreter is to render the message from one language to the other. The art of interpreting in many ways depends on the interpreter's skills in translating the message that is conveyed verbally and nonverbally. As Gile (1995) states,

> There are no formal sets of rules to provide a systematic list of the meanings of a culture's nonverbal code systems. But, we cannot ignore that nonverbal messages can be used to accent, complement, contradict, regulate, or substitute for the verbal message. (p. 226)

As was noted in the chapter, cultures differ greatly in their pragmatic rules, and interpreters face challenges that transcend form, content, and use of language (Cheng, 1998, 1999). The interpreting process takes place in a structured situation where one of the speakers is usually the SLP or audiologist with possibly a teacher or another allied health professional and the client (often from a culturally perceived less prestigious language). The interpreter is the participant who supposedly has command of both languages (Roy, 2000). Often, there is no social equality between the participants and the recipient of the service, and there is a high likelihood that the team of professionals and the interpreter have not been trained to work with one another. As Englund Dimitrova (1997) indicated, very few people are used to or trained for communicating through another individual. In this situation, the interpreter becomes "the actor solving not only problems of translation, but problems of mutual understanding" (Roy, 2000, p. 30). Although the interpreter needs to remain neutral (interpret faithfully and accurately), the conversational flow must be maintained, and it is the interpreter who manages this flow. The success of the interpretation process is highly dependent on how the interpreter is able to coordinate the combination of verbal and nonverbal communication in two languages, a very complex task.

Essentially, the interpreter needs to convey the cultural knowledge and ways of speaking in a given situation and, "in the end all participants jointly produce the event, and all are responsible, in differing degrees for its communicative success or failure" (Roy, 2000, p. 100). The professionals collaborating with an interpreter should be mindful of the many demands on the interpreter and help in any way possible.

SLPs and audiologists should also be aware of the cultural beliefs that affect a family's reaction to a diagnosis or treatment recommendation. A cultural definition of what constitutes an impairment is critically dependent on the values of each particular cultural group. Chapter 3 covers extensive information on cultural values on a number of issues that pertain to the professions of SLPs and audiologists, such as beliefs and attitudes about specific speech and communication disorders and their possible causes, the definition of what constitutes a disability, and different types of treatment plans and relationships between professionals and clients, among other issues. Child-rearing practices and communication expectations of children also vary widely within and across various cultures (Heath, 1983; Lubell, Lofton, & Singer, 2008; van Kleeck, 1994; Vigil & Hwa-Froelich, 2004). There are differences in how parents and other persons respond to their children's language and how families encourage children to initiate and continue a verbal exchange. Socioeconomic and individual differences must always be considered as well as differences in educational practices. Some families understand and support bilingual education, while others have no options or opinions because they believe that schools know best about how to educate their children. Among those families, there are a variety of attitudes toward the first and second language and culture, various levels of formal education in the first or second language, and differing expectations for their children. Families' perceptions also vary regarding the use of assistive technology (Huer, 2000; Parette, Brotherson, & Huer, 2000).

In addition to verbal, nonverbal, and cultural variables, interpreting is dependent on particular situations or contexts. Some situations are more complex than others, for example, when the I/T needs to assist in assessing the speech and language of a child, which is less predictable compared to taking a background history. A counseling session about results of a hearing evaluation may also be more complex because of the nature of the hearing problem and the follow-up that needs to take place. The interpreting process may be further complicated because the context of what is being interpreted may be totally foreign to one of the parties. For example, in the United States, rights must be disclosed to individuals before they sign a contract or agree to a procedure; this is unknown to many people from other countries. Informing someone of his or her rights is done in educational and medical contexts.

In this section of the chapter, we have reviewed some of the challenges faced by interpreters during the process of interpreting. This process consists of taking into account verbal, nonverbal, cultural, and contextual elements.

DISCUSSION ITEMS AND ACTIVITIES

1. The SLP or audiologist and interpreter are going to assess a student who speaks language XXX (select a language in your group). The SLP or audiologist knows very little about the language. Where and how should the information about that language be gathered?

2. Role-play interpreting the following situations with an interpreter who speaks a given language—both interpreter and SLP/audiologist take notes about verbal and nonverbal communication features. At the end, discuss what was the same or differ-

ent in each language, English and language XXX.

a. The parent says, "I have been very worried about my son's speech ever since he was 2 years old, but no one listened to me!" (angry, anxious-looking face)

b. Father comments, "I don't agree with what the SLP said, because P. [3 years old] is very clear at home, and he can understand all we say to him."

c. Mother says, "I can't help M. because I don't speak English. Am I confusing her if I speak XXX at home with her?"

d. "When I was pregnant with T., I had a car accident and I had to stay in the hospital for 3 days. I think it is this that caused the problem" (mom sobs).

e. "I don't understand what you are saying—in my country there are no services for children, and do I have to pay for all of this?" (parent has a very worried look on her face).

3. What should an SLP and interpreter be aware of about code-switching and language loss?

4. What methods could an SLP or audiologist use to make sure he or she is not overlooking or misunderstanding nonverbal communication from a client?

5. How would you explain the following situations to a parent who is unfamiliar with any of the following procedures? Also, request the I/T to translate these phrases into the target language:

a. Parents' rights for special education

b. Permission to obtain medical records (parent is confused about the need for that data for a speech-language evaluation)

c. Goals and objectives of an IEP

d. Least restrictive educational environment

REFERENCES

Abreu, R., Adriatico, T., & DePierro A. M. (2011, November). ¿Qué pasa? "What's happening" in overcoming barriers to serving bilingual children? *ASHA Leader, 16*, 12–15.

Anderson, R. (2004). First language loss in Spanish-speaking children: Patterns of loss and implications for clinical practice. In B. Goldstein, (Ed.), *Bilingual language development and disorders in Spanish-English speakers* (pp. 193–212). Baltimore, MD: Brookes.

Baker, C., & Jones, S. P. (1998). *Encyclopedia of bilingualism and bilingual education*. Clevedon, UL: Multilingual Matters.

Berman, R. (2001). Cross-linguistic perspectives on narrative development: Epilogue. In L. Verhoeven & L. Strömqvist (Eds.), *Narrative development in a multilingual context* (pp. 419–428). Amsterdam, the Netherlands: John Benjamins.

Bliss, L., & McCabe, A. (2008). Personal narratives: Cultural differences and clinical implications. *Topics in Language Disorders, 28*(2), 162–177.

Bliss, L., & McCabe, A. (2011). Educational implications of narrative discourse. In S. Levey & S. Polirstok (Eds.), *Language development: Understanding language diversity in the classroom* (pp. 209–227): Los Angeles, CA: Sage.

Bloom, L., & Lahey, M. (1978). *Language development and language disorders*: New York, NY: Wiley.

Bureau of Labor Statistics, U.S. Department of Labor. (2014). *Occupational outlook handbook, 2014–15 edition, interpreters and translators*. Retrieved November 4, 2014, from http://www.bls.gov/ooh/media-and-communication/interpreters-and-translators.htm

Burgoon, J. K., Buller, D. B., & Woodall, W. G. (1996). *Nonverbal communication: The unspoken dialogue*. New York, NY: McGraw-Hill.

Burling, R. (1973). Language development of a Garo and English-speaking child. In C. A. Ferguson & D. A. Slobin (Eds.), *Studies of child language development* (pp. 69–90). New York, NY: Rinehart & Winston.

Campbell, G. L., & King, G. (2011). *Concise compendium of world's languages* (2nd ed.). London, UK: Routledge.

Carr, S. E. (1997). A three-tiered healthcare interpreter system. In S. E. Carr, R. P. Roberts, A. Dufour, & D. Steyn (Eds.), *The critical link: Interpreters in the community* (pp. 271–276). Amsterdam, The Netherlands: John Benjamins.

Cheng, L.-R. L.(1998). Beyond multiculturalism: Translators make it happen. In V. O. Pang & L.-R. L. Cheng (Eds.), *Struggling to be heard* (pp. 105–122). Albany, NY: SUNY Press.

Cheng, L.-R. L. (1999). Moving beyond accent: Social and cultural realities in living with many tongues. *Topics in Language Disorders, 8*(3), 293–310.

Crystal, D. (1997). *The Cambridge encyclopedia of language* (2nd ed.). New York, NY: Cambridge University Press.

Echevarría, J., Vogt, M. E., & Short, D. (2012). *Making content comprehensible for English learners: The SIOP model* (4th ed.). New York, NY: Pearson.

Ekman, P. (1975, September). The universal smile: Face muscles talk every language. *Psychology Today, 9*, 35–39.

Englund Dimitrova, B. (1997). Degree of interpreter responsibility in the interaction process in community interpreting. In S. E. Carr, R. Roberts, A. Dufour, & D. Steyn (Eds.), *The critical link: Interpreters in the community* (pp. 147–164). Philadelphia, PA: John Benjamins.

Florián, L. (2010). *A comparative and dialectical lexicon of variations in modern Spanish vocabulary: Tracking linguistic differences across cultural, national and dialectical differences.* Lewiston, NY: Edwin Mellen Press.

Fontes, L. (2008). *Interviewing clients across cultures: A practitioner's guide.* New York, NY: Guilford.

Genesee, F., & Sauve, D. (2000, March 12). *Grammatical constraints on child bilingual code-mixing.* Paper presented at the Annual Conference of the American Association for Applied Linguistics, Vancouver, British Columbia, Canada.

Gile, D. (1986). La reconnaissance des kango et la perception du discours japonais. *Lingua, 70*(2/3), 171–189.

Gile, D. (1995). *Basic concepts and models for interpreter and translator training.* Philadelphia, PA: John Benjamins.

Gillam, R., Peña, E., & Miller, J. (1999). Dynamic assessment of narrative and expository discourse. *Topics in Language Disorders, 20*, 33–47.

Graves, D. (2014). *The nonverbal dictionary of gestures, symbols and body language cues.* Spokane, WA: Center for Nonverbal Studies Press.

Greenlee, M. (1981). *Specifying the needs of a "bilingual" developmentally disabled population: Issues and case studies.* Los Angeles, CA: National Dissemination and Assessment Center.

Grosjean, F. (1982). *Life with two languages: An introduction to bilingualism.* Boston, MA: Harvard University Press.

Grosjean, F. (2012). *Bilingual: Life and reality.* Boston, MA: Harvard University Press.

Grossman, H. (1995). *Teaching in a diverse society.* Needham Heights, MA: Allyn & Bacon.

Hall, E. T. (1977). *The hidden dimension.* Garden City, NY: Anchor.

Heath, S. B. (1983). *Ways with words.* New York, NY: Cambridge University Press.

Hudley, A., & Mallinson, C. (2011). *Understanding English variation in U.S. schools.* New York, NY: Teachers College University Press.

Huer, M. B. (2000). Examining perceptions of graphic symbols across cultures: A preliminary study of the impact of culture/ethnicity. *Augmentative and Alternative Communication, 16*(3), 180–185.

Knapp, M. L. (1972). *Nonverbal communication in human interaction.* New York, NY: Holt, Rinehart, and Winston.

Kramer, K., Mallett, P., Schneider, P., & Hayward, D., (2009). Dynamic assessment of narratives with Grade 3 children in a First Nations community. *Canadian Journal of Speech-Language Pathology and Audiology, 33*(3), 119–128.

Langdon, H. W. (2008). *Assessment and intervention of communication disorders in linguistically and diverse populations.* Clifton Park, NY: Cengage.

Leopold, W. (1970). *Speech development of a bilingual child* (Vols. 1–4). New York, NY: AMS Press.

Lippi-Greene, R. (2004). Language ideology and language prejudice. In J. Rickford & E. Finegan (Eds.), *Language in the USA: Themes for the 21st century* (pp. 289–304). Cambridge, UK: Cambridge University Press.

Lippi-Greene, R. (2012). *English with an accent: Language, ideology and discrimination in the*

United States (2nd ed.). New York, NY: Taylor and Francis.

Lubell, K. M., Lofton, T., & Singer, H. H. (2008). *Promoting parenting practices across cultural groups: A CDC Research Brief*. Atlanta, GA: Centers for Disease Control and Prevention, National Center for Injury Prevention and Control.

Lustig, M. W., & Koester, J. (1999). *Intercultural competence: Interpersonal communication across cultures*. New York, NY: Longman.

Martin-Jones, M. (1995). Code-switching in the classroom: Two decades of research. In L. Milroy & P. Muysken (Eds.), *One speaker, two languages* (pp. 90–110). New York, NY: Cambridge University Press.

Mayer, M. (2003a) . *Frog, where are you?* (Hardcover) New York, NY: Dial Books for Young Readers.

Mayer, M., & Mayer, M. (2003b). *One frog too many*.(Hardcover) New York, NY: Dial Books for Young Readers.

McLeod, S. (2007). *The international guide to speech acquisition*. Clifton, NY: Delmar Learning-Cengage.

McLeod, S., & Goldstein, B. (2012). *Multilingual aspects of sound disorders in children*. Clevedon, UK: Multilingual Matters.

Milroy, L., & Muysken, P. (Eds.). (1995). *One speaker, two languages*. New York, NY: Cambridge University Press.

Morris, D. (1994). *The human animal*. New York, NY: Crown.

Myers-Scotton, C. (1992). Comparing code-switching and borrowing. *Journal of Multilingual and Multicultural Development, 13*(1–2), 19–39.

Nicholson, N. S., & Martinsen, B. (1997). Court interpretation in Denmark. In S. E. Carr, R. Roberts, A. Dufour, & D. Steyn (Eds.), *The critical link: Interpreters in the community* (pp. 259–270). Philadelphia, PA: John Benjamins.

Omniglot: The online Encyclopedia of Writing Systems and Language. Omniglot.com (Simon Ager, author) (1998–2015). Retrieved, October 24, 2014, from http://www.omniglot.com/index.htm

O-net online. (2014). *Summary report for: interpreters and translators*. Retrieved October 24, 2014, from http://www.onetonline.org/link/summary/27-3091.00

Paradis, J., Genesee, F., & Crago, M. (2011). *Dual language development & disorders: A handbook on bilingualism and second language learning* (2nd ed.). Baltimore, MD: Brookes.

Parette, H. P., Brotherson, M. J., & Huer, M. B. (2000). Giving families a voice in augmentative and alternative communication decision-making. *Education and Training in Mental Retardation and Developmental Disabilities, 35*(2), 177–190.

Penney, C., & Simmons, C. (1997). Training the community interpreter: The Nunvut Artic college experience. In S. E. Carr, R. Roberts, A. Dufour, & D. Steyn (Eds.), *The critical link: Interpreters in the community* (pp. 55–64). Philadelphia, PA: John Benjamins.

Ramkissoon, I., Proctor, A., Lansing, C. R., & Bilger, R. C. (2002). Digit speech recognition thresholds (SRT) for non-native speakers of English. *American Journal of Audiology, 11*(1), 23–28.

Roy, C. B. (2000). *Interpreting as a discourse process*. New York, NY: Oxford University Press.

Shi, L., & Sánchez. D. (2010). Spanish/English bilingual listeners on clinical word recognition tests: what to expect and how to predict. *Journal of Speech, Language and Hearing Research, 53*, 1096–1110.

Smith, C. S. (2001, April 9). Collision with China: The semantics. *The Washington Post*, p. 2B.

Swan, M., & Smith, B. (2001). *Learner English: A teacher's guide to interference and other problems* (2nd ed.). Cambridge, UK: Cambridge University Press.

Uba, L. (1994). *Asian Americans: Personality patterns, identity and mental health*. New York, NY: Guilford.

van Kleeck, A. (1994). Potential bias in training parents as conversational partners with their children who have delays in language development. *American Journal of Speech Language Pathology, 3*(1), 67–78.

Vigil, D. B., & Hwa-Froelich, D. A. (2004). Interactional styles in minority caregivers: Implications for intervention. *Communication Disorders Quarterly, 25*(3), 119–126.

Vihman, M. (1981). Phonology and the development of the lexicon: Evidence from children's errors. *Journal of Child Language, 8*, 239–264.

Vihman, M., & McLaughlin, B. (1982). Bilingualism and second language acquisition in preschool children. In C. C. Brainerd & M. Pressley (Eds.), *Verbal processes in children: Progress in cognitive development research* (pp. 35–57). New York, NY: Springer Verlag.

Westby, C. (1994). The effects of culture on genre, structure, and style of oral and written texts. In G. P. Wallach & K. G. Butler (Eds.), *Language learning disabilities in school-age children and adolescents* (pp. 180–218). New York, NY: Merrill.

Wolfram, W., & Schilling-Estes, N. (2006). *American English: Dialects and variations.* Malden, MA: Blackwell.

Zentella, A. C. (1999). *Growing up bilingual: Puerto Rican children in New York.* Malden, MA: Blackwell.

Chapter 3

Cultural Elements

Terry Irvine Saenz

CHAPTER GOALS

- Provide a discussion of *culture* and different types of *acculturation*
- Provide definitions of *disability*, *handicap*, *illness*, and *pain*
- Describe issues of confidentiality
- Describe cross-cultural beliefs about the causes of disabilities
- Describe differences between visible and invisible disabilities
- Describe differences in access and exposure to resources
- Describe the varying role of various family members as decision makers for services
- Describe the influence of formal educational variables
- Describe the role of the interpreter/translator (I/T) as a *cultural broker*

The degree of similarity between the larger society and the culture of a family may have a decisive impact upon the ability to easily communicate and convey meaning among the participants of an intercultural interaction (Fontes, 2008). Both verbal and nonverbal (such as gestures and personal distance) aspects of communication, which were reviewed in Chapter 2, if highly dissimilar, will make it more difficult to convey meaning among participants in a conference, meeting, or an evaluation. Consequently, it is important to consider cultural aspects of any intercultural interaction.

DEFINING CULTURE

Culture is a complex concept to define as it includes such components as language; political, economic, and educational systems; technology; religious patterns; values; social structures; interaction patterns; and more that are transmitted from generation to generation but also evolve and are unique to a group of people (Banks & McGee Banks, 2010; Triandis, 1989). Within any society, individuals fit into a cultural continuum, with some of them orienting themselves more to their home culture and others to the culture of the larger society. In addition to identifying ways of living that have been effective in the past, a given culture outlines strategies for coping with social situations and methods of thinking about social behavior and the self that have been reinforced

55

before. When individuals have been socialized in a particular culture, they may use custom to substitute for thought (Triandis, 1989).

Understanding the role of culture in working with culturally diverse children and families is particularly important now, as many countries are becoming increasingly diverse. For example, in the United States, one out of five children is currently an immigrant or a child of an immigrant (Nguyen, 2006). The growth of culturally diverse children in the United States is primarily due to immigration patterns, with the fastest growing group in the population of children under 18. From 1996 to 2002, the majority of growth in immigrant children came from Mexico, then remained steady for a few years and subsequently decreased slightly from 37% to 28%. In 2012, statistics indicated that first-generation children came from three primary locations, including China, India, and the Philippines, at 5% each (Child Trends, 2013).

In addition, when a speech-language pathologist (SLP) or audiologist works with an I/T, the professional and I/T frequently are from different cultures. Cultural differences may come up during interaction between the professional and the I/T in terms of perceptions of the purpose of testing or meetings or how to best interact with parents, children, and other members of the community. SLPs and audiologists increase their effectiveness in working with I/Ts when they study cultural differences in general and become aware of differences between specific cultures.

Assimilation/Acculturation Issues

Acculturation is a key concept to consider when working with children and families of other cultures. One definition of acculturation is that it is a process in which individuals from one cultural group adopt the behaviors and beliefs of another group (Hazuda, Stern, & Haffner, 1988). Alternatively, it may be defined as a process of psychological and cultural change resulting from the continuing contact of people from different cultural backgrounds (Berry, 2006a). After initial contact between cultures, most contact situations turn into the development of societies with more than one linguistic, cultural, or religious entity within them. Usually, the greatest amount of change may occur in the minority culture (Organista, 2007). In addition, acculturation is not necessarily static across one's lifetime but can be a continuous process (López-Class, Castro, & Ramírez, 2011).

A frequently cited model of acculturation is Berry's (2003) model of acculturation strategies by minority cultures. He characterizes the process of acculturation as a three-step process: contact, conflict, and adaptation. Contact involves the ways in which two cultural groups meet, including by immigration, seeking refuge, or invasion. Conflict is the tension that results when one cultural group attempts to dominate another cultural group. Conflict may not result in all cases of cases of acculturation, but it is common (Organista, 2007). Adaptation is the final form of accommodation reached between groups where the purpose is to reduce conflict (Berry, 2003).

Berry (2003) has cited four types of acculturation strategies of minority cultures, including *integration, assimilation, separation,* and *marginalization*. In the *integration* strategy, individuals have an interest in maintaining their group culture when interacting with members of other cultural groups, yet they additionally wish to participate in the larger society. In the *assimilation* strategy, people do not wish to preserve their cultural identity and attempt to have daily interactions with those of other cultures. In the *separation* strategy, individuals attempt to maintain their own culture and prefer to avoid interacting with those of other cultures. In the *marginalization* strategy, people have little possibility or interest in the preservation of their original culture (often because cultural loss has been enforced by the larger society) and additionally have little interest in interacting with those of other cultures (often because of exclusion or discrimination) (Berry, 2003, 2006a).

One measure of acculturation is language proficiency in the native language and the dominant language of the country (Horevitz & Organista, 2012; López-Class et al., 2011). A number of researchers have implied that language proficiency in the second language can be associated with adaptation to a new culture (Masgoret & Ward, 2006). Additionally, knowledge of the language spoken by the larger society is important in learning about another culture, as language is the primary way through which cultural information is communicated (Masgoret & Ward, 2006). For example, individuals who have chosen an integration strategy may have fluency in both their native language and the larger society's language. In contrast, individuals who have chosen an assimilation strategy may have substantially better fluency in the larger society's language than in their native language, while individuals who have chosen a separation strategy may be more fluent in their native language. The relationship between two cultures and two languages is represented in Figure 3–1.

There are a number of other acculturation factors, including the acquisition of culturally related behaviors of the larger culture, such as relational behaviors, making friends with or marrying individuals of another culture, and acquiring membership in groups from the larger society (López-Class et al., 2011). The location where individuals live, their social networks, their immigration history, and the type of institutions they may encounter influence the process of acculturation. Thus, a family living in a part of a community with individuals who share the same language and culture and participate in the same events may be less acculturated than individuals who live outside of an ethnic enclave. Similarly, individuals who participate with members of their own culture in a number of organizations, including churches, synagogues, or mosques, may be less acculturated than their peers. When there is ongoing immigration, as well as frequent trips to the country of origin, it is easier to maintain ties with an individual's original culture (Nguyen, 2006).

Migration status also may have considerable impact upon a family's acculturation. Individuals who voluntarily come to the United States for economic reasons, such as many people from Mexico, may have different acculturation experiences than individuals who were forced to immigrate as political refugees, including many people from Southeast Asia, Cuba, and Central America south of Mexico. In such cases, there is a difference between voluntary and involuntary immigration (Berry, 2006a). In addition, some individuals, such as some Mexican nationals, periodically travel back and forth from their native country, undergoing a cyclical process of acculturation that is different from the typical acculturation process (López-Class et al., 2011).

Other areas in which acculturation may occur include the cultural value of

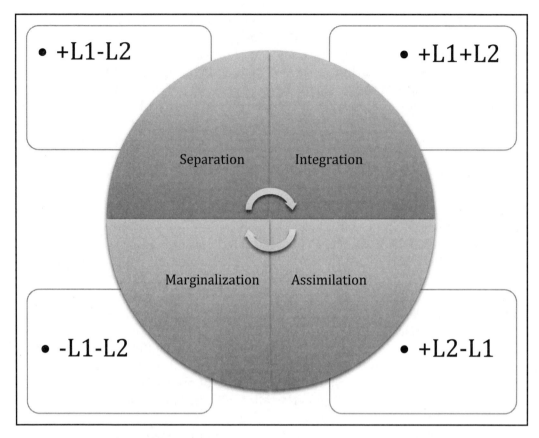

Figure 3–1. Relationship between two cultures and two languages. Adapted from Berry, 2003. L1: first language; L2: second language (here English).

familism, or emphasis upon the nuclear or extended family, gender roles, children's need for achievement, and parenting practices (Chun & Akutsu, 2003; Marín & Gamba, 2003). Acculturation has no consistent effect upon familism, with more acculturated individuals not consistently having decreased family ties. Researchers have found conflicting results of acculturation on familism, with negative, positive, and no effects upon it (Chun & Akutsu, 2003). However, maintenance of a minority culture consistently has a positive effect on family relationships (Birman & Taylor-Ritzler, 2007).

Greater acculturation may result in more equal gender roles between spouses. For example, in traditional Latino families, there may be strict gender roles, yet more acculturated Latino women have moved beyond their traditional roles into more egalitarian relationships (Chun & Akutsu, 2003).

In terms of children's need for achievement, many traditional Asian students see it as their responsibility to academically achieve to please their parents. Students of Mexican immigrants in the United States may have a somewhat complicated reaction to the need for achievement (Roche, Ghazarian, & Fernández-Esquer, 2012). Such students are more likely to achieve if they have more ability in the English language and strong familism. At the same time, they may be less likely to achieve if their parents have social ties in the United States and the students value early paid work.

Parenting practices can be complicated by the fact that children often are more acculturated to the larger culture than their parents (Pawliuk et al., 1996; Santisteban & Mitrani, 2003), with the second generation gravitating more readily towards assimilation or integration (Schwartz & Zamboanga, 2008). In extreme cases, this may be reflected in language use, in which children speak only a larger society's language, while parents exclusively speak their native language (Santisteban & Mitrani, 2003). In addition, children's acceptance of majority cultural values and attitudes, when contrasted with parents' more traditional expectations, can result in powerful family conflicts (López-Class et al., 2011; Santisteban & Mitrani, 2003).

Acculturation differences between older generations may play a role during family meetings and in sharing information with professionals. For example, a family meeting may include a grandparent, who may not be very acculturated to the larger society and may have poor mastery of English, as well as one or more parents who may have more of an integrative orientation and stronger English skills. Therefore, when working with professionals, some older family members may be reluctant to share personal information or to agree to perform recommended interventions due to lack of trust for the larger culture's values (Fontes, 2008). This may be especially true of refugee families who have fled from repressive regimes

and who consequently may be wary of government institutions and the need to provide information that is typically elicited from parents in a speech-language assessment, such as pregnancy or birth history. For example, even Native American families in the United States may be less trusting of government institutions given a history of repression by the government (Clay, Seekins, & Castillo, 2010). Due to similar experiences in Australia, indigenous Australians may have a fear of authority and of governmental institutions (Hollinsworth, 2013).

Another area of potential difference in acculturation is the issue of *collectivism* versus *individualism*. Individuals from *individualistic* cultures are less oriented toward the needs and goals of their group (Triandis, 1995; Trumbull, Rothstein-Fisch, Greenfield, & Quiroz, 2001). They feel freer to pursue their individual goals without regard for their group's objectives; they may feel that they only need to care for themselves and their nuclear family (Hofstede, 2001). They may have a relatively positive attitude toward individuals who are not of their group (Triandis, 1989). Additionally, they have a lower *power distance* index, or the degree to which less powerful members of organizations and institutions accept and expect that power is unequally distributed (Hofstede, 2001). That is, inequality between those in power and those who are dependent on that power is smaller. This index is 80 in several Arab countries, whereas it is only 40 in the United States and only 11 in Austria. Thus, compared to societies that are more collectivistic, parenting in individualistic societies is more likely to emphasize independence, self-reliance, and creativity (Triandis, 1989, 1995). European countries, Australia, Canada, and the United States are higher in individualism, and therefore, their power distance index tends to be lower compared to other countries (Hofstede, 2001).

Individuals of *collectivistic* cultures value fitting in and being a part of one or more groups (Triandis, 1989). They often pursue the goals of their group to reach interpersonal harmony among group members. Depending on the group they are part of, these individuals may be expected to share the norms and behaviors of their group and to provide loyalty to the group in return for ongoing protection (Hofstede, 2001). Relationships with members of their group are positively perceived, but such individuals may be more suspicious of those who are not of their group (Triandis, 1989). Parents in collectivistic cultures often emphasize obedience, conformity, and reliability in their child rearing. Parents also may not expect independent self-help behaviors in some cultures as early as in Western cultures (Cohen, 2013; Fontes, 2008). In addition, members of collectivistic cultures often have a higher power distance index (Hofstede, 2001; Triandis, 1989). Hence, Latin American, Asian, African, and Arab countries are lower in individualism than other countries (Hofstede, 2001).

There are a number of implications of differences in the individualistic versus collectivistic continuum and differences in power distance. Parents from individualistic cultures may be more likely to make their own decisions regarding the speech-language pathology services of their child, whereas individuals of collectivistic cultures may be more likely to consult with other family members. Furthermore, individuals from collectivistic cultures may be more suspicious of institutions of the larger culture while at the same time having greater respect for

professionals in the school setting. As a consequence, it may be somewhat more difficult to gain individuals' trust if they come from a collectivistic culture, yet they may be more hesitant to disagree with professionals.

Another potential aspect of acculturation is *acculturative stress*, or the response of people to life events that occur with intercultural contact, and experiences that occur during the process of acculturation that are harmful and disruptive to the individual and cultural group (Berry, 2006b; Organista, 2007). Families experiencing conflict between family members due to different levels of acculturation are undergoing acculturative stress, with many families of immigrants experiencing this type of difficulty. Young children may personally experience little acculturative stress if exposed to the second culture at an earlier age, but older children may have difficulties (Berry, 2006b). Depression and anxiety often result from acculturative stress (Berry, 2006b), and the higher the degree of acculturative stress, the lower the level of social welfare (Organista, 2007).

One cause of acculturative stress is the prejudice experienced by immigrants (Guimond et al., 2013). The official policy of countries can differ in the degree to which it espouses assimilation or integration of culturally diverse groups. Berry (2003) proposes four different strategies that a larger, more dominant society may take toward a minority group. The society may favor *multiculturalism*, where other cultural groups are encouraged to keep their own culture and to adapt to the larger society, *the melting pot*, in which they are encouraged to assimilate to the larger society, *separation*, in which they are forced to remain separate from the larger society, and *exclusion*, in which the larger society imposes marginalization upon the other culture. When the larger society facilitates integration of a minority culture, the acculturation strategy of integration produces the least acculturative stress, while the acculturation strategy of marginalization results in the highest level of acculturative stress (Berry, 2003). In addition, attempts to assimilate to the larger culture without maintenance of one's original culture or separation from the larger culture can have adverse effects (Nguyen, 2006), although acculturation to any culture may have beneficial effects for some populations (Gupta, Leong, Valentine, & Canada, 2013).

The United States has been described as following an official policy and having cultural norms with elements of the melting pot as well as multiculturalism (Guimond et al., 2013). Nonetheless, at least some cultural groups have historically experienced prejudice and discrimination and have not been encouraged to acculturate to the larger society, all of which have affected their acculturation (Organista, 2007) and their acculturative stress.

Acculturative stress is highest when the behavioral and cultural similarity between two groups is lowest and pressure is greatest on a minority cultural group to acculturate because of a larger society's low tolerance for cultural and racial diversity (Berry, 2003). Discrimination is often highest for members of the first generation of immigrants, whose differences in clothing, accent, and customs are more apparent (Phinney, 2003). Individuals who are visibly and identifiably different than the larger society also are more likely to experience discrimination (Phinney, 2003). European immigrants to North America have historically experi-

enced lower rates of acculturative stress (Organista, 2007). In contrast, Native Americans have been especially subject to acculturative stress, given their history of invasion and forced relocation and subsequent policies of separation from mainstream society on reservations (Organista, 2007).

The implication for professionals working with cultural minority families is that it is important to be mindful of the fact that family members may be undergoing considerable stress in their acculturation to the larger society. As previously noted, different members of a family may be undergoing different types of acculturation with different levels of acculturative stress. The additional stress of a speech-language and/or hearing and possible learning disorder upon members of an immigrant family is not to be underestimated, given that a family may already be under considerable acculturative stress in attempts to acculturate to the larger society.

Another issue in terms of acculturation is a family's attitude toward institutions. Individuals who are less acculturated and who come as refugees from other countries may distrust institutions, including the school system. Alternatively, some individuals may feel that it is not their position to challenge large institutions, and they are less like to assert themselves in interactions with school personnel (Santisteban & Mitrani, 2003). The implications are that, on the one hand, SLPs and audiologists may need to deal with distrust on the part of immigrant families. On the other hand, they may need to do their best to ensure that the concerns of each family are expressed and heard.

Children of immigrant families face their own challenges in acculturation.

They have the task of acculturating to the school setting, often the primary location for their initial contact with the larger culture. However, these children may be more acculturated to the larger society than their parents, and because of their exposure to the second culture and language in school, they participate in two worlds, the larger world and the home world (Fontes, 2008; Pawliuk et al., 1996). As a result, they may be caught between two worlds, not being able to articulate their difficulties and approach their parents with their concerns and problems, thinking that their parents do not understand the larger society and its institutions sufficiently to assist them (Birman & Taylor-Ritzler 2007). Depending on the child's native culture, expectations for social participation in the classroom and with peers may vary widely from expectations for participation within the family (Vedder & Horenczyk, 2006). For example, classroom expectations may include the implicit rule that students should verbally participate in classroom discussions, whereas some families may expect children to be respectfully silent unless addressed. For adolescents, there may be a conflict between the home culture and the norms of a society that advantages individuals who conform to dominant styles of language, clothing, and lifestyles, and peers, who may advocate a different set of values than those of a minority culture (Fontes, 2008; Kunst & Sam, 2013).

There are different opinions about the impact of proficiency in the native language and the second language upon bilingual children's adaptation and adjustment. Some researchers believe that maintenance of the child's native language and a good understanding of his or her culture contributes to his or her ethnic identity, which in turn should support healthy adaptation (Vedder & Horenczyk, 2006). Alternatively, some researchers believe that proficiency in the second language is related to social participation (Vedder & Horenczyk, 2006). Yet others believe that immigrant students with proficiency in both their native languages and the national language have more positive social adjustment (Portes & Rumbaut, 2006; Vedder & Horenczyk, 2006).

There are a number of seemingly problematic behaviors that some children may engage in when they are from an immigrant family that may be due to their acculturating to the classroom in their new country (Fontes, 2008). They may appear unfriendly and aloof if they feel as if they are being left out or have limited second-language proficiency. If children have difficulties in the language of instruction, they may have difficulty focusing their attention or systematically approaching tasks. They may be slow to begin or complete tasks and be perceived as forgetful because of a lack of language proficiency. Their answers to teachers' questions or comments may be produced slower if they have been taught to value reflective thinking rather than quickness. When learning a second language or any new material, for that matter, children and adults need more time to process information and compose answers; this is referred as wait-time. Some children with little formal schooling, including some refugees, may have difficulty keeping track of assignments or school supplies. They may appear to be hyperactive or impulsive if they misunderstand instructions or do not understand classroom rules or may seem undisciplined in class because of stricter classroom rules in their country of origin. Children may be used to collaborating on classroom tasks, and therefore, appear to be cheating.

Children, as well as adults, may experience prejudice and discrimination (Vedder & Horenczyk, 2006), which may vary in different environments (Potochnick, Perreira, & Fuligni, 2012). Positive contact with children of other cultures in the school setting can be an important means of reducing such discrimination and prejudice for immigrant children. However, as many schools continue to include ethnically segregated populations, immigrant children frequently congregate with those of other immigrant groups and not necessarily members of the larger society (Potochnick et al., 2012).

To summarize, families and children may face a variety of circumstances in their immigration to the host country. They may adopt a specific acculturation strategy, either of their own volition and/or in reaction to the attitude of the host society toward their culture (Berry, 2003). There is a greater probability of acculturation to the host society with successive generations in the host country, but some cultures experience prejudice and discrimination from the larger society (Organista, 2007). These circumstances are the cause of many elements of acculturative stress.

Children are often acculturated through their contacts with other cultures in the schools. They frequently are more acculturated than their parents and other older family members, but they may experience acculturative stress when faced with differences between their own and their parents' acculturation. Some of their behaviors may be misperceived in negative ways due to their lack of proficiency in the second language or classroom expectations, and feelings of prejudice and discrimination may not be unusual.

RESPONDING TO THE CLIENT'S/FAMILY'S VOICES

Defining a Disability

The International Classification of Functioning, Disability and Health (ICF) defines *disability* as a term for activity limitations, participation restrictions, and impairments (World Health Organization, 2002; ICF, cited in World Health Organization, 2011). According to the ICF, disability refers to negative aspects of interaction between individuals with health conditions (such as Down syndrome, depression, and cerebral palsy) and environmental and personal factors (such as limited social support, inaccessible public buildings and transportation, and negative attitudes).

However, there are a variety of definitions of disability in the literature, each with its own emphasis and implications. The medical model of disability focuses on the biological aspects of a disability and its difference from the norm (Fraser, 2013; Roscigno, 2013). Other researchers believe in a social model of disability, in which such labels as *disabled* and *nondisabled* are socially constructed. According to such researchers, the issue of disability as a problem results from the attitudes of the larger society and is used to marginalize individuals with disabilities (Fraser, 2013).

There is considerable evidence that the concept of what constitutes a disability varies among cultures. For example, South Asian Muslim families believe that the ability of a person to function with a disability is more important in one's community than the specific disability label (Hasnain & Leung, 2010). Similarly, a Native American child who functions well at home and does not have physical evidence of a disability may not be considered as having a disability (Joe, 1997).

What Constitutes Confidential Information? Disclosure to Strangers

When working with immigrant families using the services of an interpreter, the concept of confidential information may be an issue. Refugees from other countries may have adopted a strategy of not trusting other people, having come from a country where information disclosed about them led them to flee (Tribe & Keefe, 2009). Immigrants who come from countries with dictatorships and secret police also may distrust the safety of personal information (Fontes, 2008). Given a history of oppression or marginalization by the government, some Native Americans may be hesitant to trust the government and its representatives (Lomay & Hinkebein, 2006).

In some cultures, individuals have a general reluctance to talk about personal matters and prefer that one speaks about them indirectly because the information may be considered the collective property of a group and should not be divulged without the group's permission (Fontes, 2008)—for example, when information may be considered to bring shame to the family or the family's cultural group. Among some East Asian cultures, keeping sensitive information private is considered a virtue, because it allows individuals to save face (Fontes, 2008). Nowak (2005) reports that for Vietnamese, there may be the belief that divulging personal information may jeopardize their legal status. In other cultures, including Latino and Native American, a strong personal relationship is required before secrets are shared with an interviewer. When individuals are using traditional medicine to treat a disability, they may be reluctant to share this or other folk practices with an interviewer (Fontes, 2008).

The opportunity for distrust is even higher when an interview involves an interpreter. Family members may need reassurances about confidentiality, as they may fear gossip being spread about their family (Fontes, 2008). Family members may need to know the reasons for personal questions and the elicitation of personal information. The fear of confidentiality may vary depending on the background of the interpreter. A professional interpreter may elicit less fear than a member of the family's community or family, as secrets may be difficult to keep in some small tightly knit ethnic communities (Fontes, 2008; Jackson, 1998; Norbury & Sparks, 2013). In fact, family members, especially children or minors, should not interpret for a family because of the issue of family secrets. In general, it may be stated that trained interpreters are associated with better clinical care (Karliner, Jacobs, Chen, & Mutha, 2007). In addition, collaboration with untrained interpreters is more associated with breaches of confidentiality (Phillips, 2010). Remote interpretation, in which the interpreter is not physically present, may even be preferred in some cases because of increased confidentiality (Gany et al., 2007). Because of these concerns, it is always important to caution any I/T about the importance of confidentiality and explain the concept to him or her.

Compounding issues of confidentiality and trust is the dilemma when an interpreter is not of the same ethnic group as the family and there is a history of antipathy between the cultural groups of the interpreter and the family (Tribe & Keefe, 2009). In such cases, it is preferable to obtain the services of a different interpreter. To avoid difficult situations, I/Ts can be introduced to a family at the outset of a meeting, and the family can be asked if they are agreeable to the I/T interpreting for the meeting.

Cross-Cultural Beliefs as a Need to Pinpoint Causes for a Disability

Cultural beliefs about a disability can vary across cultures, and in some cases, modern Western beliefs about disability may coexist with traditional beliefs. It is important to emphasize that cultural beliefs can be changed, modified, or strengthened in families who are immigrants (Ravindran & Myers, 2012). These beliefs can be changed by the availability of resources, perceptions of disabilities in the new country, and the family's ability to access these resources. However, some cultural differences have been found in attitudes toward disabilities.[1]

Latino Attitudes[2]

Latino attitudes toward disability vary depending on a specific geographic area and socioeconomic status. For example, professionals in Peru are aware of the biological bases of developmental disability, while low-income community members are more likely to attribute it to economic insecurity, domestic problems, drug and alcohol abuse, and parental violence (O'Shea, Girón, Cabrera, Lescano, & Taren, 2012). Community members' attitudes toward an individual with a developmental disability are strongly influenced by the reputation of his or her family. Some families react by sending the child to a public school or special education center, while others shut their children inside their homes, but there is no evidence that community members or professionals have discriminatory attitudes toward developmental disabilities. For other Latinos, disability may be seen as God's will and a way of demonstrating worthiness for a spiritual reward (Hanson & Kerkhoff, 2007). Spirituality is often involved in health and healing, with an emphasis on interdependence, respect, and harmony. Prayers and the use of religious symbols may be seen to promote healing. In addition, *curanderismo*, or Mexican folk healing, may involve rituals to promote recovery (Hanson & Kerkhoff, 2007).

East Asian Attitudes

There are some similarities in the attitudes of East Asian cultures. The religions and philosophies of Buddhism, Confucianism, and Taoism allow for punishment with disabilities for transgressions in a former life as well as for a present life (Chiu, Yang, Wong, Li, & Li, 2013). Middle-class South Korean mothers are expected to provide a high level of support to their children, and disability, including autism, is considered shameful for both children and their families (You & McGraw, 2011). In some cases of autism, spouses or in-laws may blame the mother for the child's problem (You & McGraw, 2011), and the mother may even blame herself, although some mothers may resist these prejudices.

---

[1]The reader will find that the various topics may not be discussed for all the same groups, as information was not readily available.

[2]The designation *Latino/Hispanic* is used interchangeably in this guide.

In China, not only the person with disabilities but also family members lose face (Chiu et al., 2013). The more concerned a family member is with face, the more perturbed he or she is at stigma from others. However, some Asian Americans may see a disability as a blessing or a sign of good fortune (Hasnain & Leung, 2010).

Southeast Asian Attitudes

In Vietnam, families and children with intellectual disabilities may be stigmatized and may respond to possible rejection with secrecy or concealing the condition and withdrawing from social activities (Ngo, Shin, Nhan, & Yang, 2012). In rural Cambodia, the Buddhist conception of karma is also invoked as an explanation for disabilities, with the role of the person who is disabled to endure his or her suffering (Gartrell & Hoban, 2013).

East Indian Attitudes

In eastern India, many individuals may adhere to medical reasons as well as sometimes nonmedical reasons for some disabilities, such as misdemeanors in a past life, or karma (Staples, 2012). A disability may be considered to give an individual the chance to resolve mistakes from a past life, and the suffering of a family allows the family to fulfill duties in this life (Ravindran & Myers, 2012). Individuals may try whatever is available to treat disabilities, with the poor willing to try medical interventions but hindered by cost or difficulties in accessing care (Staples, 2012). Some culturally based treatments for autism may include Ayurveda, a form of Indian medicine, and homeopathy, and even highly educated immigrant parents may combine both traditional and Western approaches (Ravindran & Myers, 2012).

Filipino Attitudes

In the rural Philippines, some individuals believe that developmental disabilities occur to those who have encountered and have been possessed by a bad spirit (Brolan et al., 2014). At times, traditional healers are contacted to help the individual with a disability.

Muslim Attitudes

Some Muslims believe that a disability is an act of God and is an individual's fate (Al-Aoufi, Al-Zyoud, & Shahminan, 2012). When a family has a child with disabilities, it may be seen as a test of faith (Al-Aoufi et al., 2012). All groups, according to Islamic tradition, including those with disabilities, have their own rights, including the right to be treated equally, to be included in society, and to have an education. There is also an emphasis on the protection of the weak (Schuelka, 2013). However, some families may try to avoid stigma by not having their children participate in social activities (Al-Aoufi et al., 2012). They may feel that the disability may be a punishment from God or a result of the evil eye or envy. Spiritual remedies may be resorted to, including prayer (Al-Aoufi et al., 2012). Even highly educated individuals may subscribe to supernatural beliefs for such disabilities as developmental disability (Scior, Hamid, Mahfoudhi, & Abdalla, 2013).

African Attitudes

In Africa, some individuals may attribute the cause of disabilities to witchcraft or the power of offended ancestral spirits (Munsaka & Charnley, 2013) or, alternatively, a curse (Stone-MacDonald, 2012), although many understand the role of medical and health issues. Individuals with disabilities may be excluded from leadership positions (Munsaka & Charnley, 2013). In some cases, children are hidden at home (Stone-MacDonald, 2012). In other instances, individuals may believe that God has a plan and that having a child with disabilities is part of that plan (Stone-MacDonald, 2012). In such cases, it is believed that parents should feel blessed, and, for some parents, it may be a way to demonstrate God's love to the community. Children with disabilities may be taken to medical doctors and traditional healers or taken to a church for prayers (Stone-MacDonald, 2012).

Native American Attitudes

There also are differences in the conceptualization of disabilities for some Native Americans. In addition to modern medical explanations, causes of developmental disabilities may be attributed to the violation of a tribal taboo, in some cases a violation that has occurred before a child's birth, or witchcraft (Joe, 1997). As with other cultures, family members may use a medical explanation with outsiders and reserve a traditional explanation for the kin group. Traditional tribal interventions, like healing ceremonies, may be used to address the reason for the disability. In some cases, Native Americans have converted to Christianity; in others, they have blended their traditional beliefs with mainstream Western religions; and yet in others, they have adhered to traditional tribal beliefs (Lomay & Hinkebein, 2006).

Implications of Attitudes

There are a number of implications of these differing cultural beliefs about disability. Families, depending on their degree of acculturation, are more likely to adhere to Western explanations for disability or to traditional cultural explanations, although these may not be mutually exclusive in many cases. Families who adhere to traditional beliefs about disabilities or who use traditional healing methods are not invariably open with Western professionals about their beliefs and practices. Traditional healing practices and Western interventions are frequently not deemed mutually exclusive, but instead, families may use both types of interventions.

Definitions of Handicap, Illness, and Pain

There are a number of definitions of *handicap*, *illness*, and *pain*. *Handicap* was used in the 20th century to refer to the impairments of individuals (Amundson, 2006). The World Health Organization (WHO) introduced the definition of handicap as not the impairment itself but the disadvantages resulting from social discrimination that affected individuals with impairments. However, the term has fallen into disfavor.

Illness can be defined as "the state of being sick. A sickness, disease, or disorder" ("Illness," 2014). *Pain* can be defined as an "unpleasant feeling that is conveyed to the brain by sensory neurons . . . it also includes perception, the subjective interpretation of the discomfort" (Barrett & Odle, 2006, p. 2754).

Although these terms have standard definitions, there may be considerable differences between cultures in terms of how they cope with illness and pain. As previously noted, individuals of different cultures may have culturally influenced concepts of disability, and differences may be evident in conceptualizations of illness and pain. These differences may be increased by the fact that there may not be equivalent terminology for some types of illness or disability in different languages, and the connotations of some types of illness or disability may be quite different for the family or client and the professional (Jackson, 1998). This can be an issue when the reactions of a family or client seem unexpected to the professional, and the family judges the symptoms with suspicion (Altschuler, 2013).

In addition, differences between some disabilities and illness may be blurred in some cultural contexts. For example, some Latino individuals visit *curanderos* (Mexican folk healers) for help with illness or trauma (Hanson & Kerkhoff, 2007). In the Philippines, some individuals go to traditional healers for treatment of developmental disabilities (Brolan et al., 2014). Some Native Americans also consult with tribal healers in cases of disability (Joe, 1997). The implication is that there may be a fine line between illness and disability in some cultures, and individuals may use alternative means to attempt to alleviate or cure a disability.

Differences Between a Visible and an Invisible Disability (i.e., Deafness or Physical Impairment vs. Learning Disability)

Latino Attitudes

There may be a considerable difference in attitude toward visible and invisible disabilities. Latino families may have different criteria in determining if a child has a disability. There may be an emphasis on being *bien educado*, or having respectful behavior toward elders and an appropriate social demeanor (Cohen, 2013). Children who do not meet normal developmental milestones may not be of concern due to the concept of *añoñar*, or nurturing or pampering. It may be considered the duty of parents to create a pleasant environment for their child and to protect him or her from illness or injury. Consequently, parents may have different expectations of a child than service providers.

It not unusual for some Latino families to refer to their child with developmental delays or more severe disabilities as *enfermo/enfermito* (sick) and misunderstand the importance of a less visible handicap such as a language and/or learning disability For example, the first author of this guide has heard parents refer to those children as being a *burro* (a donkey). The latter remark has been observed more commonly in parents or families who may not have attained a higher level of formal education.

Asian Attitudes

Invisible disabilities may be equally stigmatized and evident in other countries as well. In Vietnam, a widespread emphasis on academic achievement makes developmental disabilities particularly stigmatized (Jamieson, 1993). In Korea, mothers of children with autism may have to deal with public disapproval of their children's behavior (You & McGraw, 2011), as their children's inappropriate behavior is surprising to onlookers given their normal appearance. Some South Asian immigrant students may be confused about the definition of a mild developmental disability (Coles & Scior, 2012). Therefore, it will be important for professionals to provide examples for the parents and families about the implications of a client's disorder for successful performance both at home and at school.

Muslim Attitudes

Similarly, for some South Asian Muslim families, a person's functionality, emotionally, cognitively, and physically, is more important than the specific label of disability (Hasnain & Leung, 2010). Some Middle Easterners may have difficulty identifying that an individual has a mild developmental disability (Scior et al., 2013).

Native American Attitudes

Joe (1997) reports that among Native American families, there are those who may not believe a child with Down syndrome has a disability if he or she has all body parts and can eat, walk, and help others at home.

Implications

The clinical implications of differences in attitudes toward visible and invisible disabilities are important. Speech-language disorders, when unaccompanied by visible signs of disorders, may not be considered disabilities within a family's culture. If a child is able to perform basic day-to-day functions, parents may be skeptical of the diagnosis of a disorder. Alternatively, the diagnosis of a disorder without visible signs may be shameful for parents, as the child appears normal but does not act according to societal expectations, or his or her disabilities may be misunderstood because of their own level of and experience with formal education.

It is very important for the SLP or audiologist to discuss these potential differences in attitudes toward disabilities

with the I/T before meeting with a family. If the I/T is of the same culture as the family, he or she can provide insight on how to approach the subject with the family. When the SLP or audiologist and I/T have a coordinated strategy in working with the family, it can make the meeting run much more smoothly.

Experience and Exposure to Resources (Special Education Services, Medical Examinations, Procedures, Referrals to Other Specialists, Etc.)

The United States, through the Americans With Disabilities Act of 1990 (Ne'eman, 2009), provides a free appropriate public education to all children with disabilities. However, many other countries, notably in the Third World, do not have the same level of services for individuals with disabilities, and families may be unfamiliar with the services available.

Latino

For Hispanic parents, there may be a conflict between the schools and the parents about their children with disabilities' need for independence (Shogren, 2012). Educators may perceive them as overprotective, and parents may disagree with educators when they try to communicate their views about goals for the future. Parents may also perceive that educators have violated their trust. In a low-income urban neighborhood in Peru, children with developmental disabilities may go to a local public school without charge or pay tuition to attend a special education center, although no centers are local (O'Shea et al., 2012). However, this may not be so in other countries of Latin America, including Mexico. Although legislation protects the rights of children with disabilities to education in Guatemala, the majority of children with disabilities are not in school (McFadden, 2013).

East Asian

For individuals with developmental disabilities in China, there is a mixed system of special education and integrated education, but facilities are limited and generally urban (Chiu et al., 2013). In South Korea, children have the right to a free and appropriate public education, and the number of special schools for children with disabilities has increased (You & McGraw, 2011).

South Asian

In terms of medical interventions, many in India are very willing to seek such interventions, although medical costs are prohibitive, and individuals must sometimes travel long distances to access care (Staples, 2012).

Islamic

In Saudi Arabia, special education is based on Islamic rules that state that education should be for all children (Al-Aoufi et al., 2012). In Brunei Darussalam, an independent Malay Islamic Sultanate, children with disabilities are taught in regular schools. Pakistan has special education centers, but there is a shortage of special education teachers (Khatoon, 2003, cited in Patka, Keys, Henry, & McDonald, 2013).

African

Zimbabwe in Africa has a policy of universal education, although some children with disabilities may never attend school (Munsaka & Charnley, 2013).

The Case of Immigrants to the United States

Latino. Immigrants may have mixed experiences with the services they receive in their host country. For Latinos in the United States, if trust is gained, there is a great deal of respect for teachers, SLPs, and audiologists as well as for the system, once they gain confidence in the people they are working with. In this regard, trust is key. However, Latino families may not be aware of the services available to them and have difficulty advocating for their family member effectively for services (Cohen, 2013). This is due to the fact that procedures and regulations are often a novelty or different, and lack of sufficient English language proficiency may be a barrier in finding services that are available. In addition, the first author of this book has often witnessed that parents are surprised that assessments and intervention in the public schools are free of charge.

South Asian. Ravindran and Myers (2012) report that well-educated eastern Indian parents of children with autism living primarily in the United States may be dissatisfied with the services that their children receive or feel that they do not receive enough services. Parents indicate using both conventional therapies, such as applied behavior analysis (ABA) and traditional speech-language therapy, and also may follow other treatments such as special diets, chelation, supplements, and biofeedback as well as complementary therapies like auditory integration. Still, some other parents use additional treatments from their Indian culture, such as Ayurveda (an Indian medicine system) and homeopathy.

Likewise, Croot (2012) reports that Pakistani families of children with developmental disabilities experience dissatisfaction with professionals. Some parents are concerned that professionals have not been honest with them in the past, have at times treated their concerns abruptly, and/or do not fully understand the complexity of the child's problems or their concerns. In some cases, parents do not follow professionals' advice after weighing the relevance of treatment goals to their family life.

Even though these groups of immigrants report being dissatisfied with the services provided for their children with various disabilities, it would be unfair to state that those coming from certain locations within South Asia may not be satisfied with services or tend to be more dissatisfied. There are not many reports on attitudes from this wave of immigrants, and, therefore, generalizations should be avoided.

Native American

For Native American families, there may be a conflict between the values of the Native American culture and the larger society (Joe, 1997). Parents may withdraw from interaction with outside agencies or refuse services if there is a conflict about how services will be provided or the identification of the service provider.

In sum, immigrants from various corners of the world have had varying experiences with special education services and their providers. Some immigrant families have had limited exposure to special education and medical resources in their home countries because of issues of distance, cost, or lack of availability. Some families have used unconventional and alternative treatments for their child's dis-

order. Families that have received services in the United States or United Kingdom have sometimes found them inadequate for a number of reasons. Some families have received what they perceive as insufficient services, while other families have felt that professionals have betrayed their trust or not treated them as equal partners in the process of helping their child. At times, there can be cultural conflicts, in which the values and expectations of the larger society clash with those of a family. However, generalizations regarding a particular group need to be avoided at all costs, and all professionals should keep an open mind to the various families and their children. There are always exceptions, and each case is unique.

Role of the Family in the Identification and Treatment Process: Who Has the Ultimate Voice for Approval for Suggested Programs or Procedures?

The ultimate authority for providing consent for programs or procedures may vary with each family. It is not invariably the mother or the parents who make the final decision. In some families, the extended family plays a greater role than in others.

In traditional Hispanic/Latino families, there may be traditional gender roles, with the mother the nurturer and caregiver (Hanson & Kerkhoff, 2007). Hispanic families may be very close, and it is advantageous to involve the entire family in treatment planning (Sharma & Kerl, 2002). However, more traditional Hispanic families may defer to professionals and should be encouraged to participate in decision making.

For South Koreans, the father is the head of the household, and the mother is expected to sacrifice her own desires and needs to raise her children (Cho, 1998). For Native Americans, family can include the nuclear family and the extended family, including grandparents, aunts, uncles, cousins, and clan members (Lomay & Hinkebein, 2006).

The type of culture, collectivistic or individualistic, may have an impact on who serves as a decision maker. Both Chinese and Arabic communities in Australia may be more collectivistic than Anglo communities, with a greater emphasis on dependence on, and sacrifice for, the extended family (Westbrook & Legge, 1993). In such families, decision making may be more of an extended family process.

The implication for determining a decision maker for services in a meeting is that it is not invariably the mother or even the father who makes the final decision. Sometimes decision making is a group process, and sometimes family members will consult with outside traditional specialists, although they may not share such consultations with the professionals in the schools. Consequently, it is important for SLPs and audiologists to not assume that parents are invariably the decision makers and to address all family members in a meeting as if they are potential decision makers. In a few cases, it may be necessary to have a second meeting to allow all necessary consultations to occur before the final decision is made or to allow an important decision maker to be present.

Client's Formal Education Variables: Do They Make a Difference?

There is evidence that the level of family members' formal education may be sometimes related to the level of accep-

tance of individuals with disabilities. In Vietnam, more highly educated parents of children with intellectual disabilities perceive fewer restrictions on their social life. More educated parents' greater reluctance to accept karma as a cause of their child's disability may reduce the impact of stigma on their social activities, although parents with a higher socioeconomic status may perceive a higher degree of restriction (Ngo et al., 2012). In contrast, Chinese caregivers with a higher socioeconomic status may be less concerned about the stigma associated with disabilities (Chiu et al., 2013). More highly educated individuals in Pakistan may be more accepting of individuals with developmental disabilities (Patka et al., 2013).

There is some evidence that more highly educated individuals are more likely to be familiar with the actual causes of disabilities. Few highly educated residents from India in the United States believe in traditional explanations of autism, although many supplement conventional therapies with alternative and traditional Indian treatments (Ravindran & Myers, 2012). Paradoxically, lower income individuals in India may be less likely to endorse supernatural causes for disabilities (Staples, 2012). However, many highly educated students in Kuwait endorse supernatural causes for developmental disabilities (Scior et al., 2013).

The implications of the educational level of the family are not conclusive. In some instances, more educated families are more accepting of disabilities, which makes them more accepting of their child's diagnosis. However, education is not conclusive in terms of the understanding of disability causes. Individuals without a high level of education may be aware of conventional explanations for disabilities, while individuals with a high level of education may endorse supernatural causes.

Consideration of Families' Dietary Preferences

As more physically involved children are integrated into the public school setting, SLPs may be asked to be on the team in treating children with various dysphagia disorders. It will be important for everyone involved to consider the families' dietary needs. Some families may have very strong dietary preferences for their children, preferring home foods to those provided in the school setting (Croot, 2012). In other cases, a family's religion may dictate the avoidance of certain foods. For example, most Buddhists and Hindus are vegetarians with diets of grains and vegetables (Davis, Gentry, & Hubbard-Wiley, 2002). Muslims avoid pork (Davis et al., 2002) and fast, including not drinking water, during daylight hours during the religious holiday of Ramadan (Tonkovich, 2002). Orthodox, Conservative, and some Reform Jews do not eat pork or shellfish and do not eat meat at the same meal with dairy products (Davis et al., 2002). Observant Catholics abstain from meat on Ash Wednesday and all Fridays during Lent (Tonkovich, 2002). Additionally, some cultures believe that certain conditions are due to an imbalance of hot and cold. Hot conditions are treated with foods that are described as cold, and cold conditions are treated with foods that are described as hot (Davis-McFarland, 2008). Some families may hand-feed children until they transition into the schools and may have different preferences for the use or lack of use of utensils. When these preferences are not respected, it can be a source of contention for parents.

It is important to allow parents to choose the foods that their children consume and to respect all families' dietary guidelines. The first step is to establish communication with the parents and find out in detail what their food preferences are (Davis-McFarland, 2008). The second step is to collaboratively design a swallowing program that incorporates family preferences. The school staff should be open to allowing the parent's participation in assisting with the child's feeding while in school. Many children will need the support of their parent to eat, and this might be especially important when they transition into different foods and different consistencies.

THE INTERPRETER/ TRANSLATOR AS A CULTURAL BROKER

The issue of *cultural brokering* is an important one. A *cultural broker*, or go-between, works with the professionals on one side and the family and the child on the other to make sure that both sides understand procedures according to their view of the world (Hasnain & Leung, 2010). Bicultural interpreters potentially bring an understanding of the culture of the family as well as comprehension of the procedures involved in the assessment and conferencing processes. Some of the many factors that an interpreter may consider are the individuals' gender, age, social class, and educational level (Langdon & Quintanar-Sarellana, 2003) in order to ensure the culturally appropriate level of respect for each participant (Rosenberg, Seller, & Leanza, 2008). Given the many potential differences in worldview between the family and SLP or audiologist, this information is invaluable, and the way that the I/T shares it is crucial to success.

All individuals participating in a meeting have a goal (Fontes, 2008). One of the functions that an interpreter may serve as is as support to the family or child, through social interaction or his or her presence alone (Hsieh & Hong, 2010). Family members may perceive an interpreter as a friend (Rosenberg, Leanza, & Seller, 2007). However, the interpreter is sometimes pulled between serving the needs of the institution that employs him or her and serving the interests of family members (Hsieh, 2006). In addition, sometimes interpreters have another role in the work setting and may be torn between the expectations of the other role, often as that of an advocate, and the neutrality of interpreting (Hsieh, 2006). Because of these potential conflicts, and for a variety of other reasons, interpreters may embellish, delete, de-emphasize, emphasize, and edit what other parties say (Davitti, 2013; Dubslaff & Martinsen, 2005; Fontes, 2008; Hsieh, 2007, 2010; Merlini & Favaron, 2005). More on this topic is discussed in Chapter 6 in conjunction with assessment issues.

Because of interpreters' cultural knowledge, it may be occasionally appropriate for an interpreter to stop a meeting or an assessment and talk briefly to an SLP or audiologist (Fontes, 2008). For example, if a background question asked is potentially culturally inappropriate, it is wise to allow the interpreter to briefly stop the meeting and talk to the professional before translating the question, and in fact, some interpreters may do so (Hsieh, 2010). Furthermore, if a family member or child's nonverbal communication is not understood by the SLP or audiologist, it is appropriate for the interpreter to tell the professional the meaning of the nonverbal communication (Langdon & Quintanar-Sarellana, 2003). Similarly, if a bilingual test includes alternative terms for a child's given dialect, it is appropriate to briefly stop testing and provide the correct term. According to Hsieh (2006), the most culturally appropriate way of eliciting information from a family or child or conveying bad news to a family is through an interpreter. Even better, it is recommended to review all assessment measures and/or background information questions or information beforehand with the interpreter to determine the appropriateness of all test items and/or questions. However, it is advised that the SLP or audiologist be present to answer specific questions and to ensure that the parent/family understands the information. Ultimately, it is the SLP and audiologist who are responsible for the information that has been given to the parent/family.

However, although interpreters have invaluable cultural and linguistic knowledge of the family's culture and language, it is important to make sure that interpreters' independent attempts to mediate cultural differences do not interfere with the effective or accurate transmission of information or the ability of parents to ask questions or advocate for their positions (Davitti, 2013; Hsieh, 2007).

Because of the crucial position of interpreters and their ability to enhance or hinder interaction between the SLP or audiologist and the family or child, it is essential that professionals receive training in their use. However, in a survey of SLPs, only 21% of SLPs who worked in urban areas and 5% of SLPs in settings with little client diversity reported having training in the use of interpreters (Hammer, Detwiler, Detwiler, Blood, & Qualls, 2004). In a survey carried out 3 years later, only 70% of SLPs had collaborated with interpreters in the assessment of bilingual children (Caesar & Kohler, 2007). As few as 21% of SLPs had training in collaborating with an interpreter, and 60% had worked with an interpreter for assessment or treatment, but only 25% reported feeling competent in evaluating a child's language development in collaboration with an interpreter (Guiberson & Atkins, 2012). Consequently, the scant research conducted thus far has indicated that many SLPs have not received training in collaborating with interpreters and do not always work with interpreters in the evaluation of bilingual children. This is further confirmed by a recent doctoral dissertation carried out by Palfrey (2013).

Therefore, there is an important need to train SLPs and audiologists in best practices as we know them today for collaborating with interpreters in both the assessment and intervention with bilingual children and in meetings with family members. In addition, training I/Ts in appropriate interpretation and translation techniques will enable them to convey words and concepts of one language to another more accurately and will be very instrumental in rendering cultural concepts from one culture to another.

SUMMARY

In this chapter, we reviewed how cultural aspects may influence parents' perceptions of their child's given disability and how we, as professionals, can assist in this process by adequately preparing the I/T to assist us in conveying both our questions and concerns to best assess if indeed the child has a disability. Also, for us to understand how parents perceive what

we say, it is important to prepare the interpreter to bridge the communication gap that may exist between us and the family due to a language barrier. We also have reviewed some variables such the origin of families and their education. However, we need to consider each case as unique and avoid overgeneralizations. We have also discovered that despite 30 years of the American Speech-Language-Hearing Association's recommendations for SLPs and audiologists to collaborate with I/Ts, very few professionals feel adequately prepared, and this appears to be more prevalent in the public school setting.

DISCUSSION ITEMS AND ACTIVITIES

1. When have you experienced cultural differences in your own life? As an individual? As a professional? What were those cultural differences?

2. Describe some ways in which a family's acculturation can affect your provision of services.

3. How can differences in attitudes toward disabilities affect your professional relationship with a family?

4. How can you work with a family that has differences in attitudes toward disabilities?

5. List three areas that were most surprising to you as you read the chapter. Discuss the reason for each of the areas.

6. Role-play a scenario with individuals taking the part of an SLP and one or more parents. Pretend that the parents' child has just been diagnosed

with a language disorder, but the parents are worried about the stigma of the diagnosis in their community.

7. Interview a member of a different linguistic and cultural group and ask him or her about where he or she sees him- or herself fit within the various quadrants shown in Figure 3–1. Ask him or her to state reasons for his or her comments.

8. Imagine a parent who is illiterate in Spanish who states that her youngest son of six children, a kindergartener, does not have any problems in Spanish, because she can understand him at all times. The bilingual teacher, who is a native speaker, cannot understand him, and other children shy away from him because he cannot be understood in either English or Spanish. The parent is convinced there is nothing wrong with her son. She has another child who was like him, and now he is doing well in school. How would you prepare the I/T to work with this case? What would you say as an SLP?

REFERENCES

Al-Aoufi, H., Al-Zyoud, N., & Shahminan, N. (2012). Islam and the cultural conceptualization of disability. *International Journal of Adolescence and Youth, 17,* 205–219. doi:10.1080/02 673843.2011.649565

Altschuler, J. (2013). Migration, illness and health care. *Contemporary Family Therapy, 35,* 546–556. doi:10.1007/s10591-013-9234-x

Amundson, R. (2006). Handicap. In G. Albrecht (Ed.), *Encyclopedia of disability* (Vol. 2, p. 816). Thousand Oaks, CA: SAGE Reference.

Banks, J., & McGee Banks, C. (Eds.). (2010). *Multicultural education: Issues and perspectives.* Danvers, MA: John Wiley.

Barrett, J., & Odle, T. (2006). Pain. In J. Longe (Ed.), *The Gayle encyclopedia of medicine* (3rd ed., Vol. 4, pp. 2754–2757). Detroit, MI: Gale.

Berry, J. W. (2003). Conceptual approaches to acculturation. In K. Chun, P. Organista, & G. Marín (Eds.), *Acculturation: Advances in theory, measurement, and applied research* (pp. 17–37). Washington, DC: American Psychological Association.

Berry, J. W. (2006a). Contexts of acculturation. In D. Sam & J. W. Berry (Eds.), *The Cambridge handbook of acculturation psychology* (pp. 27–42). Cambridge, UK: Cambridge University Press.

Berry, J. W. (2006b). Stress perspectives on acculturation. In D. Sam & J. W. Berry (Eds.), *The Cambridge handbook of acculturation psychology* (pp. 43–57). Cambridge, UK: Cambridge University Press.

Birman, D., & Taylor-Ritzler, T. (2007). Acculturation and psychological distress among adolescent immigrants from the former Soviet Union: Exploring the mediating effect of family relationships. *Cultural Diversity and Ethnic Minority Psychology, 13,* 337–346. doi:10.1037/1099-9809.13.4.337

Brolan, C., van Dooren, K., Taylor Gomez, M., Fitzgerald, L., Ware, R., & Lennox, N. (2014). Suranho healing: Filipino concepts of intellectual disability and treatment choices in Negros Occidental. *Disability & Society, 29,* 71–85. doi:10.1080/09687599.2013.771899

Caesar, L., & Kohler, P. (2007). The state of school-based bilingual assessment: Actual practice versus recommended guidelines. *Language, Speech, and Hearing Services in Schools, 38,* 190–200. doi:0161-1461/07/3803-0190

Child Trends. (2013). *Immigrant children.* Retrieved September 16, 2014, from http://www.child trends.org/?indicators=immigrant-children

Chiu, M., Yang, X., Wong, F., Li, J., & Li, J. (2013). Caregiving of children with intellectual disabilities in China—an examination of affiliate stigma and the cultural thesis. *Journal of Intellectual Disability Research, 57,* 1117–11129. doi:10.1111/j.1365-2788.2012.01624.x

Cho, H. (1998). Male dominance and mother power: The two sides of Confucian patriarchy in Korea. In W. H. Slote & G. A. Devos (Eds.), *Confucianism and the family* (pp. 187–208). Albany, NY: State University of New York Press.

Chun, K., & Akutsu, P. (2003). Acculturation among ethnic minority families. In K. Chun, P. Organista, & G. Marín (Eds.), *Acculturation:*

Advances in theory, measurement, and applied research (pp. 95–119). Washington, DC: American Psychological Association.

Clay, J., Seekins, T., & Castillo, J. (2010). Community infrastructure and employment opportunities for Native Americans and Alaska natives. In F. Balcazar, Y. Suárez Balcazar, T. Taylor-Ritzler, & C. Keys (Eds.), *Race, culture, and disability: Rehabilitation science and practice* (pp. 137–158). Boston, MA: Jones and Bartlett.

Cohen, S. (2013). Advocacy for the "abandonados": Harnessing cultural beliefs for Latino families and their children with intellectual disabilities. *Journal of Policy and Practice in Intellectual Disabilities, 10*, 71–78. doi:10.1111/jppi.12021

Coles, S., & Scior, K. (2012). Public attitudes towards people with intellectual disabilities: A qualitative comparison of White British and South Asian people. *Journal of Applied Research in Intellectual Disabilities, 25*, 177–188. doi:10.1111/j.1468-3148.2011.00655.x

Croot, E. (2012). The care needs of Pakistani families caring for disabled children: How relevant is cultural competence? *Physiotherapy, 98*, 351–356. doi:10.1016/j.physio.2011.05.001

Davis, P. N., Gentry, B., & Hubbard-Wiley, P. (2002). Clinical practice issues. In D. Battle (Ed.), *Communication disorders in multicultural populations* (3rd ed., pp. 461–486). Boston, MA: Butterworth-Heinemann.

Davis-McFarland, E. (2008). Family and cultural issues in a school swallowing and feeding program. *Language, Speech, and Hearing Services in Schools, 39*, 199–213.

Davitti, E. (2013). Dialogue interpreting as intercultural mediation: Interpreters' use of upgrading moves in parent-teacher meetings. *Interpreting, 15*, 168–199. doi:10.1075/intp.15.2.02dav

Dubslaff, F., & Martinsen, B. (2005). Exploring untrained interpreters' use of direct versus indirect speech. *Interpreting, 7*, 211–236.

Fontes, L. (2008). *Interviewing clients across cultures: A practitioner's guide.* New York, NY: Guilford.

Fraser, B. (2013). *Disability studies and Spanish culture: Films, novels, the comic and the public exhibition.* Liverpool, UK: Liverpool University Press.

Gany, F., Leng, J., Shapiro, E., Abramson, D., Motola, I., Shield, D., & Changrani, J. (2007). Patient satisfaction with different interpreting methods: A randomized controlled trial. *Journal of General Internal Medicine, 22*, 312–318. doi:10.1007/s11606-007-0360-8

Gartrell, A., & Hoban, E. (2013). Structural vulnerability, disability, and access to nongovernmental organization services in rural Cambodia. *Journal of Social Work in Disability & Rehabilitation, 12*, 194–212. doi:10.1080/1536710X.2013.810100

Guiberson, M., & Atkins, J. (2012). Speech-language pathologists' preparation, practices, and perspectives on serving culturally and linguistically diverse children. *Communication Disorders Quarterly, 33*, 169–180. doi:10.1177/1525740110384132

Guimond, S., Crisp, R., de Oliviera, P., Kamiejski, R., Kteily, N., Kuepper, B., Zick, A. (2013). Diversity policy, social dominance, and intergroup relations: Predicting prejudice in changing social and political contexts. *Journal of Personality and Social Psychology, 104*, 941–958. doi:10.1037/a0032069

Gupta, A., Leong, F., Valentine, J., & Canada, D. (2013). A meta-analytic study: The relationship between acculturation and depression among Asian Americans. *American Journal of Orthopsychiatry, 83*, 372–385. doi:10.1111/ajop.12018

Hammer, C. S., Detwiler, J., Detwiler, J., Blood, G., & Qualls, C. D. (2004). Speech-language pathologists' training and confidence in serving Spanish-English bilingual children. *Journal of Communication Disorders, 37*, 91–108. doi:10.1016/j.jcomdis.2003.07.002

Hanson, S., & Kerkhoff, T. (2007). Ethical decision making in rehabilitation: Consideration of Latino cultural factors. *Rehabilitation Psychology, 52*, 409–420. doi:10.1037/0090-5550.52.4.409

Hasnain, R., & Leung, P. (2010). Cross-cultural issues for Asian Pacific Americans with disabilities in the vocational rehabilitation system. In F. Balcazar, Y. Suarez-Balcazar, T. Taylor-Ritzler, & C. Keys (Eds.), *Race, culture, and disability: Rehabilitation science and practice* (pp. 185–204). Boston, MA: Jones and Bartlett.

Hazuda, H. P., Stern, M. P., & Haffner, S. M. (1988) Acculturation and assimilation among Mexican Americans: Scales and population-based data. *Social Science Quarterly, 69*, 687–706.

Hofstede, G. (2001). *Culture's consequences: Comparing values, behaviors, institutions, and organizations across nations* (2nd ed.). Thousand Oaks, CA: Sage.

Hollinsworth, D. (2013). Decolonizing Indigenous disability in Australia. *Disability & Society, 28*, 601–615. doi:10.1080/09687599.2012.717879

Horevitz, E., & Organista, K. (2012). The Mexican health paradox: Expanding the explanatory power of the acculturation construct. *Hispanic Journal of Behavioral Sciences, 35*, 3–34. doi:10.1177/0739986312460370

Hsieh, E. (2006). Conflicts in how interpreters manage their roles in provider-patient interactions. *Social Science & Medicine, 62*, 721–730. doi:10.1016/j.socscimed.2005.06.029

Hsieh, E. (2007). Interpreters as co-diagnosticians: Overlapping roles and services between providers and interpreters. *Social Science & Medicine, 64*, 924–937. doi:10.1016/j.socscimed.2006.10.015

Hsieh, E. (2010). Provider-interpreter collaboration in bilingual health care: Competitions of control over interpreter-mediated interactions. *Patient Education and Counseling, 78*, 154–159. doi:10.1016/j.pec.2009.02.017

Hsieh, E., & Hong, S. J. (2010). Not all are desired: Providers' views on interpreters' emotional support for patients. *Patient Education and Counseling, 81*, 192–197. doi:10.1016/j.pec.2010.04.004

Illness. (2014). In *Access science*. Retrieved from http://www.accessscience.com/search?q=illness&rows=10&mode=AND0

Jackson, C. (1998). Medical interpretation: An essential clinical service for non-English-speaking immigrants. In S. Loue (Ed.), *Handbook of immigrant health* (pp. 61–79). New York, NY: Plenum Press.

Jamieson, N. L. (1993). *Understanding Vietnam.* Berkeley: University of California Press.

Joe, J. (1997). American Indian children with disabilities: The impact of culture on health and education services. *Family, Systems, & Health, 15*, 251–261.

Karliner, L., Jacobs, E., Chen, A., & Mutha, S. (2007). Do professional interpreters improve clinical care for patients with limited English proficiency? A systematic review of the literature. *Health Services Research, 42*, 727–754. doi:10.1111/j.1475-6773.2006.00629.x

Kunst, J., & Sam, D. (2013). Relationship between perceived acculturation expectations and Muslim minority youth's acculturation and adaptation. *International Journal of Intercultural Relations, 37*, 477–490. doi:10.1016/j.ijintrel.2013.04.007

Langdon, H. W., & Quintanar-Sarellana, R. (2003). Roles and responsibilities of the interpreter in interactions with speech-language pathologists, parents, and students. *Seminars in Speech and Language, 24*, 235–244. doi:10.1055/s-2003-42826

Lomay, V., & Hinkebein, J. (2006). Cultural considerations when providing rehabilitation services to American Indians. *Rehabilitation Psychology, 51*, 36–42. doi:10.1037/0090-5550.51.1.36

López-Class, M., Castro, F., & Ramírez, A. (2011). Conceptions of acculturation: A review and statement of critical issues. *Social Science & Medicine, 72*, 1555–1562. doi:10.1016/j.socscimed.2011.03.011

Marín, G., & Gamba, R. (2003). Acculturation and changes in cultural values. In K. Chun, P. Organista, & G. Marín (Eds.), *Acculturation: Advances in theory, measurement, and applied research* (pp. 83–93). Washington, DC: American Psychological Association.

Masgoret, A.M., & Ward, C. (2006). In D. Sam & J. W. Berry (Eds.), *The Cambridge handbook of acculturation psychology* (pp. 58–77). Cambridge, UK: Cambridge University Press.

McFadden, E. (2013). The impact of government on quality of life for people with disabilities in the United States and Guatemala. In N. Warren & L. Manderson (Eds.), *Reframing disability and quality of life: A global perspective* (pp. 211–231). Dordrecht, the Netherlands: Springer.

Merlini, R., & Favaron, R. (2005). Examining the "voice of interpreting" in speech pathology. *Interpreting, 7*, 263–302.

Munsaka, E., & Charnley, H. (2013). 'We do not have chiefs who are disabled': Disability, development and culture in a continuing complex emergency. *Disability & Society, 28*, 756–769. doi:10.1080/09687599.2013.802221

Ne'eman, A. (2009). Disability politics. *New Atlantis: A Journal of Technology and Society, 24*, 112–116.

Ngo, H., Shin, J., Nhan, N., & Yang, L. (2012). Stigma and restriction on the social life of families of children with intellectual disabilities in Vietnam. *Singapore Medical Journal, 53*, 451–457.

Nguyen, H. (2006). Acculturation in the United States. In D. Sam & J. W. Berry (Eds.), *The*

Cambridge handbook of acculturation psychology (pp. 311–330). Cambridge, UK: Cambridge University Press.

Norbury, C., & Sparks, A. (2013). Difference or disorder? Cultural issues in understanding neurodevelopmental disorders. *Developmental Psychology, 49*, 45–58. doi:10.1037/a0027446

Nowak, T. (2005). Vietnamese. In J. Lipson & S. Dibble (Eds.), *Culture & clinical care* (pp. 446–460). San Francisco, CA: UCSF Nursing Press.

Organista, K. (2007). *Solving Latino psychosocial and health problems: Theory, practice, and populations.* Hoboken, NJ: John Wiley.

O'Shea, M., Girón, J., Cabrera, L., Lescano, A., & Taren, D. (2012). Public perceptions of intellectual disability in a shantytown community in Lima, Peru. *International Health, 4*, 253–259. doi:10.1016/j.inhe.2012.07.001

Palfrey, C. L. (2013). *The use of interpreters by speech-language pathologists conducting bilingual speech-language assessments* (Doctoral dissertation). Washington, DC: Georgetown University.

Patka, M., Keys, C., Henry, D., & McDonald, K. (2013). Attitudes of Pakistani community members and staff toward people with intellectual disability. *American Journal on Intellectual and Developmental Disabilities, 118*, 32–43. doi:10.1352/1944-7558-118.1.32

Pawliuk, N., Grizenko, N., Chan-Yip, A., Gantous, P., Mathew, J., & Nguyen, D. (1996). Acculturation style and psychological functioning in children of immigrants. *American Journal of Orthopsychiatry, 66*, 111–121.

Phillips, C. (2010). Using interpreters: A guide for GPS. *Australian Family Physician, 39*, 188–195.

Phinney, J. (2003). Ethnic identity and acculturation. In K. Chun, P. Organista, & G. Marín (Eds.), *Acculturation: Advances in theory, measurement, and applied research* (pp. 63–81). Washington, DC: American Psychological Association.

Portes, A., & Rumbaut, R. (with Fernández-Kelly, P., & Haller, W.). (2006). Growing up American: The new second generation. In A. Portes & R. Rumbaut (Eds.), *Immigrant America: A portrait* (3rd ed., pp. 244–284). Berkeley: University of California Press.

Potochnick, S., Perreira, K., & Fuligni, A. (2012). Fitting in: The roles of social acceptance and discrimination in shaping the daily psychological well-being of Latino youth. *Social Science Quarterly, 93*, 173–190. doi:10.1111/j.15406237.2011.00830.

Ravindran, N., & Myers, B. (2012). Beliefs and practices regarding autism in Indian families now settled abroad: An Internet survey. *Focus on Autism and Other Developmental Disabilities, 28*, 44–53. doi:10.1177/1088357612458970

Roche, K., Ghazarian, S., & Fernández-Esquer, M. E. (2012). Unpacking acculturation: Cultural orientations and educational attainment among Mexican-origin youth. *Journal of Youth and Adolescence, 41*, 920–931. doi:10.1007/s10964-011-9725-8

Roscigno, C. (2013). Challenging nurses' cultural competence of disability to improve interpersonal interactions. *Journal of Neuroscience Nursing, 45*, 21–37.

Rosenberg, E., Leanza, Y., & Seller, R. (2007). Doctor-patient communication in primary care with an interpreter: Physician perceptions of professional and family interpreters. *Patient Education and Counseling, 67*, 286–292. doi:10.1016/j.pec.2007.03.011

Rosenberg, E., Seller, R., & Leanza, Y. (2008). Through interpreters' eyes: Comparing roles of professional and family interpreters. *Patient Education and Counseling, 70*, 87–93. doi:10.1016/j.pec.2007.09.015

Santisteban, D., & Mitrani, V. (2003). The influences of acculturation processes on the family. In K. Chun, P. Organista, & G. Marín (Eds.), *Acculturation: Advances in theory, measurement, and applied research* (pp. 121–135). Washington, DC: American Psychological Association.

Schuelka, M. (2013). A faith in humanness: Disability, religion and development. *Disability & Society, 28*, 500–513. doi:10.1080/09687559.2012.717880

Schwartz, S., & Zamboanga, B. (2008). Testing Berry's model of acculturation: A confirmatory latent class approach. *Cultural Diversity and Ethnic Minority Psychology, 14*, 275–285. doi:10.1037/a0012818

Scior, K., Hamid, A., Mahfoudhi, A., & Abdalla, F. (2013). The relationship between awareness of intellectual disability, causal and intervention beliefs and social distance in Kuwait and the UK. *Research in Developmental Disabilities, 34*, 3896–3905. doi:10.1016/j.ridd.2013.07.030

Sharma, P., & Kerl, S. (2002). Suggestions for psychologists working with Mexican American individuals and families in health care settings.

Rehabilitation Psychology, 47, 230–239. doi:10 .1037//0090-5550.47.2.230

Shogren, K. (2012). Hispanic mothers' perceptions of self-determination. *Research and Practice for Persons with Severe Disabilities, 37*, 170–184.

Staples, J. (2012). Culture and carelessness: Constituting disability in south India. *Medical Anthropology Quarterly, 26*, 557–574. doi:10.1111/maq.12007

Stone-MacDonald, A. (2012). Cultural beliefs about disability in practice: Experiences at a special school in Tanzania. *International Journal of Disability, Development and Education, 59*, 393–407. doi:10.1080/1034912X.2012.723947

Tonkovich, J. (2002). Multicultural issues in the management of neurogenic communication and swallowing disorders. In D. Battle (Ed.), *Communication disorders in multicultural populations* (3rd ed., pp. 233–265). Boston, MA: Butterworth-Heinemann.

Triandis, H. (1989). The self and social behavior in differing cultural contexts. *Psychological Review, 96*, 506–520.

Triandis, H. (1995). *Individualism and collectivism.* Boulder, CO: Westview Press.

Tribe, R., & Keefe, A. (2009). Issues in using interpreters in therapeutic work with refugees. What is not being expressed? *European Journal of Psychotherapy & Counseling, 11*, 409–424. doi:10.1080/13642530903444795

Trumbull, E., Rothstein-Fisch, C., Greenfield, P. M., & Quiroz, B. (2001). *Bridging cultures between home and school: A guide for teachers.* Mahwah, NJ: Erlbaum.

Vedder, P., & Horenczyk, G. (2006). Acculturation and the school. In D. Sam & J. W. Berry (Eds.), *The Cambridge handbook of acculturation psychology* (pp. 419–438). Cambridge, UK: Cambridge University Press.

Westbrook, M., & Legge, V. (1993). Health practitioners' perceptions of family attitudes toward children with disabilities: A comparison of six communities in a multicultural society. *Rehabilitation Psychology, 38*, 177–185.

World Health Organization. (2002). *Towards a common language for functioning, disability and health: ICF.* Retrieved from http://www.who. int/classifications/icf/icfbeginnersguide. pdf?ua=1

World Health Organization. (2011). *Summary: World report on disability.* Retrieved from http://whql:bdoc.who.int/hq/2011/WHO_ NMH_VIP_11.01>eng.pdf

You, H.-K., & McGraw, L. (2011). The intersection of motherhood and disability: Being a "good" Korean mother to an "imperfect" child. *Journal of Comparative Family Studies, 42*, 570–598.

Chapter 4

Interpreting and Translating in Speech-Language Pathology and Audiology

Terry Irvine Saenz

- Review the Code of Ethics for speech-language pathologists (SLPs) and audiologists as it applies in collaborating with interpreters and translators (I/Ts)
- Provide information on recruiting I/Ts
- Describe the preparation of I/Ts by SLPs or audiologists
- Describe the importance of SLPs or audiologists updating their information on working with I/Ts
- Describe ways to evaluate I/Ts' performance
- Describe ways to assess I/Ts' bilingual skills
- Describe the multiple functions of I/Ts, including message converter,

message clarifier, cultural clarifier, and patient (client) advocate
- Describe the I/T Code of Ethics
- Describe the importance of I/Ts'
  - Knowledge of two cultures and modes of verbal and nonverbal communication
  - Ability to convey the same meaning in two languages, knowing technical terminology, and being familiar with dialectical differences
  - Skill in adapting to the speech and language patterns of clients with communication disorders
  - Maintenance of neutrality and confidentiality and interpreting faithfully
  - Maintenance of linguistic skills, participation in ongoing learning, and remaining flexible

RESPONSIBILITIES OF SLPS AND AUDIOLOGISTS

Following a Code of Ethics

In reviewing the Code of Ethics of the American Speech-Language-Hearing Association (ASHA, 2010), at least six rules of ethics that apply directly to working with I/Ts were found:

1. Under rule of ethics I.A., "individuals shall provide all services competently."
   a. Rule of ethics I.A. has the implication that, even when using the services of an I/T, SLPs and audiologists must provide competent services.
2. Under rule of ethics I.B., "individuals shall use every resource, including referral when appropriate, to ensure that high-quality service is provided" (ASHA, 2010).
   a. This rule clearly implies that I/Ts should be involved in the assessment, intervention, and individual education plan (IEP) or individual family service plan (IFSP) process when needed to communicate effectively with a child and/or the family. It is essential that SLPs and audiologists do not try to conduct assessments, intervention, or meetings in a language other than English unless they are strong speakers of the language, as poor language skills increase the possibility of miscommunication (Fontes, 2008). To avoid such a situation, it is important to tell a family that they may request an interpreter at any time (Fontes, 2008).
3. Rule of ethics I.F. indicates that "individuals who hold the Certificate of

Clinical Competence (CCC) may delegate tasks related to provision of clinical services to assistants, technicians, support personnel, or any other persons only if those services are appropriately supervised, realizing that the responsibility for client welfare remains with the certified individual" (ASHA, 2010).
   a. This rule implies that SLPs and audiologists are responsible for the supervision of services provided by I/Ts, even if those services are provided in a language other than English.
4. Rule of ethics I.N. indicates that "individuals shall not reveal, without authorization, any professional or personal information about identified persons served professionally" (ASHA, 2010).
   a. Therefore, according to this rule, in conjunction with rule of ethics I.F., SLPs and audiologists must honor confidentiality as part of their own actions and must ensure that I/Ts under their supervision must also do so.
5. Rule of ethics II.B. spells out that "individuals shall engage in only those aspects of the professions that are within the scope of their professional practice and competence, considering their level of education, training, and experience" (ASHA, 2010).
   a. This has implications for the importance of SLPs and audiologists becoming conversant with standards and procedures for working with I/Ts as well as for ensuring that I/Ts do not overstep their level of competency.
6. Rule of ethics IV.B. states that "individuals shall prohibit anyone under their supervision from engaging in

any practice that violates the Code of Ethics" (ASHA, 2010).

Consequently, the responsibility of SLPs and audiologists is to ensure that I/Ts under their supervision follow the ASHA Code of Ethics. While I/Ts have additional responsibilities and ethics, the main responsibility for any interpreted interaction lies clearly with the SLP and audiologist. They are responsible for training the I/T, teaching him or her the ethics of interpretation, and ensuring that the interpreted interaction follows the ASHA Code of Ethics.

These responsibilities are important ones, and they are the ones that are not always easily implemented. In a study of SLPs, including bilingual SLPs, the majority of those surveyed responded that they were not competent or only somewhat competent to evaluate an individual's language development, even using the services of an I/T, when they did not speak or understand the language of the individual (Kritikos, 2003). Similarly, the majority believed that most SLPs were not competent or only somewhat competent to assess this population. In another survey by Guiberson and Atkins (2012), only 25% of SLPs reported feeling competent in evaluating a child's language development using the services of an interpreter. This is an important area of concern for many SLPs and audiologists.

Participating in Recruiting Interpreters/Translators

Whenever possible, SLPs and audiologists should participate in the recruitment of I/Ts, preferably I/Ts whose services will be used many times in assessments and conferences. Table 4–1 lists some of the questions that may be asked of the I/T during the interview process. Also, the I/T's languages, including English, need to be assessed. This aspect is further discussed in this chapter on pages 89 to 96.

One of the first steps that professionals can take when working at a new site is to find out about resources available in language interpreting and translating. A pool of I/Ts may be found in several school districts or other professional settings such as clinics and hospitals (the latter are paid for their service compared to public schools, where they might need to offer their services for free or a minimal fee) (Karliner, Jacobs, Chen, & Mutha, 2007). In other school districts, SLPs may be able to work with other bilingual professionals, such as school psychologists, general education or special education teachers, and classroom aides. However, when an I/T holds a different position in addition to serving as an interpreter in an educational or medical setting, it can create a role conflict (Hwa-Froelich & Westby, 2003). For example, the first author of this guide, who is a bilingual SLP, has been asked to act both as the SLP for the team and the I/T. Unless there was no I/T available, it would have been a conflict of interest, but in several instances, she found herself needing to take on a double role. Therefore, this is not advisable; administrators must make an effort to hire a person who will act as an I/T.

It is important for I/Ts to adhere to the interpreting role while functioning as an interpreter (National Council on Interpreting in Health Care [NCIHC], 2004, 2005) and to advise those present when functioning in a role other than that of interpreter. All team members working with a bilingual individual must keep in mind that this individual must be trained to do the job; it is not enough to be fluent

Table 4–1. Questions to Assess the Competence and Performance of an I/T

Question	Answer
1. Where were you born?	
2. If you were born outside of this country, how old were you when you arrived in this country?	
3. If you were born outside of this country, what level of education did you attain in your former country?	
4. How long have you lived in the United States?	
5. If you were born in the United States, where did you learn your other language?	
6. Have you spent time outside of vacations in another country where your other language is spoken? If so, how long? How do you maintain your oral and reading skills in your language?	
7. How would you rate your ability? 1 = poor; 2 = below average; 3 = average; 4 = good; 5 = excellent	A. Your ability to speak your language? ____ B. Your ability to read the language? ____ C. Your ability to write the language? ____
8. Have you received formal training as an I/T? If you did, where and how long ago?	
9. What type of interpreting/translating work have you done before?	Please Circle: Deaf International Medical Legal Community
Comments:	

in two languages. A bilingual individual is not necessarily a competent interpreter, but there are exceptions, and each situation where the I/T is performing two different roles needs to be considered individually.

In a study of bilingual school psychologists' assessment practices, the sources of their interpreters were through a district-provided list, hospitals, or school staff (71.9%); outside agencies (18.4%); family or religious groups (5.3%); and university contacts or colleagues (4.9%) (O'Bryon & Rogers, 2010). In exceptional circumstances, an adult family member or friend may be asked to serve as an I/T, but this may be awkward. There is always the issue of family secrets and confidentiality when a family member or friend is used (Fontes, 2008; Jackson, 1998; Norbury & Sparks, 2013). Family and community members may expect favors or special consideration from such I/Ts, and they may be subject to considerable social pressure. In addition, there may be insufficient time to train a family member or friend in the ethics and procedures of interpretation, and consequently, testing may be compromised. However, in some instances, family and community members may be the only recourse. In such instances, it is necessary to brief the person acting as the I/T on the ethics and procedures of interpretation/translation and to debrief the I/T after the meeting or assessment.

Adequately Preparing the I/T for a Given Assignment

There are six steps that an SLP or audiologist can take to prepare an I/T for a given assignment. The first step, if the assignment involves written translation, is to determine whether the I/T feels comfortable and competent in translating from one language to the other. Some individuals may be very adequate interpreters but may lack the knowledge of writing in their native language to produce effective translations. There are two common types of translation (see Chapter 1 page 10 for a brief definition). *Sight translation* involves the oral production of a text written in one language into another language, typically in the moment (NCIHC, 2009). I/Ts use sight translation when rendering a written document in English or any language verbally into another language. The second type of translation is referred to as a *prepared translation*, in which a written text is rendered from one language into the written text of another language.

The second step, if the I/T is not an experienced I/T, is to review the code of ethics for I/Ts. These ethics will be discussed in the section on the "Responsibilities of Interpreters and Translators," "Following a Code of Ethics."

The third step is to define the role of the I/T in the interpreted interaction, whether that be a conference to obtain and/or verify information, complete an assessment, report results of the assessment, or conduct intervention. The SLP or audiologist should provide information on the educational and socioeconomic status as well as the dialect used by the family and the child so that the I/T can attempt to match the anticipated register, formality, and dialect of the family's language during the interpreted interaction (Isaac, 2002). Similarly, the SLP and audiologist should define his or her own role as a practitioner with the ultimate responsibility for the interaction. The I/T's understanding of the SLP or the audiologist's aims and goals in an interpreted interaction may aid him or her in providing a more effective interpretation (Isaac, 2002).

The fourth step is to develop a system for instances in which the I/T must step out of the interpreting role during the interaction. Some of these instances may be when speakers in the interaction are talking too quickly, not pausing, interrupting one another, or inadvertently engaging in side conversations, thus rendering it difficult to produce an accurate interpretation (NCIHC, 2005). In such instances, the I/T can ask the parties to slow down or pause more frequently. Alternatively, the I/T may not understand a particular term or word and should be able to ask for clarification (NCIHC, 2005). At times, I/Ts may make errors in interpretation, such as omitting, adding, or substituting information, and it should be emphasized to them that they should immediately correct any mistakes (NCIHC, 2005). Often, the I/T may not be aware of these mistakes, and it is the responsibility of the SLP or audiologist to listen to and observe what is being said by each party. For example, the SLP or audiologist may observe that the I/T interpretation may take longer than expected. It is appropriate to stop the process and ask for clarification if and when all that is said is interpreted by the I/T for all parties included in the interaction (Langdon & Cheng, 2002). Finally, there may be times when cultural differences between the SLP or the audiologist and the child or the child's family may result in misunderstanding, and the I/T should be encouraged to bring that to the immediate attention of the SLP or audiologist. I/Ts additionally may observe some nonverbal behaviors of the family or child missed by the SLP or audiologist and may need to share them with the SLP or audiologist during or after the interpreted interaction (Isaac, 2002).

The fifth step in preparation is to review all relevant documents, assessments, and information that will be presented to the child or family during an assessment or meeting whenever possible. If it is an assessment, the I/T should be able to look over every test beforehand and to be trained in its administration,

including basals and ceilings and the ability to repeat test items or not. Whenever possible, if it is a meeting, the I/T should be able to look over any diagnostic reports, IEPs or IFSPs, and other paperwork. The purpose of the assessment or meeting also should be detailed. For example, it is important to tell an I/T that a child is not expected to get all items of a diagnostic test correct. These dilemmas will be more prevalent when using Spanish-adapted tests, as tests in languages other than Spanish are frequently not available. More discussion on this topic can be found in Chapter 6.

Finally, the I/T should be informed of any special conditions or circumstances to observe in the assessment, intervention, or meeting. For example, the I/T can be told to be especially observant of disfluencies in the assessment of a child who may stutter. Disfluencies may need to be defined for the I/T and examples given. In addition, if the SLP or audiologist is going to give a diagnosis of a speech-language or hearing disorder in a meeting, the I/T should be informed beforehand so as to discuss the most culturally appropriate way to present the information.

Updating the I/T Process

SLPs and audiologists should keep abreast of principles and procedures in the training of I/Ts. For many I/Ts, the only formal training they will receive on the ethics and procedures of interpretation and translation will come from the SLP or audiologist. Consequently, the more information the SLP or audiologist can obtain from self-study or workshops, the more effective he or she can be in training I/Ts.

In addition, there are a number of actions that an SLP or audiologist can take during the actual interpreted inter-action that will improve the quality of the interaction (Fontes, 2008). There may be occasions when a child or family may ini-tially appear to be relatively competent in the second language, but that competency slips with distress (Phillips, 2010). In such cases, it may be helpful to bring in an I/T after a conference or assessment has started. In addition, conferences involve the conveyance of information that is sometimes complicated, and frequently, a need to consent to clinical intervention, which are additional reasons why an interpreter may be needed (Phillips, 2010). Also, a family member may request the services of an I/T to ensure that he or she is able to understand all the information presented and can more easily respond when needed.

Greetings and Leave Takings

Greetings and leave takings may be much more important in some cultures, and every effort should be made by the team members to greet individuals in the order of status or seniority, which may mean starting with the grandfather or father. It can be useful for SLPs and audiologists to give the family their business card for contact purposes.

Talking to the Family or Client

The child or the family member(s) should be talked to directly instead of talking to the I/T. It is also helpful to establish a warm personal relationship directly with the student/child or family by looking at them rather than the I/T (Langdon & Quintanar-Sarellana, 2003). If possible, it is better to avoid abbreviations and techni-cal jargon, as these may confuse the family. In addition, the SLP or audiologist should

attempt to provide information that the family can easily understand without the I/T having to explain the terminology (Langdon & Quintanar-Sarellana, 2003). Professional terms should be explained by the SLP or audiologist by providing a def-inition and supporting statements with everyday examples. Similarly, it is better to avoid using colloquial language, say-ings, and proverbs (Tribe & Lane, 2009), as these may be confusing.

Verbal and Nonverbal Communication

The process of interpreting can be facili-tated by speaking in a voice that is loud enough without yelling and talking slowly, while using short phrases and pausing for interpretation (Fontes, 2008). It is essential to assure families explicitly of the *confidentiality* of the interpreted interaction. Given the cultural variabil-ity of gestures, it is wise to limit gestures during an interpreted interaction and to attempt to express ideas in words (Fontes, 2008). It may also be important to ask the child or family about facial expressions and unfamiliar gestures to clarify the meaning of unfamiliar nonverbal com-munication. Since expressions of distress and concern can vary widely culturally, and difficult information can be elicited or discussed in an interpreted interaction, it is important not to assume that a child or family's expression of emotion is inap-propriate. Some of this information was covered in Chapter 2.

Exploration of Issues and Alternatives

It is helpful to discuss alternatives and invite correction of one's perceptions. SLPs and audiologists should also explore issues indirectly raised by families, as some cultures may express concerns through storytelling. Therefore, listening to those accounts may be important as they may include information about the child's development and the dynamics of interactions between family members. Providing copies of reports or IEPs written in the family's language may be very helpful in many cases. Also, repetition of critical points may be useful. The first author of this guide has found that asking the parent to state what he or she found most important and helpful assists in determining if the information has been conveyed in a clear manner.

In some cases, it may be apparent that a family is uncomfortable with the gender or background of the I/T when asked to discuss personal issues. In such cases, the services of a different I/T should be used. Even though this may appear to be a subjective judgment, the members of the team should watch for nonverbal signs of discomfort on the part of the parent or family member, including a lack of interaction or signs of inattention.

Debriefing

Once the meeting or assessment has concluded, debriefing with the I/T about the interpreted interaction should take place. Debriefing is a time to give the I/T feedback about his or her performance and to share observations of the child or of the family. After stressful meetings with a family, it may also be a time to provide the I/T with reassurance and perspective about a meeting (d'Ardenne & Farmer, 2009).

Evaluating the I/T's Performance

Evaluating all aspects of an I/T's performance is difficult given that the SLP or audiologist does not speak the language used by the I/T in the interpretation or translation process. However, some initial questions can be asked to ascertain the probable mastery of the interpreted language.

Ongoing evaluation of an I/T's skills can be very helpful to both the SLP or audiologist and the I/T. The I/T's level of formal education and skills are variables to consider. For example, a fellow professional who is already familiar with confidentiality and testing procedures may be able to at least initially perform better than an I/T who is familiar with neither. Nonetheless, with ongoing evaluation and feedback, any I/T can improve his or her skills and knowledge.

Although the SLP or audiologist cannot speak the other language of the I/T, he or she can make many observations of the I/T's performance. During an assessment, there are a number of indications that the I/T is following testing protocols. For example, the SLP can determine whether the I/T is following the basals and ceilings of a standardized test by his or her marking of the test protocol. During the administration of a hearing test, the audiologist may notice that the child is not responding correctly even though he or she was given instructions to either raise a hand or drop a block in the bucket even when the sound was very faint. Better yet, when using an informally translated test, it is appropriate to administer all test items unless the child is unable to perform the task, or it is apparent that the child has missed many consecutive test items.

Signs of difficulty may be noted if the I/T appears to be repeating instructions or test items that should not be repeated or providing additional cueing. These observations are most relevant when using tests that have been normed into one of a few languages, including Spanish. A list of adapted Spanish-normed tests available for bilingual Spanish-speaking individuals living in the United States is available in Table 6–1.

There are additional ways to evaluate an I/T in the testing situation. His or her nonverbal behavior and ability to establish rapport with children is evident without understanding the words used in an interaction. In addition, during formal and informal assessments, the I/T can be encouraged to and observed writing relevant notes about the child's responses. The quality of these notes can be discussed with the I/T during his or her debriefing.

During meetings, there are many other ways to observe the quality of interpretation without being fluent in the second language. Never underestimate the importance of nonverbal language in a meeting situation. If an I/T's body language is not congruent with the message theoretically being interpreted, that is a cause for concern. Similarly, if the body language of family members indicates discomfort, that, too, can be a cause for concern, although it depends on the content of the message being interpreted.

If there are extensive side conversations with the child or the child's family that the I/T does not interpret, these may indicate a problem in the I/T's skills. If an I/T does not maintain an empathic but professional demeanor, that also is a cause for concern. Similarly, if an I/T appears to react to a child's answers during assessment or appears to coach a child without the consent of the SLP or audiologist, this may be an issue.

If the I/T notifies participants when a word is not easily interpreted or if an error of interpretation has been made, those are signs of a conscientious I/T. If the I/T

indicates that a question or comment may be culturally inappropriate, that is again an indicator of a competent I/T.

Concerns about interpretation and translation can be addressed with the I/T during a debriefing following each conference or assessment session. The debriefing offers an opportunity to provide additional training as needed. Such feedback may assist an I/T in improving his or her skills. Table 4–2 includes various aspects that can be used to evaluate an I/T's interpreting and translating skills proposed by Langdon (2002).

RESPONSIBILITIES OF INTERPRETERS AND TRANSLATORS

I/Ts have a number of responsibilities. These include the faithful and accurate interpretation or translation of one language to another to allow other parties to know what each speaker has said (NCIHC, 2005). Other responsibilities are to be impartial and to maintain confidentiality (NCIHC, 2005). I/Ts also have the responsibilities of facilitating communication across cultural differences and clarifying the limits of the interpreting role to avoid conflicts of interest (NCIHC, 2005). Most important, I/Ts have the responsibility of preventing harm to the individuals involved in the interpreted interaction (NCIHC, 2005). Table 4–3 summarizes the roles of interpreters.

Defining and Assessing the I/Ts' Skills

The NCIHC (2001) has developed a guide for the initial assessment of interpreters'

Table 4–2. Evaluation of the I/T's Skills

Key: 0 = Not Applicable; 1 = Always; 2 = Often; 3 = Sometimes; 4 = Rarely; 5 = Never						
General Behaviors						
1. Does the interpreter ask questions to find out what is planned for a given meeting?	0	1	2	3	4	5
2. Does the interpreter seek clarification when something is ambiguous?	0	1	2	3	4	5
3. Does the interpreter listen carefully to what is said by all parties?	0	1	2	3	4	5
4. Does the interpreter share insights about a given culture in a manner that facilitates the process?	0	1	2	3	4	5
5. Does the interpreter appear to be respectful of both cultures and seem well-respected by the community and the families that need the interpreter's services?	0	1	2	3	4	5
6. Is the interpreter willing to acquire new skills to perform the job more effectively?	0	1	2	3	4	5
7. Is there evidence that the interpreter maintains neutrality and confidentiality throughout the process?	0	1	2	3	4	5
8. Does the interpreter accept feedback from parents and other parties involved in the process?	0	1	2	3	4	5
9. Is the interpreter punctual?	0	1	2	3	4	5
10. Does the interpreter follow the Code of Ethics?	0	1	2	3	4	5
Specific Translation Skills						
1. Does the interpreter appear to convey a given message clearly?	0	1	2	3	4	5
2. Does the interpreter retranslate something when it is unclear to any participant?	0	1	2	3	4	5
3. Does the interpreter use different methods of conveying the same information?	0	1	2	3	4	5
4. Does the interpreter appropriately use different levels of formality?	0	1	2	3	4	5
5. Does the translator appropriately use back translation to ensure that a given document has preserved the original meaning?	0	1	2	3	4	5
Comments:						

Table 4–3. *Summary of Interpreters' Roles*

DO	DON'T
Act ethically	Assume you need to help whenever called
Show respect for all members involved	
Remain neutral as well as flexible and maintain professional boundaries[a]	Take over the role of the SLP or audiologist
	Discuss a case outside a given setting
Respect confidentiality	Provide cues when not called for, advice or counseling
Follow test/activity administration accurately	
	Provide repetitions when not called for
Interpret faithfully	Accept jobs that are too difficult at a given time
Become a life learner	

[a]This role may vary but needs to be clarified to all parties involved in an interpreting process. Please refer to Chapters 4 and 6 for more detail on this topic.

qualifications (NCIHC, 2001). The guide advocates the assessment of the following components: basic language skills; an ethical case study; cultural issues; professional terminology; integrated interpreting skills, measured by a role-play; and translation of simple instructions.

The measurement of basic language skills involves the measurement of English oral comprehension and production as well as non-English language oral comprehension and production. An informal approach to assessment can be an unstructured oral interview with a rater who speaks both languages (NCIHC, 2001). It may not be necessary to measure the I/T's oral skills in a non-English language if he or she has a college-level education earned in another country or if he or she has recently arrived in the new country as an adult. When no one is available who can assess the potential I/T's skills in her or her native language, this may be the best way of ensuring that the potential I/T has sufficient fluency in the non-English language.

Ethical principles and decision making can be assessed by an oral or a written case study involving ethical principles, such as confidentiality, accuracy, respect, conveying cultural information, and impartiality (NCIHC, 2001). An evaluation of the ability to deal with cultural issues can be achieved through the discussion of case studies involving potential cultural barriers, in which potential I/Ts are asked to indicate the way they would deal with such barriers (NCIHC, 2001). Questions to ask when scoring this section include the following: (a) Did the I/T understand the influence of cultural issues, (b) did the I/T share the observation of a miscommunication and state that he or she was able to assist the SLP or audiologist with the miscommunication, or (c) did the I/T take over (NCIHC, 2001)?

An oral or a written exam or a role-play that incorporates professional terms in the text or the script can be helpful in assessing the I/T's knowledge in this area. An individual familiar with both languages and professional terminology can give and/or assess the test (NCIHC, 2001). Terms can include names of formal and informal tests, speech-language and hearing symptoms and disorders, and descriptions of interventions.

To assess integrated interpreting skills, a role-play could be used to simulate an interpreted family conference and/or assessment of a child (NCIHC, 2001). The role-play should be videotaped or audiotaped for future reference and can include problematic situations in which an interpreter might be expected to intervene, such as terminology the I/T might not understand, cultural issues, or a speaker talking too long or too quickly. The I/T's evaluation of the interaction may include the following: (a) the completeness and accuracy of interpretation, (b) the maintenance of the role of interpreter, (c) management of the flow of communication (asking for pauses or clarification when needed), and (d) handling of cultural issues (NCIHC, 2001).

To assess written translation, potential I/Ts can be asked to perform sight translation of simple instructions or parts of individual education plans (IEPs) and written-to-written translation of simple text (NCIHC, 2001). Scoring for this section can include (a) accuracy of translation, (b) dealing with ambiguous terms and requesting clarification of unknown words and concepts, and (c) the I/T's ability to convey the intended meaning of the text if the non-English language lacks equivalents of English terms. The success of the translation could be rated by a rubric from 1 to 5, where 5 is excellent, 4 is very good, 3 is adequate, 2 is below average, and 1 is poor. Again, this needs to be scored by an individual fluent in both languages.

In many instances, another individual who speaks the same language as the potential interpreter may not be available. However, information can be obtained about the I/T's understanding of professional ethics and ability to deal with cultural issues without comprehending the I/T's other language. Similarly, if an individual has grown up in another country, his or her fluency in the language and knowledge of culture of the other country can frequently be assumed, provided that the language was spoken in the home. Additionally, questions such as those under "Evaluating the I/T's Performance" can and should be asked initially of all potential I/Ts.

Table 4–4 offers some suggested topics for oral interviews in English and the target language with a scoring rubric. Table 4–5 includes a sample letter and portion of a report the I/T can translate/adapt into the target language. The assessor may rate the success of the translated assignment on a rubric from 1 to 5, where 5 is excellent, 4 is very good, 3 is adequate, 2 is below average, and 1 is poor.

The I/T's Multiple Functions

According to the California Healthcare Interpreting Association (CHIA, 2012), there are four main roles that an I/T can play within an interpreted interaction: message converter, message clarifier, cultural clarifier, and patient (client) advocate. I/Ts can potentially play more than one role during an interpreted interaction (Isaac, 2002). As a message converter, I/Ts observe body language and listen to both speakers, converting the message's meaning from one language to another without unnecessary deletions, additions, or changes in meaning (CHIA, 2012). As part of this role, an I/T should intervene when individuals speak too fast or give the I/T insufficient time to interpret.

Table 4–4. Suggested Topics for Oral Interviews

Proposed Scoring Rubric:

Note: The oral examination proposed is similar to that of the Foreign Service Institute (FSI), which is based on a scale of 1 to 5, with 3 being the minimum standard accepted to perform a given professional task. Ideally, native speakers of both English and the target language will interview the candidate. The oral interview may take place in the group session or different sessions for each language. A suggested collection of topics appears below (Language Proficiency Definitions, n.d.).

1 = **Elementary level of proficiency.** Routine travel needs; minimum courtesy requirements. Reads signs, names of places, some words/phrases in the language.

2 = **Limited working language proficiency.** Can satisfy some basic social demands and work requirements and can read simple contextually based information.

3 = **Minimum Professional Proficiency.** Speaks the language with sufficient accuracy and vocabulary to participate in formal and informal conversations in most practical, social and professional topics. Can read newspapers, reports and technical reports in a designated professional field.

4 = **Full Professional Proficiency.** Can fulfill communication on all levels within a given professional field. Can read all styles and forms of material in a given professional field.

5 = **Native or Bilingual Proficiency.** Has the oral and reading language skills of an educated person in that language.

Note: The assessment could yield an intermediate score between one level and another. For example, 3+ would indicate skills between 3 and 4.

The following questions are grouped. The first set can be asked in both languages; the second group is designed to assess English and the target language more specifically. It is suggested the interviewers select two scenarios from each group. This is based on the first author's experience in interviewing bilingual Spanish-speaking individuals.

English	Target Language
This is a two-part question:	This is a two-part question:
Provide a short summary of your experiences or training as an interpreter, and what experiences do you have in working with school-age children?	*Provide a short summary of your experiences or training as an interpreter, and what experiences do you have in working with school-age children?*
The following is a two-part question:	The following is a two-part question:
What does bilingualism mean to you? And, please tell me two advantages and two disadvantages of being bilingual.	*What does bilingualism mean to you? Also, please tell me two advantages and two disadvantages of being bilingual.*
If you have been an interpreter, what are one or two situations that have been the most difficult for you, and how did you resolve them?	*If you have been an interpreter, what are one or two situations that have been the most difficult for you, and how did you resolve them?*

continues

Table 4–4. *continued*

English	Target Language
This is a three-part question: *What do you read most frequently in English, and what has been your favorite book or article you have read lately? Please give me two reasons.*	This is a three-part question: *What do you read most frequently in English, and what has been your favorite book or article you have read lately? Please give me two reasons.*
You have lost the test that the SLP or the audiologist has lent you. *Describe what you would do.*	A parent came with her son at the wrong time to the speech and language assessment appointment because you forgot to call her to remind her (The SLP had requested this from you). The parent had to take time off from work and is unhappy; she will lose income. *What would you do and what would you say to her?*
You do not agree with the SLP with what he/she asks the parent to do at home because in the parent's culture this activity is carried out by the professional. *How would you explain this to the SLP?*	A client has a progressive hearing loss and you need to tell him he needs to consult with an otolaryngologist/ENT. *How would you do this?* (Suppose the client is very frightened and is worried about losing his hearing entirely, but the audiologist just said she is not sure of the reason but is not convinced the client should worry about losing his hearing entirely).
The parent of a child tells you on the phone that he/she does not want the child to receive a label. *How would you respond to the parent?*	The SLP tells the parent that the child needs therapy. The parent is very worried the child is intellectually challenged; the SLP just said he/she is not. *How would you convey this information to the parent?*
You are doing a sight translation for an IEP, and you notice the teacher and the psychologist are not paying attention. *What would you do?*	The SLP is asking you to translate the IEP, and you notice the mother begins to cry because she hears her child has cognitive delays. *What would you do?*

Source: Language Proficiency Definitions. (n.d). *U.S. Department of State: Careers representing America.* Retrieved June 24, 2015, from http://careers.state.gov/gateway/lang_prof_def.html

Table 4–5. *Translation Exercises*

This translation exercise consists of two parts:
(1) A sample letter from English to the Target Language
(2) A portion of a Speech and Language Evaluation Report

(1) Letter

Dear Mr. and Mrs. XXX,

Ms. YYY talked to you on the phone about our meeting to review the results of your son, KK's, speech and language evaluation. The meeting will be held at Martin Luther King Elementary school on February 22nd at 2 p.m. in Room 11. The meeting will last approximately 1 hour. You will meet with me, Mrs. D, KK's classroom teacher, the nurse, and Mr. WW, the principal. You may bring a friend or relative to this meeting if you wish. Ms. YYY will interpret the conference so that you feel more at ease understanding the content of the meeting. If you have any questions, please contact Ms. YYY at 555-1212.

Please sign the bottom of the page and circle Yes or No if you plan to attend the meeting. I look forward to seeing you.

Sincerely,

HWL, Ed. D., CCC-SLP
Bilingual Speech and Language Pathologist

Please circle

Yes, we will be at the meeting

No, we cannot be at the meeting. Please call me (indicate date and time)

_____

Signature

(2) Portion from a Speech and Language Evaluation Report

Paul is a 14-year-old adolescent who comes from a bilingual home where Tagalog is spoken in addition to English. His parents don't speak English fluently, but Paul speaks English with his two younger siblings, ages 10 and 7. At home, he communicates in Tagalog with his parents and now prefers English.

Paul has never been assessed for speech and language because all of his teachers have assumed he was still learning English. He has been living in the United States for 3 years. He attended school regularly in Manila and was learning English as a second language, but most classes were taught in Tagalog. His grades in all subjects were average and some were above average, like math and science.

continues

Table 4–5. *continued*

Paul is a cooperative and motivated young man who tries his best. His greatest challenge is comprehending what he reads in textbooks that are written in English, especially social studies and literature. His conversational skills in English are adequate, but he stills experiences problems in understanding more complex ideas and may not always convey opinions with ease. His math and science skills are adequate. He does not receive any extra support. Since Paul has been enrolled in a total immersion English program for only 3 years and demands at the high school level are high, the team recommended extra tutoring after school to teach him specific strategies for reading comprehension. A reevaluation of his academic skills is suggested at the beginning of the following semester.

Proposed Rubric for Scoring Translations:

Area	Level 1 Poor	Level 2 Below Average	Level 3 Average	Level 4 Above Average	Level 5 Excellent
MEANING	1 or more incorrect meanings	Some meanings unclear	Some imprecision but adequate meaning overall	All meanings accurate	All meanings precise
GRAMMAR	3 or more errors that are distracting or confusing	1–2 errors that cause confusion	Some errors, but only mildly distracting	Some errors that do not affect meaning	No errors
SPELLING	More than 5 errors	4–5 errors	2–3 errors	1 error	No errors
PUNCTU-ATION	More than 3 errors	3 errors	2 errors	1 error	No errors

Similarly, I/Ts must manage turn-taking to ensure that individuals speaking simultaneously will be heard in order or that an individual is allowed to finish speaking.

As message clarifier, I/Ts stay alert for words or concepts that may lead to misunderstanding (CHIA, 2012). When that occurs, I/Ts may interrupt the communication process, alert all parties that the I/T is seeing signs of confusion from one or more individuals and identify the confusing word or concept, request or assist the speaker of the unfamiliar word or concept to restate it or describe the unfamiliar word in a simpler way, and find ways to assist speakers to describe concepts using analogies or descriptions when there are no linguistic equivalents in either language. In this role, the interpreter needs to state clearly to all individuals that the message is from the interpreter. In this role, the I/T preferably waits until an individual asks for the interpreter's help in clarifying words or concepts unless communication is seriously impaired (CHIA, 2012).

As cultural clarifier, I/Ts are alert to cultural words or concepts that may lead to a misunderstanding, as cultural beliefs about illness and disability may vary significantly, and some beliefs and practices may lack equivalent terms in different languages (CHIA, 2012). In some cases, a child or client may perceive the questioning by an SLP or an audiologist as inappropriate, or the reverse may be true. In addition, nonverbal language among individuals of different cultures may vary, and both SLPs and audiologists as well as children and families may be confused by culture-specific gestures or facial expressions. When there is evidence that any party to the interaction is confused by cultural differences, interpreters can (a) interrupt the communication process, (b) alert both parties to a potential misunderstanding or miscommunication, (c) suggest concerns of culture that may be impeding understanding, and (d) assist the client in explaining the cultural concept to the SLP or audiologist or the reverse (CHIA, 2012). However, it is important to be mindful that the I/T's description of his or her culture is his or her own perspective and is not always typical, unbiased, or correct (Fontes, 2008).

The role of patient advocate is a potentially controversial one. However, an I/T could suggest that a family be given an I/T for follow-up appointments or provide information about linguistically appropriate available services (CHIA, 2012). During an interpreted session in which providers discriminate against a family or child, an I/T can take the following steps: (a) remind parties of the ethical principle of interpreting everything in the interaction; (b) ask parties to explain intentions of actions or comments, to clear up a potential misunderstanding; (c) provide the family or child with appropriate information or resources, or refer them to other staff; or (d) if the above strategies are ineffective, document the incident and contact his or her supervisor (CHIA, 2012).

Following a Code of Ethics

I/Ts should follow a code of ethics. One nationally based code of ethics is "A National Code of Ethics for Interpreters in Health Care" (NCIHC, 2004) (Table 4–6). With minor revisions, it can be adapted to a code of ethics for interpreters/translators with SLPs and audiologists. Some I/Ts may already be familiar with some or many of the principles of ethics. However, if they are not, it is the responsibility of the SLP or audiologist to introduce and explain these principles to the I/T.

The following is a review of the individual code of ethics, principle by principle.

"1. The interpreter treats as confidential, within the treating team, all information learned in the performance of their professional duties, while observing relevant requirements regarding disclosure" (NCIHC, 2004, p. 10). Confidentiality is the cornerstone of the interpretation process. Families and children must feel comfortable and safe in sharing private information with the SLP and audiologist. To ensure that families and children understand that the concept of confidentiality applies to the interpreted interaction, it is appropriate to state as much at the beginning of the interpreted interaction. At the

Table 4–6. Proposed Code of Ethics for Interpreters Collaborating With SLPs and Audiologists

The Interpreter:
1. Treats as confidential, within the treating team, all information learned in the performance of their professional duties, while observing relevant requirements regarding disclosure.
2. Strives to render the message accurately, conveying the content and spirit of the original message, taking into consideration its cultural context.
3. Strives to maintain impartiality and refrains from counseling, advising, or projecting personal biases or beliefs.
4. Maintains the boundaries of the professional role, refraining from personal involvement.
5. Continually strives to develop awareness of her/his own and other (including biomedical) cultures encountered in the performance of their professional duties.
6. Treats all parties with respect.
7. May be justified in acting as an advocate when the patient's health, well-being, or dignity is at risk. Advocacy is understood as an action taken on behalf of an individual that goes beyond facilitating communication, with the intention of supporting good health outcomes. Advocacy must be undertaken only after careful and thoughtful analysis of the situation and if other less intrusive actions have not resolved the problem.
8. Strives to continually further his/her knowledge and skills.
9. Must at all times act in a professional and ethical manner.

Source: Reprinted with permission from "A National Code of Ethics for Interpreters in Health Care," by The National Council on Interpreting in Health Care, 2004, retrieved from http://www.ncihc.org/

same time, it is important to emphasize that everything said by the families or child will be interpreted for the SLP or audiologist and vice versa (NCIHC, 2004).

There is an exception to the principle of confidentiality. Many states mandate the disclosure of information by SLPs or audiologists when an individual is being abused or when an individual is threatening harm to herself or himself or others (NCIHC, 2004). In such cases, information that would otherwise be confidential may need to be reported to the appropriate authorities. There may also be other times when a family or child reveals important information in confidence to the I/T. The I/T should make every effort to encourage the family or child to disclose the information to the SLP or audiologist. If the family or child still does not wish to disclose the information, it should be shared with the SLP or audiologist if it is pertinent to the child's speech-language-hearing disorder (NCIHC, 2004).

"2. The interpreter strives to render the message accurately, conveying the content and spirit of the original message, taking into consideration its cultural context" (NCIHC, 2004, p. 13). The responsibility of the I/T is to render messages from one language to another without making judgments as to what is important, acceptable, or relevant. It is not the responsibility of the I/T to edit what the SLP or audiologist conveys or, conversely, the speech of the family or of the child. The I/T does not censor what is said and conveys everything that is said without distorting, omitting from, or adding to the message (NCIHC, 2004, 2005). As part of a commitment to accuracy, I/Ts should immediately correct and rectify any mistakes in interpretation (NCIHC, 2005). In addition, it is recommended that the I/T speak during interpreting in the first person, as if he or she is giving the message directly (Dubslaff & Martinsen, 2005).

In service of this aim, it is appropriate that the I/T advise everyone in an interpreted interaction that everything said will be interpreted (NCIHC, 2005). As needed, the I/T can take on the roles of message converter, message clarifier, and cultural clarifier to ensure the accuracy of the interpretation (CHIA, 2012). As much as possible, the I/T should replicate the style, tone, and register of the speaker (CHIA, 2005). Instead of using simpler terms for a word with no equivalent in the child or family's language, the I/T can ask the speaker to use language more appropriate for the level of understanding of the other party. It is through their use of language that SLPs and audiologists build a relationship with the child or family; therefore, it is important for their remarks to be interpreted as faithfully as possible (NCIHC, 2004). In addition, a family's culturally based explanations or concerns should be interpreted directly and accurately by the I/T so that the SLP or audiologist obtains a better idea of the family's perspective.

"3. The interpreter strives to maintain impartiality and refrains from coun-

seling, advising or projecting personal biases or beliefs" (NCIHC, 2004, p. 15). Synonyms for *impartial* include equitable, fair, objective, unbiased, and unprejudiced (NCIHC, 2004). Impartiality means that I/Ts do not judge the content of messages to determine what to transmit or how to transmit the message. I/Ts also do not judge parties in the interpreted interaction, do not take sides, and do not attempt to persuade either party (NCIHC, 2004). If an I/T has a potential conflict of interest, such as interpreting for a family member or close friend, he or she notifies the SLP or audiologist and may need to withdraw from the interpretation assignment (NCIHC, 2005).

When I/Ts take on a role beyond message converter in an interpreted interaction, it is for the purpose of being a communication facilitator of the mutual understanding of meaning (NCIHC, 2004). However, although an I/T cannot take sides in an interaction, it is appropriate to respond to a child or family with comfort and reassurance as the response of a caring person (NCIHC, 2004).

"4. The interpreter maintains the boundaries of the professional role, refraining from personal involvement" (NCIHC, 2004, p. 16). At times, I/Ts may have other roles in the work setting. When interpreting/translating, the I/T should refrain from acting in another role unless all present know that the I/T will do so (NCIHC, 2004). When switching roles, the I/T should notify all that the switch is occurring in an interpreted interaction.

At times, an I/T will not have the qualifications for the particular role or setting in which he or she has been called to interpret. In such cases, the I/T can withdraw or, if no one else is available, can notify all parties of his or her capabilities (NCIHC, 2004).

In terms of conflicts of interest, in close-knit communities, it is essential not to share confidential information with community members (NCIHC, 2004). Being part of a close-knit community may also subject an I/T to some expectations of special consideration (Hwa-Froelich & Westby, 2003; NCIHC, 2004). Consequently, while being friendly and caring, it is important that I/Ts maintain a professional boundary that minimizes personal involvement with the family and child.

"5. The interpreter continually strives to develop awareness of her/his own and other (including biomedical) cultures encountered in the performance of their professional duties" (NCIHC, 2004, p. 18). There is a purpose in I/Ts understanding their own cultural basis for how they make sense of the world. By developing their awareness of their own culturally based understandings, I/Ts are less likely to intrude with their own cultural biases.

In addition, the more that an I/T is aware of the characteristics of his or her own cultural background, the better that he or she can facilitate communication across cultural differences and avoid misunderstandings (NCIHC, 2004). This insight allows the I/T to take on the role of cultural clarifier (CHIA, 2012). Thus, when cultural misunderstandings occur, an I/T, with the consent of all parties, can share cultural information or develop explanations that all can understand (NCIHC, 2004)

When I/Ts have access to information related to cultural aspects regarding various aspects of speech, language, hearing, and learning, they can (a) understand better the messages of speakers, (b) hypothesize about how cultural factors may affect a lack of communication between parties, and (c) assist parties in negotiating a shared meaning (NCIHC, 2004).

"6. The interpreter treats all parties with respect" (NCIHC, 2004, p. 19). I/Ts should treat all parties with respect and equality, including using preferred titles for both SLPs and audiologists and family members (NCIHC, 2005). Interpreters, as much as is feasible, should make sure that family members have the opportunity to express their opinions during the interpreted interaction (Davitti, 2013). An additional integral part of the process is that families have the right to decide what is best for them after they have received relevant and appropriate information (NCIHC, 2004).

"7. When the patient's health, well-being, or dignity is at risk, the interpreter may be justified in acting as an advocate. Advocacy is understood as an action taken on behalf of an individual that goes beyond facilitating communication, with the intention of supporting good health outcomes. Advocacy must be undertaken only after careful and thoughtful analysis of the situation and if other less intrusive actions have not resolved the problem" (NCIHC, 2004, p. 19).

As previously stated, the role of patient advocate is a controversial one and may seem to be contradicted by the ethics principle of impartiality. However, it should result from consistent and clear observation that something is wrong, and action needs to be taken to correct it. (NCIHC, 2004). It stems from the principle of upholding the well-being (physical, emotional, and social) of families and children to make sure that no harm is done.

If an I/T observes something that is likely to have a serious negative consequence for a child or family, it is his or her responsibility to try to resolve the issue with the involved parties (NCIHC, 2004). If that is unsuccessful, he or she may want to consult a supervisor or colleagues while maintaining the anonymity of the parties involved in an effort to determine the correct course of action (NCIHC, 2004).

"8. The interpreter strives to continually further his/her knowledge and skills" (NCIHC, 2004, p. 20). There are a number of ways that I/Ts can continue to further their skills. They can stay current on technical terminology and procedures (NCIHC, 2005) used in the fields of speech-language pathology and audiology as well as common terms from different dialects of the non-English language that they speak. Additionally, an I/T should strive to learn to match the register, or the degree of formality used in the family's language (Isaac, 2002) to make the family more comfortable with the interpreted interaction. Finally, the more knowledge the I/T can continue to acquire about cultural attitudes toward speech-language-hearing disorders, the better he or she will be able to interpret during cultural misunderstandings (NCIHC, 2004).

Also, continued practice in language skills in English and the other language will enable the I/T to become more proficient in his or her interpretation performance in the two languages. (NCIHC, 2005).

"9. The interpreter must at all times act in a professional and ethical matter" (NCIHC, 2004, p. 21). There are a number of actions that an I/T can take to act in a professional manner. An ethical I/T is prepared for assignments and discloses accurately his or her credentials and limitations in regard to certain assignments (NCIHC, 2005). An I/T does not discriminate against anyone in the provision of his or her interpretation (NCIHC, 2004). An I/T avoids sight translations if lacking sight translation skills (NCIHC, 2005) and acts with dignity (NCIHC, 2004). Finally, an I/T does not accept more than small tokens of appreciation from families or children (NCIHC, 2004).

Knowledge of Two Cultures and Two Modes of Verbal and Nonverbal Communication

As previously stated, it is important that the I/T has knowledge of the two cultures associated with the two languages he or she speaks. It is not enough to speak the two languages, as frequently there will be cultural differences in conceptions of disability and intervention. Such differences may be confusing to an SLP or audiologist without a knowledge of such cultural differences, and in such circumstances, it is possible to have a cultural misunderstanding (CHIA, 2012).

In addition, individuals of different cultures may have different ways of nonverbally indicating discomfort, disagreement, or other emotions. When an SLP or audiologist is unfamiliar with culturally specific ways of nonverbally communicating negative emotions, there can again be a cultural misunderstanding. In many cases, the I/T is the only individual in an interpreted interaction that is familiar with the cultures of the family and child, as well as those of the SLP or audiologist.

In the role of a cultural clarifier, the I/T can play a crucial part in clarifying cultural misunderstandings (CHIA, 2012). In that role, the I/T interrupts the communication process, alerts both parties to a potential miscommunication or misunderstanding, suggests cultural concerns that could be harming understanding, and assists the SLP or audiologist or family in communicating the concept (CHIA, 2012).

The role of cultural clarifier may be of great use in communicating with families of diverse language and cultural backgrounds. Using the LEARN process (Berlin & Fowkes, 1983), SLPs and audiologists can obtain a better understanding of the perspective of families toward disabilities and negotiate a way to come to agreement about a suggested intervention program for a child.

The first step in LEARN is *LISTEN* with understanding and sympathy to the family's perception of the child's disability (Berlin & Fowkes, 1983). The second step is to *EXPLAIN* the professional perception of the problem. The third step is to discuss and *ACKNOWLEDGE* the similarities and differences between the two models of disability. It is crucial at this point to not denigrate the family's cultural perceptions of their child's disability. The fourth step is to *RECOMMEND* treatment within the constraints of the SLP's or audiologist's and family's model of disability. There may be steps that the family wishes to take that are consistent with their cultural values. Finally, the last step is to *NEGOTIATE* agreement on the treatment plan, which may include some options from the family's cultural perspective. Such a process is more likely to gain more buy-in and participation from the family.

Ability to Convey the Same Meaning in Two Languages

It is not enough to speak two languages with a degree of fluency. I/Ts have to be able to convey the same meaning in both languages. At times, there are no equivalents for concepts or words in one language or the other language. For example, *tu* and *Usted*, which are the informal and informal words for *you* in Spanish, have no exact equivalent in English. In other cases, grammatical differences need to be accounted for. For example, "*Está comiendo la galleta*" ("He/she/it is eating the cookie") in Spanish does not have a subject, yet it is correct in Spanish, a prodrop language.

In addition, the meanings of certain disorders may be very different for individuals of another culture. According to Good (1977), the significance of "a disease category cannot be understood simply as a set of defining symptoms. It is rather a 'syndrome' of typical experiences, a set of words, experiences, and feelings which typically 'run together' for the members of a society" (p. 27). Such sets of words, experiences, and feelings constitute a semantic network of meanings that may not be understandable or have direct equivalents in another language (Good, 1977). Alternatively, the semantic network of a disorder may also suggest culturally based behaviors as ways of coping with that disorder (Jackson, 1998), behaviors that may be unfamiliar to individuals of another culture.

Different types of equivalence (Jackson, 1998) must be negotiated in an interpreted interaction. *Vocabulary equivalence* is finding the equivalent word with the right connotations to carry meaning. Some languages have no equivalent words for the technical terms used by SLPs and audiologists. *Grammatic equivalence* includes parts of speech that are absent, problematic, or present in certain languages, such as *tu* and *Ud.* in Spanish. *Idiomatic equivalence*, the equivalence of idioms, is rare across languages. *Conceptual equivalence* includes the multiple linguistic associations of words, such as the use of the heart in English for both an organ and the seat of emotion. *Experiential equivalence* means that meaningful phrases or words must refer to real experiences and objects that are familiar to both cultures. In speech-language-hearing disorders, the symptoms of a disorder are often equivalent in both languages, while terminology may not be.

Words also have *referential value* as well as *performative value* (Jackson, 1998). The referential value of a word occurs when a word refers to a concept or element in the speaker's world. The performative value of a word indicates that the use of a word implies certain behaviors in certain contexts. For speakers of different languages, both the referential value and performative values of words may differ, requiring the I/T to act as a message clarifier or cultural clarifier (CHIA, 2012).

A skillful I/T will be able to identify differences between languages during and after an assessment. This is crucial in terms of determining whether a child makes a true error in his or her language or whether it is a language difference. In addition, an I/T must be ready and able to work with an SLP or audiologist and a family as a message clarifier or cultural clarifier when terminology in one language does not have an exact equivalent in a second language (CHIA, 2012).

Knowledge of a Specialty's Terminology

The knowledge of a specialty's terminology can refer to terminology both in English and in the non-English language. The fields of speech-language pathology and audiology have a variety of terms specific to the field, some of which are not familiar to an untrained listener. The skilled I/T can learn both some of the most important technical terminology and the meanings of the terminology in simpler words in English. In that way, I/Ts can help SLPs or audiologists simplify terminology with the permission and knowledge of the SLP or audiologist if family members or chil-

dren do not know the technical terms in their non-English language. Similarly, I/Ts should know terminology names in the non-English language as well as ways of explaining the terms using simpler words.

There are a number of times during the assessment and conferencing process that I/Ts may need to use technical terminology. One such circumstance is during the intake of background information. In more complicated cases, questions eliciting the medical and developmental background of the child may require the understanding of considerable technical terminology in both languages. Technical terminology may also be required during a family conference to explain the results of formal and informal assessments and also to provide a diagnosis and to explain the type of intervention proposed, including specific goals and objectives. Once again, the skilled I/T can act as a message clarifier or cultural clarifier when there is a potential misunderstanding.

Familiarity With Dialectical Differences

The I/T should also be informed of the country or area of origin of the child or of the family in order to use the appropriate dialect with them. Dialectal differences can be apparent in even very basic terms that are frequently tested in formal tests of children. For example, the word for *orange* in Puerto Rico is *china*, while it is *naranja* in Mexico. Similarly, some Latin American countries use *vosotros* as a form of plural *you*, while others do not. Without knowing differences in dialects, I/Ts can make a number of errors. During an assessment, they can use terms, grammatical structures, or pronunciations that are unknown to a child, confusing the child and possibly resulting in the child producing an incorrect answer. When scoring a test, an I/T can inadvertently mark answers wrong that would be correct in a different dialect, including grammatical, semantic, and phonological differences. In interpreting at a conference, producing interpretations that are misunderstood can compromise the faithfulness of translation. For all of the above reasons, it is important to be familiar with dialectical differences or to not interpret for a child or family with a different dialect if faithfulness of the interpretation will be compromised. For example, the first author remembers she used the word *sacate* instead of *grama* in a standardized test on Spanish-speaking children from California, realizing only after the child did not respond that she was from Central America, where a different word is used for the word *grass*. Therefore, a careful background history of a child and family should be obtained prior to administering any test or task.

Ability to Adapt to the Speech and Language Patterns of Clients With Communication Disorders

I/Ts who collaborate with SLPs and audiologists need a special set of skills specific to those professions. In the case of both children and adults, some of their language will be compromised by speech-language-hearing disorders, and intelligibility and coherence may be disrupted. A skilled I/T is able, as much as possible, to determine what is said by a child or adult and to render it in both the incorrect and the correct form for analysis by the SLP or audiologist. The I/T should, in addition, be able to explain to the SLP or audiologist the errors and the correct forms.

Maintaining Neutrality and Confidentiality

As stated in the NICHC Code of Ethics (NICHC, 2004), it is essential that the I/T maintain neutrality and confidentiality. In maintaining neutrality, the I/T can still be an empathic human being. However, it is not his or her responsibility to take sides or to favor the SLP or audiologist, the family, or the child (NICHC, 2004). Both situations should be avoided and watched out for, as sometimes I/Ts ally themselves with the institution that employs them or identify closely with members of their ethnic community (Fontes, 2008). For example, an interpreter may want to help a family save face when obtaining background information by not interpreting the most problematic information of a case history, which is precisely the most important information to interpret.

Similarly, confidentiality within the educational team is key to protect the welfare of the family and child. It is a key component of trust between the SLP and audiologist, interpreter, and family and child. For that reason, family members should not be asked to interpret for the family or child except at the explicit request of the family (Fontes, 2008). Similarly, minor children should not be asked to interpret at all, and the importance of confidentiality can never be emphasized enough (Fontes, 2008).

Interpreting Faithfully

Part of the I/T's responsibility is to interpret faithfully without deleting, adding, or changing the message. Untrained interpreters sometimes overinterpret by trying to "clean up" disjointed statements and putting them together into a coherent whole, thereby trying to convey what the individual meant rather than what he or she actually said (Fontes, 2008). This is not a permissible practice.

As part of the preparation for an interpreted interaction, it is important to remind the I/T not to leave out seemingly unimportant details and to interpret word for word without summarizing and inferring (Fontes, 2008). It is also important for the I/T to ask for an explanation for any unfamiliar terms and to translate at the same level of language skill as the family or child.

When the I/T thinks that there is a problem with the quality of interpretation sufficient to make the interpretation inaccurate, he or she should inform the SLP or audiologist (Fontes, 2008). For example, if a child is not verbal in any language because of a speech-language-hearing disorder, the SLP or audiologist should be immediately notified.

There are times when the I/T as message clarifier or cultural clarifier may need to stop the interaction to indicate that there is some confusion in the communication process (CHIA, 2012), and the I/T, with the consent of both parties, may try to clarify the message. However, those are special circumstances, and the I/T is never to editorialize in the I/T role.

Maintaining Linguistic Skills

One important aspect of being an I/T is the maintenance and improvement of linguistic skills. The I/T should take opportunities to practice the speaking and writing of his or her non-English language as well as of English. In addition, the I/T should take advantage of interpreting/translating opportunities to obtain feedback and to practice interpreting/translating skills.

Participating in Ongoing Learning and Remaining Flexible

As part of ongoing learning, I/Ts should take advantage of workshops and presentations on interpretation and translation. In addition, they can confer with SLPs and audiologists to increase their technical vocabulary.

Above all, it is important for I/Ts to remain flexible. For example, an I/T may prepare to give a battery of tests to a child and may have to switch tests when the tests are not appropriate for the developmental level for the child. In addition, the I/T may have to help deal with behavior issues if a child is noncompliant and may have to decipher both incorrect responses and their correct counterparts. In meetings with families, the I/T may have to help the SLP or audiologist deal with the emotional reactions of a family member and cultural differences in perspectives. All of these situations require flexibility and ingenuity.

To summarize, SLPs and audiologists remain responsible for the actions of the I/T and need to train the I/T in procedures and ethics. At the same time, the I/T has the responsibility for a code of ethics, keeping confidentiality, and interpreting faithfully. Together, SLPs or audiologists and I/Ts can form a team that can most effectively serve children and their families.

DISCUSSION ITEMS AND ACTIVITIES

(6 and 7 adapted from Jackson, 1998)

1. What are the responsibilities and role of the SLP or audiologist in working with an I/T?

2. How can an SLP or audiologist initially gauge the skills of an I/T without speaking the I/T's language?

3. What kinds of feedback can an SLP or audiologist provide an I/T without speaking the I/T's language?

4. What roles can the I/T play in an interpreted interaction? When is it appropriate for an I/T to intervene in an interaction?

5. What are some of the principles of the Code of Ethics of I/Ts?

6. In a role-play, select one person each to be the SLP or audiologist, the I/T, and the parent. In English, have the individuals portraying the SLP or audiologist and the parent play their roles while the individual portraying the I/T restates what the other two individuals say, as in an interpreted interaction. Spend 5 minutes on this activity, then have the individuals portraying the SLP or audiologist and the parent critique the restating performance of the individual portraying the I/T. Switch roles and repeat the process, until each individual has had the opportunity to play the I/T role.

7. Imagine the following scenarios and find the best possible solutions for them.
    a. The SLP or audiologist feels the parent/client is not understanding what is said.
    b. The I/T is "editing" what the audiologist says.
    c. The I/T and parent are having their own side conversation and "seem to ignore the rest of the meeting."
    d. The SLP or audiologist does not seem to pay attention to the par-

ents'/family's or client's reactions to the dialogue (from the I/T's perspective).
    e. Your supervisor says there are no additional funds to hire a "trained-professional I/T."
    f. The I/T's interpreting seems to take much more time than the messages conveyed by the SLP or audiologist.

REFERENCES

American Speech-Language-Hearing Association. (2010). *Code of ethics*. Retrieved from http://www.asha.org/policy/ET2010-00309/

Berlin, E., & Fowkes, W. (1983). A teaching framework for cross-cultural health care: Application in family practice. *The Western Journal of Medicine, 139*, 934–938.

California Healthcare Interpreting Association. (2012). *California standards for healthcare interpreter: Ethical principles, protocols, and guidance on roles and intervention*. Retrieved from http://www.chiaonline.org/?page=CHIAStandards

d'Ardenne, P., & Farmer, E. (2009). Using interpreters in trauma therapy. In N. Grey (Ed.), *A casebook of cognitive therapy for traumatic stress reactions* (pp. 283–300). London, UK: Routledge.

Davitti, E. (2013). Dialogue interpreting in intercultural mediation: Interpreters' use of upgrading moves in parent-teacher meetings. *Interpreting, 15*, 168–199. doi:10.1075/intp.15.2.02.dav

Dubslaff, F., & Martinsen, B. (2005). Exploring untrained interpreters' use of direct versus indirect speech. *Interpreting, 7*, 211–236.

Fontes, L. (2008). *Interviewing clients across cultures: A practitioner's guide*. New York, NY: Guilford.

Good, B. (1977). The heart of what's the matter: The semantics of illness in Iran. *Culture, Medicine and Psychiatry, 1*, 25–58.

Guiberson, M., & Atkins, J. (2012). Speech-language pathologists' preparation, practices, and perspectives on serving culturally and linguistically diverse children. *Communication*

Disorders Quarterly, 33, 169–180. doi:10.1177/1525740110384132

Hwa-Froelich, D., & Westby, C. (2003). A Vietnamese Head Start interpreter: A case study. *Communication Disorders Quarterly, 24*, 86–98. doi:10.1177/15257401030240020501

Isaac, K. (2002). *Speech pathology in cultural and linguistic diversity.* London, UK: Whurr.

Jackson, C. (1998). Medical interpretation: An essential clinical service for non-English-speaking immigrants. In S. Loue (Ed.), *Handbook of immigrant health* (pp. 61–79). New York, NY: Plenum Press.

Karliner, L., Jacobs, E., Chen, A., & Mutha, S. (2007). Do professional interpreters improve clinical care for patients with Limited English Proficiency? A systematic view of the literature. *Health Services Research, 42*, 727–754. doi:10.1111/j.1475-6773.2006.00629.x

Kritikos, E. (2003). SLPs' beliefs about language assessment of bilingual/bicultural individuals. *American Journal of Speech-Language Pathology, 12*, 73–91.

Langdon, H. W. (2002). *Interpreters and translators in communication disorders: A practitioner's handbook.* Eau Claire, WI: Thinking Publications.

Langdon, H. W., & Cheng, L.-R. L. (2002). *Collaborating with interpreters and translators: A guide for communication disorders professionals.* Eau Claire, WI: Thinking Publications.

Langdon, H. W., & Quintanar-Sarellana, R. (2003). Roles and responsibilities of the interpreter in interactions with SLPs, parents, and students. *Seminars in Speech and Language, 24*, 235–244. doi:10.1055/s-2003-42826

National Council on Interpreting in Health Care. (2001). *Guide to initial assessment of interpreter qualifications.* Retrieved from http://www.ncihc.org/

National Council on Interpreting in Health Care. (2004). *A national code of ethics for interpreters in health care.* Retrieved from http://www.ncihc.org/

National Council on Interpreting in Health Care. (2005). *National standards of practice for interpreters in health care.* Retrieved from http://www.ncihc.org/

National Council on Interpreting in Health Care. (2009). *Sight translation and written translation: Guidelines for healthcare interpreters.* Retrieved from http://www.ncihc.org/

Norbury, C., & Sparks, A. (2013). Difference or disorder? Cultural issues in understanding neurodevelopmental disorders. *Developmental Psychology, 49*, 45–58. doi:10.1037/a0027446

O'Bryon, E., & Rogers, M. (2010). Bilingual school psychologists' assessment practices with English language learners. *Psychology in the Schools, 47*, 1018–1034. doi:10.1002/pits.20521

Phillips, C. (2010). Using interpreters: A guide for GPs. *Australian Family Physician, 39*, 188–195.

Tribe, R., & Lane, P. (2009). Working with interpreters across language and culture in mental health. *Journal of Mental Health, 18*, 233–241. doi:10.1080/09638230701879102

Chapter 5

Three Important Steps: Briefing, Interaction, and Debriefing (BID Process)

Henriette W. Langdon

- Review the briefing, interaction, and debriefing (BID) process for interviews, conferences, assessments, and interventions while outlining the role of the speech-language pathologist (SLP) and audiologist
- Describe the role of interpreters/translators (I/Ts) during the BID process while contrasting their roles in the fields of speech-language pathology and audiology
- Define best practices in collaborating with an I/T in speech-language pathology and audiology
- Trace a path for a future certification for I/Ts collaborating with SLPs, audiologists, and educational staff (written in collaboration with guest writer Teresa Wolf)

In Chapter 4 we reviewed the roles and responsibilities of each team member, SLP, or audiologist, as well as his or her charge in preparing the I/T. A code of ethics was also proposed since the profession of an I/T working in the educational field has not been officially defined.

In this chapter, we describe the necessary steps that the SLP and audiologist as well as the I/T should follow to ensure that the process is successful. We also will outline similarities and contrasts between the role of I/T in each of the two professions, speech-language pathology and audiology, by listing some best practices for an equitable process drawn from other professions and propose some trends for the future to certify/train I/Ts to work with SLPs, audiologists, and other educational staff.

The success of the interpreting process for conferences and interviews with families and clients, assessments, or intervention is enhanced when it includes three steps: briefing, interaction, and debriefing (BID). The three-step process should provide the SLP or audiologist a plan on collaborating with the I/T to ensure success on behalf of children and their families. However, despite some outlined practices taken from other fields like interpreting for courts or medical interpreting, no research on evidence-based practices exists to support any of them.

Briefing

During the *briefing* portion or the initial step of the meeting, the SLP or audiologist and the I/T, as a team, should take time to plan the content and process for a given interview, conference, or an assessment session. Several important decisions need to be made, which are listed below.

Interviews and Conferences

- *What is the purpose of the meeting?* Specifically, is this an interview to gather information about the child, is it to plan an assessment, or is it to report results of an assessment to draft goals and recommendations? If it is an interview, what is the information to be obtained? Table 5–1 includes questions to ask regarding various areas such as background information on motor and language developmental milestones, health, and school performance. If it is an assessment, what are the goals in conducting the assessment; what are the tests, activities, and materials to be used; and what is the function of the I/T? Chapter 6 includes more specific information on this topic for audiological and speech-language assessments. Finally, if the meeting is to report results of an assessment, what are the highlights of the information to be shared; will the I/T be asked to interpret what is said by the SLP/audiologist, the parent, and participants; and/or will the I/T be asked to do a sight translation of the individual education plan (IEP) or individual family service plan (IFSP)? In the latter case, additional preparation time for the I/T will be necessary.

- *What are some helpful strategies to ensure the success of the process?*
  - The approach should be consistent with the family's cultural values and beliefs and needs to be implemented within the context of the family and community. Here the I/T may be very helpful but needs to remain objective.
  - The SLP or audiologist and the I/T should have an ongoing dialogue. It may be difficult because the I/T may be different for each case.
  - The SLP or audiologist should keep grammatical constructions simple and clear and avoid idiomatic words or professional jargon.
  - The SLP or audiologist should *define* specific professionally related terminology such as auditory comprehension, sensorineural loss, speech-language impairment, or autism by providing concrete examples that have application to the child's home and learning environments. This is not the role of the I/T **but of the SLP or audiologist**.

Table 5–1. *Interview About a Child With a Family Member*

Language used by the Interpreter:		
Name of the Interpreter:		
Date of the Interview:		
Name:	DOB:	
Age:	Grade:	
Number and age of siblings:		
Mother's occupation:	Father's occupation:	
Mother's highest level of formal education:	Father's highest level of formal education:	
Language Use and Preferences:		
Language(s):	Country of origin:	
Has the child resided in countries where other languages were spoken?		YES NO
If yes, where?	When?	How long?
Please describe the child's experiences with other languages:		
How long has the family resided in the United States?	Father: Mother:	Child:
Language(s) of interaction between child and:	Father: Mother:	Siblings:
	Other family members:	
Is there a language the child seems to favor?		
Who converses most often with the child at home?		
What is the main language used by the adults at home?		
Does the child respond in the language used by the adults?		YES NO
If not, what language does the child use?		
Language preference in listening to the radio, CDs, or TV? (Please circle)		
Home Language	English	No Preference
Language preferred for reading and writing by the child, if applicable?		
Home Language	English	No Preference

continues

Table 5–1. continued

Education:			
Did the child attend school in the country of origin or other countries? (Please circle)			
YES NO	If yes, how many years?		
How long has the child attended school in the United States?			
Has the child attended any other U.S. schools before his or her present school? (Please circle)			
YES NO	If yes, where and for how long?		
Type of educational program: (Please circle)			
Only English (which grades)?		ESL (which grades)?	
Bilingual (which grades)?		Saturday school (which grades)?	
Did the child attend preschool/Head Start? (Please circle)		YES NO	
Has the child's education been continuous or interrupted?			
If interrupted, please describe reason(s):			
Any problems at school with: (Please circle all that apply)			
Listening to the teacher		YES	NO
Remembering what is taught		YES	NO
Following directions		YES	NO
Finishing homework		YES	NO
Participating in activities		YES	NO
Learning to read		YES	NO
Understanding what he or she reads		YES	NO
Learning math		YES	NO
Writing problems		YES	NO
Behavior		YES	NO
Making friends		YES	NO
Expressing ideas clearly		YES	NO
Others understanding the child		YES	NO
Acquiring English compared to other children		YES	NO
If you marked YES for any of the items, please describe:			

Table 5-1. *continued*

Health and Developmental Information:				
Any problems with: (Please circle all that apply)				
Pregnancy		YES		NO
Birth process		YES		NO
Hearing		YES		NO
Vision		YES		NO
Allergies		YES		NO
Health		YES		NO
Hospitalizations		YES		NO
Birth weight:	Born at: (Please circle)	Home	Clinic	Hospital
If you marked YES for any of the items, please describe:				

Family's Perception of the Child's Language Performance at Home:				
Have you noticed any difficulties the child has with? (Please circle)				
Home Language	Understanding	Speaking	Reading	Writing
English	Understanding	Speaking	Reading	Writing
Describe how the child's speech and language development in the home language compares to that of the siblings or children in the community. (Please circle)				
Same	Different	Please describe if there are problems:		
Any problems at home with: (Please circle all that apply)				
Following directions		YES		NO
Understanding what others say		YES		NO
Others understanding what the child says		YES		NO
Attention		YES		NO
Behavior		YES		NO
Making friends		YES		NO
Playing with others for a while		YES		NO
Learning new concepts		YES		NO
If you marked YES for any of the items, please describe:				

continues

Table 5–1. *continued*

Do you or any family members: (Please circle all that apply)		
Tell the child stories?	YES	NO
Read stories with the child? Or look at pictures in a book?	YES	NO
Talk to each other when engaged in any activity?	YES	NO
Comment on what you both watch on TV?	YES	NO
What reading material is available to children and adults at home?		
Which language (Please circle)	Home Language	English	Both
Child's interests and favorite activities:		
Please describe the child's typical day:		
Notes:		
Name and position of the person conducting the interview:		

Source: Adapted from Langdon (2002a).

For example, say that *autism* is a label that describes a child who has significant difficulty with communication both verbally and nonverbally. Then provide some common characteristics such as lack of interaction with others, behavioral issues due to lack of comprehension of what goes on, repetition of words or statements that are unrelated to a given situation, and so on. Indicate that children can improve with specific approaches such as behavior and speech-language therapy, consistency in schedules both at home and school, and so forth.

o *Watch for indicators of translation difficulty.* Consider the importance of nonverbal communication (NV), but avoid stereotypes! Watch for

the expression of the parent to ensure that he or she appears to comprehend what is said and that communication between participants is proceeding smoothly. Both the SLP or audiologist and I/T should watch for signs of confusion or lack of communication.

• *What are some strategies* the SLP, audiologist or I/T may implement in case the parent is reluctant to respond to some of questions on the interview? For example, the parent may hesitate to answer questions related to pregnancy or may not recall some of the information requested. How can the team ensure that the parent is feeling comfortable during the interview or the conference? If it is a conference to report results and suggest recommendations, can either one of the team members anticipate that the parent may disagree with the results or recommendations, and if so, what might be done? What may be some issues that may surface in a particular case where cultural differences might come up, and how might the I/T assist in this case, as someone familiar with the culture?

- *Important information to remember:* Family members and patients may not understand the laws and regulations that guarantee their rights. Procedures for informing them and gaining their written consent may be unfamiliar or unsettling. Requesting that these individuals summarize the main points that they understand is a helpful technique to ascertain that they indeed understand the essence of their rights. The SLP or audiologist may consider interrupting the meeting occasionally and requesting that the parent summarize some of the information provided in his or her own words to ensure that the information is accurately understood.

The authors of this guide recommend that services provided by an I/T be documented in an IEP or IFSP to ensure that fair and equitable treatment has been secured. Students 18 years and older and/or family members of minor children must understand the results of assessments, recommendations, and intervention plans.

Family members often fail to question what the school team has recommended. This attitude is common in individuals who were raised in countries where the advice of professionals is accepted unconditionally. Families and clients need to have the time and opportunity to assimilate the process, to understand the assessment or intervention, and this should be respected. Naturally, there might be situations where an agreement from the family is needed immediately (e.g., when requesting permission to perform an endoscopy in case of an emergency). In that case, the SLP should communicate very clearly the reason for urgency in making such a decision.

It is not unusual for a family to bring an advocate who is bilingual to a meeting. Establishing a positive attitude from the start is key to a successful outcome. For example, the process can be facilitated if the SLP or audiologist begins the meeting by stating the role of each member and by indicating that comments from the bilingual advocate are welcome. The I/T will continue to interpret all comments from all participants. The members of the conference team should convey that they are working as a unit. Ultimately, all parties need to understand that the interview or the conference is carried out to benefit the child and that the SLP and/or audiologist is the person who is legally responsible for the outcome of the interaction.

- *Review of preferred interpretation strategies.* Depending on the experience of both the I/T and the SLP or audiologist in working together as a team, review some helpful strategies to ensure success of an interview or conference.

○ *Type and mode of interpreting necessary*. Determine if the interpreting should be consecutive or simultaneous. The method and process will depend on the number of participants and the family's level of comprehension in English. Some bilingual family members may not need interpreting services for the entire content of a given conference. Others may not need interpretation of what is said to them in English but may prefer to make their comments and questions in the other language.

○ All participating members *should introduce themselves by name and role*. The I/T should remind everyone present that his or her role is to interpret all of the information that will be shared, even if it might be negative or offensive to anyone participating in the meeting.

○ The SLP or audiologist *should direct all comments* to the parent, student, or client, but *not* to the I/T. This allows participants to feel that all messages are addressed directly to them. However, this strategy can be difficult to implement because either party may feel uncomfortable communicating to one another through another person, the interpreter. In addition, the team members must keep in mind that in some cultures, making direct eye contact is avoided as a sign

of respect. The participating professionals should be sensitive to the family's background and culture and respond accordingly. Several of these issues have been discussed in previous chapters.

○ In some instances, *family members do understand more English* than they are willing to admit, and in all cases, they should be asked if they wish to use the I/T's services. While they may understand English, they may want to make sure they understand all of the details and may feel more comfortable speaking in the language in which they are most fluent.

○ *The I/T should interpret all statements using the first person*. For example, if a parent says, "I have been concerned about my child," the I/T presents the statement as is, without saying, "Mrs. X says that . . . "

○ *One person at a time should speak*. Side conversations between participants in an interview or a conference should be avoided. The SLP or audiologist and the I/T should be sensitive to the reactions of the family members, and they need to be certain that messages are clearly conveyed. The I/T should transmit everything that is said, including all attendees' responses, comments, questions, requests for clarification, or repetitions.

○ *Seating arrangements are also important*. All participants need to place themselves so they can see each other with no obstructions.

Assessments

The first set of suggestions applies to both an audiological and a speech-language assessment, the second set is more specific to speech and language, and the last one applies more to audiological assessments:

- *Purpose of the assessment.* Discuss the reason for the assessment, the child's relevant background information (medical, developmental and educational), and his or her general areas of strength and areas of challenge. When discussing intervention methods, include the purpose of the session and the desired outcomes.
- *Procedure to follow.* Review specific assessment materials and directions as well as the order in which they will be used. Outline plans in case there might be behavior issues, difficulties with the materials presented, or a case where the content might be too easy or will not yield the information that is sought. It is not unusual to face situations where the process turns out to be different than expected, and the team needs to change strategies accordingly.
- *To facilitate the process*, the I/T should preferably have met the child prior to an assessment, if at all possible in a casual situation such as during recess or play-conversation, to establish rapport and begin to build trust. This may occur more often in an educational setting but not in a medical facility where the child may need to be seen for an emergency like in a case of trauma. In any event, the I/T should be briefed as much as possible about pertinent aspects of a child's background and should be familiar with the assessment procedures, tests, and materials.
- *The SLP or audiologist should be present during the assessment.* Regardless of preparation, the I/T should not assess or test an individual without the presence of the SLP or audiologist. Even though the I/T may be the major person interacting during the assessment process, it is vital that the SLP or audiologist be present to observe the interaction, direct the interpreter, and be available to clarify directions or the interpretation of a test item.

In case of a speech-language assessment, the team should consider the following:

- *Test items and protocols.* Both the SLP and I/T should be familiar with the test items and protocols used in the assessment (most likely in Spanish, in which there are more normed tests). Ensure that both SLP and I/T are familiar with scoring procedures, and that the I/T has ways to communicate with the SLP about what to do if unsure of the child's responses while conducting the assessment. Knowing how to administer a given test in Spanish will require additional prior training for both SLPs and I/Ts.
  - *Method of recording.* Review the protocols and how responses need to be recorded. For example, check if the answers should be marked as correct

or incorrect and transcribed verbatim.

o *Basals and ceilings.* The SLP should guide the I/T about which test items should be administered first, including how to establish a basal and when to stop administering the test items (i.e., ceiling). This area will be most relevant if Spanish tests will be used, as other tests have not been normed on bilingual subjects in the United States.

o *Gesture use.* If standardized testing is administered, discuss the appropriateness of the use of gestures or body language that might cue the child.

- *If there are no testing/assessment materials in a language,* is it necessary to design/adapt some of them in a given language? More specific information on procedures, materials, and what to do in case there are no tests in the child's target language is discussed in Chapter 6.
- *Will the I/T need to elicit a language sample* and, if so, how will it be obtained and analyzed?

Items to consider in case of an audiological assessment:

- *Is the I/T familiar with the type of tests* that will be conducted? Will this be a screening or more in-depth testing? Will it include assessment of speech-reception thresholds (SRTs), tympanograms, acoustic

brainstem response (ABR), and/or any other specific testing? What is necessary for the child to understand to provide the desired responses?

- *Technical and professional terms need to be reviewed.* For example, translation of words that may appear to be common such as *deaf* or *hard of hearing* even in one language like Spanish should be verified, as there are many ways of expressing the terms in various dialects of various languages.[1] The word *soft* may be translated in various ways in Spanish dialects like *suave, ligero, quedito,* or *bajo,* so that the I/T must be sure to use the correct term. If the word is not translated accurately to reflect a given dialect, it could be a source of confusion for the client. This comment was made during a personal interview with a practicing audiologist.[2]

During Interaction

Interaction, the next step, includes the actual time that the SLP or audiologist and the I/T work together in a conference or assessment session. The I/T should not be left alone during the interaction, even when he or she has had prior experience. The I/T should keep in mind that the SLP or audiologist is the one who is ultimately legally responsible for the process. The SLP or audiologist may want to videotape or audiotape the interaction to facilitate reviewing the child's responses to a given test or tests and the language sample.

[1]Catherine Yoshinaga-Itano, PhD-Aud (personal communication, September 7, 2014), and Sandy Bowen, PhD (personal communication, September 8, 2014).
[2]Evelyn Merritt, MA-Aud (personal communication, September 3, 2014).

It is recommended that:

- *The SLP or audiologist should address the parent or client directly*, rather than addressing the interpreter.
- *The interpreter transmits what is said by all parties as accurately* as possible. The I/T and the SLP or audiologist should work collaboratively and maintain a united team.
- *Both the SLP or audiologist and I/T* should take notes about their observations.
- *Also, the SLP or audiologist may observe important behaviors of both the I/T and the child in his or her interactive responses.* For example:

Observing the I/T:

- I/T asks questions immediately as needed
- Uses appropriate nonverbal communication
- Seems to provide clear instructions
- Provides adequate amount of reinforcement
- Asks for information from the SLP or audiologist when needed

Observing the child during the assessment:

- The child displays general behavior problems such as perseveration, short attention span, and/or distractibility
- Needs repetition and cuing, using more gestures than needed instead of words to express ideas
- Has difficulty with language skills, evidenced by excessive pauses, hesitations, response delays, reauditorization, and short answers
- Seems to benefit from strategies such as repetition, modeling, and breaking down information

During Debriefing

The I/T should not leave immediately after the conclusion of a session. The team of the SLP or audiologist and the I/T should review the different points that were discussed, evaluate the results, and plan the necessary follow-up. Sufficient time should be allocated to review the client's assessment results and be certain that the family's questions, legal rights, and recommendations are addressed adequately. Although the I/T's role is important at every step of the process, all parties should consider that the SLP or the audiologist is the professional who is ultimately responsible for the outcome of the assessment as well as for the follow-up for speech, language, hearing, and communication services.

During the *debriefing* period, the I/T and the SLP or audiologist review the outcomes of the conference or assessment session by focusing on the dynamics of the conference or the client's responses to specific testing materials, verbal interactions, or activities like play skills. Follow-up plans are also outlined during this time. Specific areas to consider during conferences and speech-language and audiological assessments follow:

For interview and conferences:

- In what ways was the interview or conference productive?
- What are the specific aspects that facilitated the interaction?
- How could the process be improved in the future?

For assessments:

- The child's responses are reviewed for accuracy.

- The language sample is reviewed and the I/T agrees to transcribe and translate the most relevant passages to analyze the child's language skills.
- Any difficulties in the process are reviewed with sharing of ideas of how to improve the process in subsequent collaborations between the SLP and the I/T.
- What type of follow-up is necessary and how will it be completed?
- Review the strategies that were used by the I/T to facilitate the process by analyzing responses to various test items. For example, the I/T may alert the SLP that the child had multiple articulation errors, possibly explain the child's hesitation about providing verbal answers, being fatigued, needing a break, and so forth, although an SLP might note this behavior as well.
- Was the communication between the SLP and audiologist during the assessment effective or was it a cause for distraction for the child, and how could it be improved the following time?

In summary, the I/T and the SLP or the audiologist should ensure that the environment supports the parent or family member, including the older student or the child, to maximize the outcome.

The written report should document that the interview, conference, and/or assessment took place in collaboration with an I/T, and the role of each team member should be described. This includes documentation of the materials used, the procedures followed in recording results, and the statement about the validity of the results obtained. A sample report can be found in Box 5–1 for a speech and language evaluation. Box 5–2 provides an audiological evaluation conducted with an I/T.

If collaboration with an I/T is necessary during intervention, a continuous dialogue should take place between the I/T and the SLP. The I/T under the direction of the SLP can assist the child in gaining specific language and communication skills in the primary language. Here is an excellent situation where the bilingual speech-language pathologist assistant (SLP/A) can play an important role in enhancing a child's speech and language skills. Subsequently, the SLP can introduce the same concepts in English once it is determined that the child is able to comprehend sufficient English to respond to intervention in that language. The SLP should be familiar with essential information about the particular language, which can be gained by consulting sources such as McLeod (2007) or Omniglot Dictionaries (http://www.omniglot.com/links/dictionaries.htm). The I/T, under the direction of the SLP, will be asked to provide the child's family-specific suggestions for activities to follow up with at home. To ensure that parents or families understand their role in helping the child at that time, an effective method is for the SLP or audiologist to ask them to explain what they understood using their own words. The parents can also participate during the intervention sessions by modeling strategies and techniques suggested by the SLP with the assistance of the bilingual SLP/A. Additionally, this individual can assist the families of children involved in early intervention programs as well as those young children who may need hearing aids and/or cochlear implants and therapy.

BOX 5–1. SPEECH AND LANGUAGE ASSESSMENT REPORT CONDUCTED WITH THE ASSISTANCE OF AN INTERPRETER

Background Information

Ali is a 2.5-year-old only child who lives with his parents. Turkish is the only language spoken in the home. Ali is exposed to approximately 1 hour of English a day when out in the community while he attends various classes. He spends the majority of his day with his mother, attends the above-mentioned classes as well as Turkish play groups, and visits various parks, museums, and zoos.

Health and Development

No problems with pregnancy or birth were reported, and all developmental milestones have proceeded normally except for speech. His mother reports that he has a vocabulary of approximately 40 words, and he uses single words for the most part, only combining two words occasionally. Mrs. P., his mother, reported that her younger brother was late in talking (3 years), but once he began saying words, his speech developed very rapidly.

Ali has been a healthy child—his hearing was assessed 5 months ago. A full evaluation was not completed because Ali became upset in the sound booth; however, he passed the hearing screening at 25 dB. Hearing is not a concern at this time, and Ali is scheduled for another audiological assessment in the next 3 weeks.

Assessment Procedure

Ali's language skills were assessed through observation of his play skills, prelinguistic behaviors, and an inventory of his English and Turkish vocal productions and sounds. The assessment was conducted in both English and Turkish by an English and bilingual English/Turkish-speaking graduate student (GE) who served as an interpreter (I/T). The I/T was briefed prior to the assessment about Ali's background, and no further questions of the parents were needed at that time; therefore, GE met with the parent prior to the assessment to introduce herself and check if the information that had been collected was correct.

Ms. A.B., the SLP, interacted with Ali by engaging him in various activities such as playing with various toys, completing some puzzles, stringing beads, and playing with blocks. The role of the I/T was to record any utterances that may have been approximation of words in Turkish or real words. In those cases, the I/T was instructed to either ask Ali to repeat the correct word and/or expand it to determine if he would respond in Turkish. When Ms. A.B.'s main interaction with Ali was completed, GE took on the role of Ms. A.B. and played with Ali using the same or other toys and communicated with him in only Turkish.

Once the assessment was completed, Ms. A.B. and GE discussed their observations and shared some highlights with the parent. Because the parent was bilingual, GE's role was to listen and clarify anything Ms. A.B. said, which might have not been clear to the parent. Prior to the conference, GE explained her role. After the parent left, GE and Ms. A.B. decided on how they would coordinate their efforts in having GE provide a transcribed sample of Ali's utterances. GE was requested to read the final report and make any comments if needed.

Utterances spontaneously produced during assessment

English Words	Turkish Words
Fish	Baba /bɑbɑ/* (father or big)
Hep (help)	Aç /atʃ/ [atʃ] "open (it)" (imperative)
No	Araba /ɑɾɑbɑ/ [a:ba] "car"
uh-oh	Ne "what"
oh-no	Bol "ball"
Bye	Saç /satʃ/ [saʃ] "hair"
boom	/ [bu] "this"
/bʌbʌ/(bubble)	[bul] "find"
	"dadada" the firetruck noise
	Anne /anne/ "mother"

English Sounds

Sound	Initial	Medial	Final
Developmentally appropriate sounds			
/p/		Apple	Help
/b/	/ba/ (boat) Boom	/bʌbʌ/ (bubbles)	
/d/	/dʌdʌdʌ/ (fire truck noise in Turkish) "Dis" (this) "Dem" (them)	/dʌdʌdʌ/ (fire truck noise in Turkish)	
/h/	Help	Oh-no	
/m/	Moo		Boom

Sound	Initial	Medial	Final
/n/	No	Oh no!	
Other sounds			
/ɫ/		Help	Apple
/f/	Fish		
/ʃ/ as in "sh"	"Shhhh" (boat making noise)		Fish
Vowels			
/ae/ as in "hat"	Ahhhhh (cars crashing) apple		
/oʊ/ as in "go"			Uh-oh Oh-no
/ɪ/ as in it "hit"		Fish	
/u/ as in "blue"			Moo
/aʊ/ as in "now"			Now
/aɪ/ as in "bye"			Bye

Turkish Sounds

Sound	Initial	Medial	Final
/b/	Baba "father"	"A:ba" /araba/ "car"	
/d/		/dadada/ (Fire engine noise)	
/n/	Ne "what"	Anne "mother"	
/m/		Ama "but"	
/s/	Saç "hair"		
/t͡ʃ/			Aç "open"
/l/			Bul "find!"
/p/		Öpül "to be kissed"	
/Ö/	Öpül "to be kissed"		
/a/		Baba "father"	Baba "father"
/h/	Hop (intended: help)		

Ali was shy at first and did not greet the adults. However, he smiled and voluntarily accompanied them to the assessment room. He demonstrated appropriate turn-taking and proxemics throughout the assessment. His frequency of eye contact was informally observed to be slightly less than age-matched peers. However, it could be due to his shyness and being in a new environment.

Ali pointed and gestured to express himself throughout the assessment. He made sound effects for boats, crashing cars, and cars in distress. He demonstrated appropriate intonation to express distress and excitement.

Ali's fine and gross motor skills appear to be within normal limits for his age. He was coordinated and skillful in using his body to stand, squat, sit in a chair, and knock over blocks. He had no difficulty with fine motor tasks such as stacking blocks, picking up small objects, opening a box of crayons, placing puzzle pieces in their place, or scribbling on paper.

A formal oral motor exam was not conducted at this time. Additionally, he became upset near the end of the assessment and appeared unlikely to respond well to such a procedure. The following observations of Ali's oral motor skills were made during the assessment: (a) no difficulty chewing, swallowing, or drinking liquids, and no excess saliva and (b) inability to purse lips in order to blow bubbles or pretend to blow out a candle. Ali's attempt to purse lips appeared more like lip smacking. However, he was willing to attempt to imitate the movement.

Ali was interested in books and independently brought them to Ms. A.B. and GE to read. He looked and pointed at the pictures and labeled one picture ("fish"). When putting the book away, he laid it down horizontally, looked at it, realized it was the wrong orientation, and corrected it. He showed interest in crayons and independently pulled crayons from a box and began scribbling on a piece of paper.

Discussion

Language Comprehension

Ali's mother reported he understands everything she says and follows directions. During the assessment, Ali followed simple directions in English when paired with a gesture. For example, he responded to "give me the apple" with an outstretched hand. At this time, language comprehension is not a concern. However, it should be monitored over time for difficulties.

Language Expression

Ali demonstrated communicative intent and used language and gestures to communicate a variety of concepts such as sharing excitement, enacting a scenario, identifying a picture in a book, and asking for help. Ali produces all the speech sounds appropriate for his age in each language. However, he has a significantly limited vocabulary in both English and Turkish. A child Ali's age should have 200 to 300 words and be forming simple sentences. Ali has approximately 100 or fewer words between English and Turkish and rarely combines words in either language. However, his mother reports he said his first sentence the day before the assessment: "Bye bye, fish." Additionally, he produced three two-word combinations during the assessment.

Nevertheless, Ali demonstrates the foundational skills necessary for speaking. That is, he has communicative intent, symbolic play, pretend play, appropriate use of gestures, vocal inflection, and age-appropriate speech sounds. However, he rarely imitates new words and frequently disengages from interacting if an imitation or vocalization is requested of him.

Summary and Recommendations

At this time, there is no apparent cause for Ali's limited vocabulary and hesitancy to imitate new words and sounds. However, speech and language therapy is warranted, considering Ali is significantly behind his peers with regard to vocabulary and the complexity of his utterances. His speech and language delay is not due to bilingualism. There is no support in research that states that bilingual children are behind in general speech or language development compared to their monolingual peers.

Ali presents with a moderate expressive language delay, characterized by limited vocabulary and a hesitancy to imitate new words. However, he has age-appropriate speech sounds, communicative intent, and foundational language skills. Due to the significant delay in expressive language in both Turkish and English, speech-language therapy is warranted. Prognosis for improvement is excellent given his current desire to communicate, the progress he has made over the past months, and his supportive family.

Ideally, speech and language therapy should be conducted in Turkish, which is his primary language at home. However, this is impossible, as there are no available trained SLPs in Turkish. It is recommended, therefore, that therapy be conducted in English with suggestions for the parents on follow-up activities in Turkish when together. In this case, these suggestions seem feasible. If the parents were not bilingual, the intervention of a bilingual I/T would be necessary to interpret the purpose of the sessions and what the parents could do at home to help Ali.

BOX 5–2. AUDIOLOGICAL ASSESSMENT REPORT CONDUCTED WITH THE ASSISTANCE OF AN INTERPRETER

Team members: Parent, audiologist, and I/T

Samantha is a 5-year-old girl who has been exposed to both Vietnamese and English. Samantha received a full audiological evaluation and, for the first time, was identified as having a moderate sensorineural hearing loss. Dr. McC assessed her with the assistance of Ms. J.W., a trained Vietnamese interpreter/translator (I/T). The main role of the I/T was to assist in gathering background information about Samantha's health and educational history and to accurately translate the audiological findings and recommendations. A secondary role was to translate instructions for the behavioral audiological tests to Samantha.

The initial interview indicated that the family has lived in the United States for only 2 years. Samantha was born in a small village in South Vietnam. She contracted rubella when she was 18 months old and, from that episode on, her parents noted that she lost a great deal of hearing, and her language development in Vietnamese (which had been proceeding normally) regressed significantly. Due to lack of resources in the village where the family lived, Samantha was unable to be assessed or fitted with hearing aids. It has taken the family 2 years to settle in the United States, and this is the first opportunity they have had to see an audiologist.

Since Samantha is 5 years old, she was given instructions both in English (by the audiologist) and Vietnamese (the I/T) to raise her hand when she heard "beeps" in the headphones. Samantha was shy and did not seem comfortable raising her hand, so the audiologist decided to use play audiometry to obtain pure-tone thresholds. In order to do so, Samantha was reinstructed in English (audiologist) and Vietnamese (I/T) to throw a block in a bucket whenever she heard a tone. Since the audiologist demonstrated this first, Samantha easily participated in the play audiometry paradigm, and pure-tone thresholds were obtained. They revealed a mild-to-moderate sensorineural hearing loss bilaterally. Speech recognition thresholds also were obtained since Samantha was able to point to pictures of common words in English (i.e., airplane, hotdog, rainbow). Normally, children who are 5 years old are able to repeat the PB-K words, but Samantha was not familiar with the vocabulary in English. Since no recorded and standardized Vietnamese word lists were available, word recognition scores could not obtained at the initial assessment.

Hearing aids have just been fitted. With the assistance of Mrs. J.W., Dr. McC explained to the parents how to take care of the hearing aids. Samantha is supposed to wear her hearing aids at the volume 4 level as specified in the audiological report. The parent should check that the hearing aid is in running order and ensure there is no background noise such as crackling sounds or circuit noise. If there is no sound, it might be necessary to replace the battery. It is also important to check for cracks in the hearing aid case, ear mold, and tubing and ensure there is no buildup of wax or moisture and clean any that is found.

Dr. McC made arrangements to suggest some special accommodations in the classroom such as preferential seating, an auditory trainer, and better classroom acoustics. These accommodations need to be followed up by the district educational audiologist who happens to be bilingual in Vietnamese, so Dr. McC explained to the parents why the use of an FM system in the classroom, in conjunction with personal hearing aids, is imperative for Samantha. Fortunately, the district educational audiologist happened to be bilingual in Vietnamese, so she was able to follow through both on obtaining the technology and keeping the parents informed as to its benefits.

Note. The author appreciates the input offered by Dr. McCullough in composing this audiological report.

DEFINING BEST PRACTICES IN COLLABORATING WITH AN I/T IN SPEECH-LANGUAGE PATHOLOGY AND AUDIOLOGY

For the past 30 years, the American Speech-Language-Hearing Association (ASHA) has made recommendations as to the need to collaborate with I/Ts when the SLP or audiologist does not speak the same language as the child or client (refer to Chapter 1, page 9) (ASHA, 1985). To date, there has been scant research on this process, and understandably, there is still a lack of consensus on what might be best practices. A summary of current research on this topic is provided here. The areas considered include the role of the I/T, the training of the I/T and SLP or the audiologist, the carrying out of the BID process itself, and the assessment of speech and language disorders in bilingual students with the assistance of an I/T.

Role of the I/T, Training, Preparation, and Adherence to the BID Process

Most of the research has documented the training of SLPs but not the I/T, with two exceptions (Langdon, 2002b; Sánchez-Boyce, 2001). Even though her sample was very small (only three interpreters answered a questionnaire) (Langdon, 2002b), the I/Ts who completed a questionnaire felt that best practices were followed when their role was more as that of acting as a filter (could clarify), and clarification was sought in instances where the information was not easily understood. However, at times, the process of debriefing was omitted because the team of the SLP and I/T had worked together for a while and the SLP trusted the I/T could "work on their own."

Sánchez-Boyce (2001) observed dyads of psychologists or SLPs and paraprofessionals who acted as I/Ts during assessments. The researcher found that the role of the I/T was not always that of someone who remained "neutral" in the process. Instead, at times, in addition to conveying the meaning of an interaction, the I/T's role was more that of a "cultural broker," while in others, it was more like a "liaison" in the interaction. In many ways, the I/T was not only someone who interpreted but also someone who took on various roles as described in Chapter 4, namely, message clarifier, cultural clarifier and patient advocate. In addition, the role of the I/T may not always be understood by all personnel who are involved in the assessment of English-language learner (ELL) students, even within the same working environment. Hwa-Froelich and Westby (2003) found that even within one building, school personnel might have different expectations of the I/T.

Langdon (2002b) conducted a follow-up survey by 63 SLPs practicing in the schools in California who had from 1 to 35 years of experience. The SLP participants were divided into six groups. Those who had the fewest years of experience were those who had received the most academic training in collaborating with interpreters and translators (85.5%) compared to only 50% for those who had 25 to 35 years of experience. Hammer, Detwiler, Detwiler, Blood, and Qualls (2004) and Kritikos (2003) in their surveys reported that a very small percentage of SLPs had received specific training in collaborating with an I/T in assessing ELL students.

In her recent dissertation, which documents practices followed by 175 SLPs in a large mid-Atlantic district in regards to bilingual assessments conducted with the assistance of an I/T, Palfrey (2013) reported that, despite SLPs having received training in collaborating with I/Ts, the BID process could not always be followed. Therefore, the I/T was not always sure about what areas needed to be addressed during the assessment. Discrepancies in how and to what degree the SLP prepared the I/T for an assessment were also reported (Palfrey, 2013). Specifically, SLPs were not always present during the interaction session, and approximately only half of those surveyed shared background information with the I/T prior to an assessment. Only a small proportion, or 22%, shared protocols used for assessment ahead of time.

Lack of Consensus Regarding When and How to Assess an ELL Student With the Assistance of an I/T

Caesar and Koehler (2007) found that SLPs did not use services of an I/T consistently. It often seemed unclear how the results of assessments with the assistance of an I/T were interpreted to determine if a student had a true speech/language disorder. Palfrey (2013) found a variety of results regarding when and what materials were used in assessing ELL students with the collaboration of an I/T. For example, some participants felt that assessing the student in the other language was not necessary if the student appeared English dominant (or stronger in English), while others did not feel that results obtained with the assistance of an I/T were valuable, or that there was insufficient time to assess the student in the other language due to schedule constraints. Overall, respondents indicated they gathered information from teachers and families, observed the student in a couple of settings when possible, used informal assessments as well as dynamic assessment, and about 33% assessed students in both languages. Selected assessment materials that were used frequently included a language sample, the Peabody Picture Vocabulary Test 4 (PPVT-4; Dunn & Dunn, 2007), Preschool Language Scales 4 and 5 (Zimmermann, Steiner, & Pond, 2011; Zimmermann, Steiner, & Pond, 2012), and the Comprehensive Assessment of Spoken Language (CASL; Carrow, 1999). For details, the reader is referred to Palfrey's (2013) dissertation.

Most of the SLPs in the study performed their assessments using English tests, but several did administer the same test with the assistance of an I/T in the student's language (which required translation/adaptation). Interestingly, only one third of the SLPs had confidence in the comments and opinions made by the I/Ts they worked with. The researcher did not provide a reason for this impression, but it is likely due to the SLPs' lack of training and experience in collaborating with interpreters. Furthermore, the SLPs often thought that the job of the I/T was to interpret and not "assist." The majority of SLPs administered tests in English and requested assistance from the I/T to readminister the items the student failed using his or her target language.

The State of Affairs in the Field of Audiology

Thus far, the authors have not been able to locate research that focuses on the practices followed in audiology specifically.

Personal communication with five different audiologists and/or specialists with the deaf and hard of hearing who work in various settings that include university research, private practice, and school settings confirms this statement.[3] There was a consensus among the professionals interviewed that this is a global concern with our growing multilingual populations in all corners of the world. All agreed that a concerted effort needs to be made to join efforts to share new information and knowledge (please see below).[4]

SUMMARY

Even though parameters to conduct a bilingual assessment have been outlined in the literature (Goldstein, 2000; Gutiérrez-Clellen & Peña, 2001; Kohnert, 2013; Laing & Kamhi, 2003; Langdon & Cheng, 2002), collaborating with an I/T remains a very challenging task. The results of a comprehensive study conducted recently by Palfrey (2013) indicate that some preferred practices are followed while others are not. Specifically, gathering information from teachers and families, obtaining and analyzing a language sample, assessing in both languages when appropriate, and conducting a combination of formal and informal measures is commonly used. However, the observation of a child in more than one setting or using dynamic assessment is not always

---

[3]This author thanks the following individuals who graciously shared their time to share their viewpoints on this topic with her: Sandy Bowen (PhD), Susan Clark (MA-Aud), June McCullough (PhD-Aud), Evelyn Merritt (MA-Aud), and Christine Yoshinaga-Itano (PhD-Aud).

[4]Dr. Yoshinaga-Itano reported that she is trying to create a website with information on various lists in various languages that may be taped and modified according to a given dialect in the language through technologic modifications and thus disseminated worldwide (personal communication, September 7, 2014).

followed uniformly. In addition, many clinicians continue to rely heavily on formal measures that have been normed on English-speaking subjects and have been informally translated into the student's home language. Additionally, some SLPs decide it is unnecessary to assess the student in the home language because the student is considered English dominant or was transferred to an English-only teaching setting from one where English was taught using specialized second-language techniques. Another important finding was the lack of SLPs' complete confidence in the I/T's role and capability of assisting them in the assessment and interpretation of the results and the observations made during testing. Finally, the recommended practices in adequately preparing the I/T for the interpretation process were not followed appropriately.

In addition, conversation with various professionals around the country confirms that research on practices followed by audiologists collaborating with I/Ts is not readily available. Research on best practices in collaborating with language interpreters and translators in the field of audiology is practically nonexistent and deserves further attention.

RECOMMENDATIONS (WITH TERESA WOLF)

Even though the field of interpreting and translating has existed for a long time, hopefully, further research on best practices will be conducted in the context of the collaboration that takes place between the I/T and the SLP or audiologist. Therefore, SLPs and audiologists in all settings are encouraged to pursue research in these areas. Some recommendations for

further study include even more urgency in the field of audiology. If we do not have accurate data on children's hearing, we cannot prescribe the correct hearing aid, and this should also be a concern for ear, nose, and throat (ENT) physicians who consult with our growing linguistically and culturally diverse populations not only in the United States but throughout the entire world.

1. Continue conducting similar surveys to the one designed by Palfrey (2013) to explore the current status of the I/T as well as SLPs' and audiologists' perceptions of their role in interviews and conferences. Begin the survey in 10 states that have the highest numbers of culturally and linguistically diverse (CLD) populations. Collect information regarding communication disorders professionals' number of experiences working with interpreters, types of interactions (e.g., conferences, therapy, or assessments), and knowledge base in the field of working with interpreters, and languages used. Design separate questionnaires for SLPs, audiologists, and I/Ts. Observe a few of the interactions between SLPs, audiologists, and I/Ts after completion of their questionnaires to compare and contrast your findings.

2. Collect data on specific practices currently in use and document helpful strategies. Determine how many SLPs and audiologists are familiar with the BID process and how many follow this practice, with a specific focus on *assessment*. Determine what the SLPs' and audiologists' as well as I/Ts' roles are in the three steps. In addition, determine the indicators of a good and a poor performance by an

interpreter in the eyes of an SLP and audiologist.

3. Survey I/Ts in the fields of speech-language pathology and audiology. Ask them to describe their training, daily practice, and the working conditions they need to successfully fulfill their professional duties. How is it different than working with other allied health professionals?

4. Survey clients who have received services from an I/T. Use questionnaires (such as Box 7–4) to determine their effectiveness in the opinion of family members.

5. Identify specific strategies for working with interpreters in different settings (e.g., schools, clinics, hospitals, and agencies) and the training needed. Compare how the BID process is carried out in different settings, and determine if the process differs according to the age of the client or type of communication disorder. Develop guidelines that may be used in each area.

6. Research the differences in effective assessment between standardized tests and dynamic assessment for the CLD population. Share results with state and school organizations, which set guidelines for interfacing with I/Ts.

7. Compare and contrast practices used in other fields of interpreting to refine best practices in working with SLPs and audiologists. Conduct a large-scale survey to define how the BID process is implemented by various disciplines represented in a school setting. For example, what specific skills are needed by an interpreter working with a psychologist compared with a special education teacher? An SLP or an educational audiologist?

8. Work with interpreters' organizations (e.g., International Medical Interpreters Association [IMIA], Tennessee Association of Medical Interpreters and Translators [TAMIT]) to create specialized preparation programs for working with communication disorders professionals that will enable interpreters to be certified and recognized for the work they do. Implement professional development programs, as suggested throughout this entire guide, to provide SLPs, audiologists, and I/Ts a common framework of currently known best practices. Work with organizers of interpreter training courses to offer training in working with communication disorders professionals as part of the course. (Even medical interpreters need to be educated about specific terminology and procedures used in each of our fields, speech-language pathology and audiology.)

9. Offer professional development opportunities to I/Ts and SLPs or audiologists working with them. Discuss and expand a given topic according to the needs of specific groups. For example, some I/Ts may need more practice in administering specific tests and tasks, and some SLPs/audiologists may need more practice in watching the I/T assess a client or in training an I/T to help collect a language sample.

10. Create a bank of tasks in various languages that could be used by teams that are assessing a client in a given language. For example, make videos demonstrating the use of curriculum-based assessments for different age and grade levels to assess specific skills, such as general knowledge and the ability to follow directions,

comprehend paragraphs of different lengths and complexities, make verbal associations, and read various types of paragraphs in the given language.

11. An ultimate goal should be to create a training program such as the one suggested in Chapter 7, which will enable the I/T working in the school setting with either an SLP or audiologist to receive a state/national certificate that will enable him or her to be recognized as a professional, just as the I/T who works with the deaf, in international conferences, and in court and medical interpreting.

DISCUSSION ITEMS AND ACTIVITIES

1. Based on the information provided in the chapter regarding the BID process, get into teams of five persons and role-play a conference where you will need to interview a parent regarding the background of her child. One person will act as the SLP or audiologist, the other will be the parent who will share the same L1 as the I/T, and two persons will be the observers. Review the content of Table 5–1. As a team, decide the age of the child and, depending on L2, the place of origin as well as experiences and formal education, if applicable. At the conclusion of this activity, debrief about the process. What was easy and what was difficult? What might you do differently next time?

2. A similar activity may be rehearsed in the cases illustrated in Box 5–1 and Box 5–2. In this activity as the previous one, once it is completed, debrief

about the process. What was easy and what was difficult. What might you do differently next time?

REFERENCES

American Speech-Language-Hearing Association. (1985). *Clinical management of communicatively handicapped minority populations. ASHA, 7*(6), 29–32.

Caesar, L. G., & Kohler, P. D. (2007). The state of school-based bilingual assessment: Actual practice versus recommended guidelines. *Language, Speech, and Hearing Services in Schools, 38,* 190–200.

Carrow, E. (1999). *Comprehensive Assessment of Spoken Language (CASL).* Austin, TX: Western Psychological Publishers.

Dunn, L. M., & Dunn, D. M. (2007). *Peabody Picture Vocabulary Test* (4th ed.). Bloomington, MN: Pearson.

Goldstein, B. (2000). *Cultural and linguistic diversity resource guide for speech-language pathologists.* San Diego, CA: Singular/Thomson Learning.

Gutiérrez-Clellen, V. F., & Peña, E. (2001). Dynamic assessment of diverse children: A tutorial. *Language, Speech, and Hearing Services in Schools, 32,* 212–224.

Hammer, C. S., Detwiler, J. S., Detwiler, J., Blood, G. W. & Qualls, D. (2004). Speech-language pathologists' training and confidence in serving Spanish-English bilingual children. *Journal of Communication Disorders, 37,* 91–108.

Hwa-Froelich, D., & Westby, C. (2003). A Vietnamese Head Start interpreter: A case study. *Communication Disorders Quarterly, 24,* 86–98.

Kohnert, K. (2013). *Language disorders in bilingual children and adults* (2nd ed.). San Diego, CA: Plural.

Kritikos, E. P. (2003). Speech-language pathologists' beliefs about language assessment of bilingual/bicultural individuals. *American Journal of Speech Pathology, 12,* 12–91.

Laing, S. P., & Kamhi, A. (2003). Alternative assessment of language and literacy in culturally diverse populations. *Language, Speech and Hearing Services in Schools, 34,* 44–55.

Langdon, H. W. (2002a). *Interpreters and translators in communication disorders: A practi-*

tioner's handbook. Eau Claire, WI: Thinking Publications.

Langdon, H. W. (2002b). Communicating effectively with a client during a speech-language pathologist/interpreter conference: Results of a survey. *Contemporary Issues in Communication Science and Disorders, 29,* 17–34.

Langdon, H. W., & Cheng, L.-R. L. (2002). *Collaborating with interpreters and translators: A guide for communication disorders professionals.* Eau Claire, WI: Thinking Publications.

McLeod, S. (2007). *The international guide to speech acquisition.* Clifton, NY: Cengage Omniglot Dictionaries. Retrieved July 10, 2014, from http://www.omniglot.com/links/dictionaries.htm

Palfrey, C. L. (2013). *The use of interpreters by speech-language pathologists conducting bilingual speech-language assessments* (Doctoral dissertation). Washington, DC: Georgetown University.

Sánchez-Boyce, M. L. (2001). *A bridge over troubled waters: The use of Spanish-speaking interpreters during special education assessment* (Doctoral dissertation). Davis: University of California, Davis.

Zimmermann, I. L., Steiner, B. S., & Pond, M. A. (2011). *Preschool language scales* (English) (5th ed.). Bloomington, MN: Pearson.

Zimmermann, I. L., Steiner, B. S., & Pond, M. A. (2012). *Preschool language scales* (Spanish) (5th ed.). Bloomington, MN: Pearson.

Chapter 6

Assessing Bilingual/Culturally and Linguistically Diverse Children[1]

Henriette W. Langdon

In this chapter, we describe both challenges and solutions in conducting and evaluating a speech and language or audiological assessment for culturally and linguistically diverse children (CLD) up to age 21 with the assistance of an interpreter/translator (I/T).

Both speech-language pathologists (SLPs) and audiologists must feel confident in relying on the I/T to take some additional responsibilities during assessment in addition to playing the role of a bridge between the SLP or audiologist and the client and his or her parent(s). Specifically, the I/T may be requested to administer some tests in the target language of the child and/or administer a language sample. In case of an audiological assessment, the I/T may be in charge of ensuring that the child understands the directions of a given test and/or judges the child's responses for certain tests such as the speech reception threshold (SRT) in some languages where it is available. Recommendations to conduct a more seamless process will be based on current knowledge of best practices in assessing bilingual children, including this author's own experience in carrying out bilingual assessments herself. However, as indicated in Chapter 5, evidence-based practices in collaborating with an interpreter in any given situation like assessments during either a speech-language or audiological assessment have yet to be documented, tested, and validated.

The first section of the chapter discusses issues that pertain to speech-language as well as audiological assessments, the second section is more specific to speech and language, while the third section is more pertinent to audiological assessments. The following topics are reviewed:

- When should the services of a trained I/T be requested?

---

[1]In this chapter as others, *child* is used interchangeably with *student* and *client*. The terms *bilingual* or *culturally and linguistically diverse children* (CLD), are used interchangeably as well.

- Why should two languages be evaluated?
- Review of tests in languages other than English
- Preassessment considerations
- RIOT—a suggested procedure for assessment
- What to do when tests are available in the first language
- What to do when tests are not available in the first language

ASSESSMENT ISSUES THAT ARE PERTINENT TO SLPS, AUDIOLOGISTS, AND I/TS

When Should the Services of a Trained I/T Be Requested?

An I/T should assist in an assessment when the SLP or the audiologist does not share the same language as the child and/or the family and when the professional is not sufficiently proficient in the child or family's preferred language of communication. Specifically, the services of a trained I/T are necessary when the professional's proficiency in the target language does not meet the criteria set by the American Speech-Language-Hearing Association (ASHA, 1988) for self-nomination as a bilingual SLP or audiologist. For example, an SLP might speak sufficient Spanish to administer some of the subtests of a normed test in Spanish such as the Clinical Evaluation of Language Fundamentals–Preschool (CELF Preschool-2) Spanish Version (Wiig, Secord, & Semel, 2009) but may not be sufficiently proficient to collect and transcribe a language sample because the child's speech is very

difficult to understand due to multiple phonological errors.

An audiologist might be able to speak sufficient Spanish or a language other than English to provide the necessary directions for a child to complete play audiometry and to communicate with a family using the target language to report the results of an audiological evaluation where hearing is normal. However, he or she might face a challenge when needing to convey that a child has a conductive hearing loss or another problem where further elaboration and counseling are necessary. Furthermore, even when the diagnosis yields normal results, a family may have further questions or comments that the audiologist may understand but may have difficulty formulating in clear and concise language for the parents to easily comprehend. Alternatively, there may be cases where obtaining more comprehensive background information or providing more specific recommendations to the parents is necessary. For example, situations when services from an I/T might be needed include counseling the parent about follow-up recommendations, such as in the fitting of a hearing aid, the referral for a consultation with an ear, nose, and throat (ENT) specialist regarding cochlear implantation and/or accommodations to follow at home and in the learning environment. Specifically, a more comprehensive understanding of a client's daily activities enables the audiologist to prescribe a more accurate hearing device if needed.

When and Why Assess the Child's Target Language?

It is recommended that the SLP or audiologist collaborate with a trained I/T to assess the child's target language[2] whenever one of the following three main situations arises. The first one is when a child's proficiency in English is still developing and when more difficulties in acquiring English than expected are observed. Additionally, the parents may report the child's first language has or is developing more slowly compared to siblings and/or other children in the same community. The second instance is when the child responds in the home language when spoken to by the family or caregivers, and the child seems to understand peers who speak the same language while interacting informally in the classroom or playground. The third instance is when the child has been enrolled in a bilingual program at school or attends Saturday school where the other language is used.

The idea of *language dominance* needs to be reconsidered as well when determining if the child's language reflects a possible disorder. The fact that a child is more dominant in English compared to the target language does not indicate that a basic language disorder may be ruled out. Kohnert (2013) reports that bilingual children may perform differently in each language depending on the task considered as well as their age. Therefore, asking which language is dominant is not a helpful question; as Peña, Bedore, and Zlatic-Giunta (2002) comment, bilingualism should be considered "cumulative" rather than "comparative." Furthermore,

> ... different ways of combining test scores across languages were tested, combining scores in a composite or selecting combinations of better task

or language performance to use as a basis of decision-making.... classification can be more accurate when scores in both languages are combined and languages are used systematically for decision-making. (Peña & Bedore, 2010, p. 21)

These conclusions were reached by the researchers based on a sample of 2,500 children using results from various tests that assessed semantics and morphosyntax. The results indicated that the best way to differentiate children who had a true language disorder (Spanish-English) was to combine results based on the performance in both languages. If scores were evaluated separately in each language and even in the "dominant" language, the accuracy of identification of children with a true language disorder was lessened. Similar findings are reported in discussing the profile of 18 bilingual Spanish-English speaking children aged 6 to 10 years old (Kohnert, 2013). The researcher found that younger children who had been identified as having a language disorder performed better in Spanish on various tasks such as the Clinical Evaluation of Language Fundamentals–Preschool Edition (CELF-Preschool 2–Spanish) (Wiig et al., 2009), as well as other measures, including a language sample, whereas older students performed better in English. Therefore, it is necessary to test each of the two languages in addition to keeping in mind the type of task considered, the conditions of testing, and the examiner's linguistic skills in Spanish or the language in which the assessment is taking place. Other factors such as speed and accuracy, attention,

---

[2]The target language is L1—often referred to as first, primary, or home language or even dominant language.

working memory, alertness, social interactions, motivation, and play skills that are not captured by test measures should be accounted for as well. Additional information from observation in other environments, as well as reports from parents and teachers and progress over time assuming optimal teaching accommodations documented by response to intervention (RTI), is helpful in interpreting results from testing.

Reference to the *dual iceberg analogy* proposed by Cummins (1981, 1984) (Figure 6–1) may assist in understanding that each of two languages includes some components that are more apparent than others, with some that are common and others that are different for both.

As Cummins (1981, 1984) stated so many years ago, there is an underlying proficiency between two languages, which he refers to as Common Underlying Proficiency (CUP) or Central Operating System, and two visible portions of the icebergs, or surface features, that are specific to each language and are referred to Separate Underlying Proficiency (SUP). However, because dominance and proficiency in each language are continually shifting depending on the type of language task considered as well as exposure and experiences in each of the student's languages, there are never "two identical icebergs." Langdon (2011) proposed that we consider specific elements as being part of the SUP and CUP, and this is illustrated in Figure 6–1. She suggested that six elements be included in the area of SUP and three core elements in the area of CUP. Some of the elements were selected in reviewing Howard, Sugarman, Perdomo, and Adger (2005). The six elements in SUP would include (a) specific features for each language component (syntax,

grammar, phonology, morphology); (b) awareness of two languages (early skill); (c) specific personal experiences, including emotions that are attached to each language; (d) orthographic features and print; (e) cultural aspects, story structure, and rhetoric devices; and (f) experiences with each language. These areas represent universals in language and cognition. The CUP area would consist of three core components, oral language, written and thinking skills, and foundational components. These areas are common areas because each language has some form of language structure, sound system, and vocabulary made up of nouns, verbs, descriptors, word order, and pragmatics. Therefore, *the core oral language components*, elements such as language structure, sound system, words, descriptors, adjectives, concepts, pragmatics, gestures, and metalinguistic awareness, would be included. The alphabetic principle, orthographic awareness and rules, meaningfulness of print, habits and attitudes about reading and writing, higher level thinking and metacognition, and content knowledge would be part of the *core written and thinking skills component* areas. The *foundational components* would integrate general perceptions, attention, memory (short, long, working), and motivation. Taking into account elements that are part of the common and separate language proficiencies may provide the assessor with a clearer picture of the bilingual individual's overall language competence and performance. Without considering the other languages of a bi- or multilingual individual is like "assessing only one ear during an audiological evaluation, or evaluating only one eye during a vision examination" (Author).

In a recent review article, Shi (2014) discusses the importance of assessing the

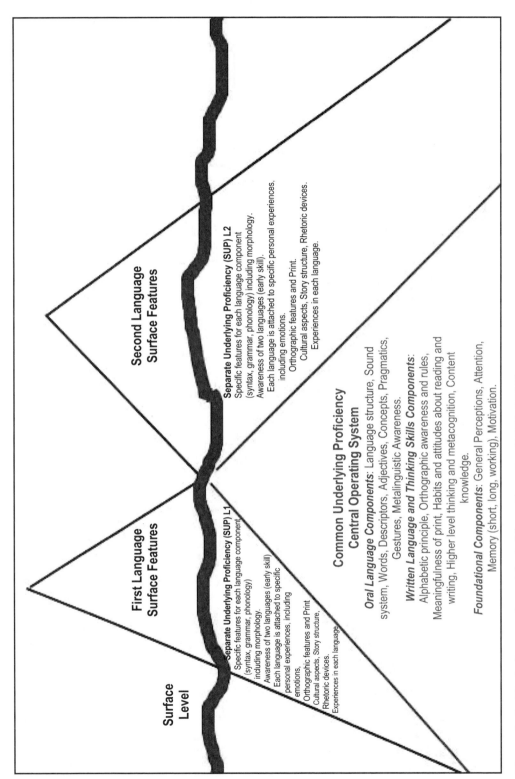

Figure 6–1. The iceberg analogy. Adapted from Cummins (1981, 1984).

speech discrimination abilities of bilingual individuals (primarily Spanish-English) in both of their languages even if these individuals appear to be dominant in English. Shi (2014) provides an up-to-date literature review on various studies that address factors influencing these individuals' performance on audiometric tests, namely, type of bilinguals (simultaneous vs. sequential at various ages), the particular dialect spoken, and conditions (quiet vs. noise). The importance of considering each bilingual's language history and daily use of each language when assessing the hearing status of the particular individual is emphasized. Even though discussion on best practices to assess young children or adolescents is not specifically addressed, it is likely that the same issues discussed in relation to speech and language assessments appear to be pertinent.

In addition, it is important to keep in mind that language loss or differences in experiences with each language might interfere with a smoother pace and proficiency in acquiring English. For example, the child might be more proficient in retelling a story in English and answering questions because of greater experience in performing tasks such as these in the school setting, or reading and writing skills in English could be stronger compared to the home language due to lack of explicit instruction in the written modality (Langdon, 2008). This is the reason it is advised to take a careful history of each language as discussed in Chapter 5.

Review of Testing Materials in Languages Other Than English

For decades, SLPs and audiologists have been struggling to find appropriate procedures to provide fair and appropriate assessments of CLD populations. Interpretation and translation are integral components of such clinical encounters. Vocabulary knowledge and the ability to understand and use linguistic concepts have been the basis of many language assessments, and these are highly dependent on accurate interpreting and translating.

Researchers and scholars in speech-language pathology and psychology have written about some of the limitations and pitfalls of translations of tests. However, many clinicians have erroneously resorted to translating tests in English given the great paucity of testing materials in languages other than English that provide specific information on hearing, speech, language, and communication skills. However, even the results of those tests that are available in Spanish need to be interpreted with care because few have been normed on individuals who have the very same experiences with and uses of the language. Therefore, alternative measures must be devised to evaluate skills in the children's primary language. Most likely, there will never be tests in any language that accurately assess the language proficiency in a bilingual individual even in his or her primary language.

Results of speech and language tests are only indicative of a small portion of the individual's language competence in any given language. In no case should normed tests in English be translated into another language for any purpose. Most often, the level of difficulty of a given item is not equivalent across languages, so norms cannot be used because they have not been developed for the second language. Even when norms have been established for a given language, they may not be entirely applicable for a given client. Dialectal differences impact meaning and are common in many languages. In addition, each client has had a very specific exposure to and experience in each language, which influences his or her linguistic and communicative competence.

Langdon and Wiig (2009) discuss some factors to consider in developing tests in other languages that may be fairer to use with a particular bilingual population. This task is possible but is extremely challenging. Three considerations need to be taken into account mentioned by the authors (p. 269). First, ensure that the "items included reflect the structure of the primary language spoken by the targeted population"; second, "test developers must hypothesize and validate which words and structures will differentiate normal learners from others who are experiencing difficulties in learning or using language"; and third, "dialectal differences in syntactic, lexical and phonological forms used by speakers of the language across several geographical regions should be included" (p. 269). For further details on how certain existing tests have been adapted and normed into Spanish, the reader is referred to the Langdon and Wiig (2009) article. Specific tests such as the Clinical Evaluation of Language Fundamentals–Preschool Spanish Edition (CELF-2 Preschool Spanish) (Wiig et al., 2009), the Clinical Evaluation of Language Fundamentals–Fourth Edition Spanish (CELF-4 Spanish) (Wiig, Semel, & Secord, 2006), and the Wiig-Assessment of Basic Concepts (W-ABC) (Wiig & Langdon, 2006), which have been adapted into Spanish, are discussed in greater detail. Specifically, a word-by-word translation even when the words have an equivalent level of complexity across two languages needed to be rephrased to reflect the structure of the language. For example, the sentence, "How are a knife and fork alike?" could not be translated into Spanish as *"¿Cómo son un cuchillo y un tenedor iguales?"* Instead, that same question needed to be translated as *"¿Cómo son iguales un cuchillo y un tenedor?"* or *"¿Cómo se parecen un cuchillo y un tenedor?"* (WABC-English/Spanish) (Langdon & Wiig, 2009, p. 270). Similarly, in adapting the Spanish version of the sentence repetition subtest of the CELF-4 Spanish (Wiig et al., 2006), the order of item difficulty had to be switched because of the performance of students during the standardization process.

The length of individual words is sometimes used as a yardstick for English language development. In contrast, Cantonese Chinese is essentially monosyllabic, so length does not play such an important role in the assessment of this language. Word length is not equivalent across languages. A Spanish language version, for example, might be slightly longer than the English version. Many common words such as *zapato* (shoe), *abrigo* (coat), *pantalón* or *pantalones* (pants), and *manzana* (apple) are longer in Spanish than in English. Therefore, length needs to be considered when translating or adapting any material because it may influence memory and language expression. The frequency of occurrence of words in one language may also differ significantly across languages, so tests based on frequency of occurrence are not directly translatable. This fact has implications when developing tests that assess receptive and expressive vocabulary. In addition to the tests in Spanish that have been named thus far, a number of other tests available have been adapted from the English versions, but not all have been normed.

Four recently published tests that are norm referenced, the Expressive One-Word Picture Vocabulary Test (Bilingual)

(Martin, 2012a) and the Receptive One-Word Picture Vocabulary Test (Bilingual) (Martin, 2012b), the Preschool Language Scales Fifth Edition Spanish (PLS-5 Spanish) (Zimmerman, Steiner, & Pond, 2012), and the Bilingual English-Spanish Assessment (BESA) (Peña, Gutiérrez-Clellen, Iglesias, Goldstein, & Bedore, 2014), are scored using the principle of *conceptual scoring*. Specifically, the child's total score compiles performance in the two languages. It includes all items in both Spanish and English. For example, on the PLS-5 Spanish version, the child is allowed to complete the items that were not answered in Spanish using English, thus yielding a more accurate score of the child's general language competence. On the BESA, scores in each language may be compared on the various subtests to determine which ones were performed better and in which language. If the SLP wishes to have normative data on language samples in both English and Spanish, he or she may administer the English version and then request the I/T to administer the Spanish-available version. However, special training on how to use and analyze the sample will need to be provided to the I/T and may need to be provided at a different time. Table 6–1 lists most commonly used speech and language tests in Spanish with annotated notes about age ranges, norming data, and scoring procedures.

Cross-linguistic and cross-cultural research data indicate many differences in language acquisition. For example, Choi (1997) reported that, unlike English speakers, Korean-speaking and Mandarin-speaking children learn verbs and nouns in a parallel manner. The generally accepted assumption that children all over the world develop nouns first may therefore need to be reexamined

and challenged. Research by Tardiff, Gelman, and Xu (1999) confirmed that indeed verbs might be more prevalent in toddlers in Mandarin compared to English. However, mothers from both groups used more nouns in certain contexts like book reading but more verbs while playing. Nevertheless, the children who spoke Mandarin used more verbs overall compared to the sample of those who spoke English. Therefore, the vocabularies of young children need to be evaluated depending on the context in which they are used by the person interacting with them. Although our understanding of language development in languages other than English is still emerging, clinicians assessing young children's vocabulary have more resources to assess those children's early lexical development. For example, the Spanish adaptation of the MacArthur Inventory of Communication Development (now the MacArthur Bates CDI inventory), first created in English by Fenson et al. (1993), was designed based on documenting words used by young children during parent-child interactions. These inventories have been adapted into another 60 different languages to include two different French dialects (Canadian and French) and various Spanish dialects (Columbian, Cuban, European, and Mexican), among many other languages. The reader is referred to an excellent resource by Dale and Penfold (2011), available at http://mb-cdi.stanford.edu/documents/AdaptationsSurvey7-5-11Web.pdf. Within the description of the research conducted on any given language, the editors cite specific article journals where the research was published. Additionally, McLeod (2007) provides resources on the speech development of various languages, including some studies that have been conducted in those languages. A recent

Table 6–1. Most Frequently Used Bilingual Spanish-English Tests

Name/Author(s)	Norms/Ages	Type of Test
Contextual Probes of Articulation Competence (CPAC-S) (Goldstein & Iglesias, 2006)	1,127 children from the United States, Mexico, and Puerto Rico Pre-K to 8:11	Assesses individual phonemes and phonological processes. Based on Secord's Contextual Articulation Tests (S-CAT) Available from: Greenville, SC: Super Duper Publications
Spanish Articulation Measures (SAM) (Mattes, 2005)	No norms 3:0 and up	Criterion referenced—assesses individual phonemes and phonological processes Available from: Oceanside, CA: Academic Communication Associates
Test of Phonological Awareness in Spanish (TPAS) (Riccio, Imhoff, Hasbrouck, & Davis, 2004)	1,000 children 4:0 to 10:11	Assesses phonological awareness skills Available from San Antonio, TX: Pearson
Clinical Evaluation of Language Fundamentals–Preschool (CELF-P2) (Spanish) (Wiig, Secord, & Semel, 2009)	More than 450 children, both monolingual in Spanish and bilingual in English 3:0 to 6:11	Assesses various areas of language comprehension and expression. A chapter is written by Henriette Langdon on how to use the test when collaborating with an interpreter. Available from San Antonio, TX: Pearson
Clinical Evaluation of Language Fundamentals (CELF-4) (Spanish) (Wiig, Semel, & Secord, 2006)	1,100 subjects 5:0 to 21:11	Like the Preschool version, CELF-4 assesses various areas of language comprehension and expression. Available from San Antonio, TX: Pearson
Receptive and Expressive One-Word Picture Vocabulary Test–Spanish Bilingual Version (ROWPVT-SBE and EOWPVT–SBE) (Martin, 2012a, 2012b)	1,200 subjects 2:0 to 70 +	Assesses receptive and expressive vocabulary skills using pictures. The subject can respond in either language. Available from: Greenville, SC: Super Duper Publications San Rafael, CA: A-R Publications

continues

Table 6–1. *continued*

Name/Author(s)	Norms/Ages	Type of Test
MacArthur Inventarios del Desarrollo de Habilidades Comunicativas (CDI) (Jackson-Maldonado et al., 2007) (See text to search other languages.)	2,000 Infants/toddlers 6 to 30 months	Evaluates receptive/expressive vocabulary in different semantic categories as per parent/caretaker report as well as basic directions. Two levels, 6 to 19 months and 18 to 30 months. Evaluates gestures and use of early syntactic structures. Available from: Baltimore, MD: Brooks Publishing Co.
Preschool Language Scale (PLS-5) Spanish Edition (Zimmerman, Steiner, & Pond, 2012)	1,150 bilingual children from the United States and Puerto Rico Birth to 7:11	Assesses various linguistic structures receptively and expressively using manipulatives and pictures. May be administered to monolingual Spanish- and/or bilingual Spanish-English-speaking children. In the latter case, children may respond in either language, and credit is given regardless of the language used in administering or responding to the different items. Available from San Antonio, TX: Pearson
Bilingual English-Spanish Assessment (BESA) (Peña, Gutiérrez-Clellen, Iglesias, Goldstein, & Bedore, 2014)	874 children. 420 completed the test in both languages; 739 completed it in Spanish and 642 completed it in English. 4:0 to 6:11	May be administered in Spanish or English or both. Includes phonology, semantics, morphosyntax, and pragmatics. For details, refer to https://2languages2worlds.wordpress.com/tag/besa/ Available from: San Rafael, CA: A-R Publications.
Wiig Assessment of Basic Concepts (Spanish) (W-ABC) (Wiig & Langdon, 2006)	685 children 3:0–7:11	Assesses receptive and expressive concepts using pictures books. Two different levels. Dialectal differences from the Spanish world are considered. Available from: Greenville, SC: Super Duper Publications

Table 6–1. *continued*

Name/Author(s)	Norms/Ages	Type of Test
Structured Photographic Elicitation Test (Spanish Version) (SPELT-3) (Langdon, 2012)	700 Spanish-speaking children exposed to English, from various Spanish-speaking countries 4:0–9:11	Assesses grammar, syntax, and use of pragmatics through elicitation of various types of questions based on various scenes. A compendium of semantic variations from the Hispanic world is available. Available from: DeKalb, IL: Janelle Publishers
Systematic Analysis of Language Sampling (SALT) (Miller & Iglesias, 2008)	4,140 subjects Urban and border Texas & Los Angeles 5:0–9:9	Analysis of transcript length, syntax, semantics, and discourse. Transcripts are taken from conversation, narration, and exposition. Available from: info@SALTSoftware.com 1-888-440-7258

publication by McLeod and Verdon (2014) is very helpful in locating tests in various languages, although the majority of the tests are normed on monolingual subjects speaking that particular language. A list of 30 tests is described by citing the language, ages, areas assessed, and number of subjects included in the norming sample. The majority of tests were designed to identify sound-speech disorders by assessing sound production and identifying phonological processes. Languages represented include Cantonese, Danish, Greek, Korean, Norwegian, Portuguese, Swedish, Turkish, and several others. A few phonological tests for bilingual clients are mentioned as well, such as Maltese-English, Spanish-English, and Pakistani-English. The authors describe in detail specific characteristics of the tests, such as the language in which the manual was written, the presentation of the test (colored or black and white photographs and the number on each page), the country where the test was developed and the particular inventory of sounds assessed. An analysis of the psychometric values of the various tests is also reported. A total of 19 languages that can be assessed using articulation measures are identified. Yet, the authors indicate that overall intelligibility and feedback from persons who know the child well need to be taken into account as well. For example, a child might be difficult to understand in connected speech in the first language, even though an articulation/phonology test that assesses single words might indicate that he or she is able to produce the sound in isolation and/or at the word level. Another website created by McLeod (2012) provides the clinician references to specific resources and testing materials in specific languages.

Even though the research mentioned above is just emerging, the results will be very helpful to SLPs and audiologists who are working with children whose first language is increasingly diverse, not only in the United States but around the globe. Because there is limited research on the development features of first languages and a lack of resources, many countries continue using translations and adaptations of many English tests in various fields, including psychology, speech-language pathology, and even audiology. Very few tests have been normed in other languages, and the process is quite complicated and lengthy. An excellent resource about the effort needed to develop fair tests in various domains such as intelligence testing, curricular achievement, and personality can be found in Hambleton, Merenda, and Spielberger (2005). The clinical implications of such cross-linguistic research are significant in guiding the translation or adaptation of tests from one language to another and for deciphering test results based on language-specific normative data and input. Langdon and Wiig (2009) caution users to critically analyze the development, reliability, and validity of each test (even when normed on Spanish-English populations) to ascertain that the individual tested matches the normed population. As reviewed in Chapter 5, relying on only test results to determine that a bilingual or even monolingual individual has a possible speech and/or language disorder or a particular hearing impairment is misleading. Using multiple sources of information, such as a careful language history, reports from teachers and family members, language samples, dynamic assessment, and progress over time with careful monitoring are important ingredients in decision making.

GUIDELINES FOR ASSESSING A CLD CHILD WITH THE ASSISTANCE OF A TRAINED INTERPRETER

Before conducting an assessment or deciding that an I/T is needed, the SLP or audiologist should consider the following seven factors:

1. *Personal factors related to the student.* Aptitude, working memory skills, attitude, motivation, anxiety, the learner's identity, and adjustment to a new culture all influence the speed and proficiency at which individuals learn a second language (Bernat & Gvozdenko, 2005; Duff, 2013; Skehan, 2013; Ushioda & Dörnyer, 2013; Williams, 2013).

2. *Use of each language.* Each language may be used in different contexts and for different purposes; therefore, knowledge of concepts and performance may vary as well. The idea proposed by Cummins (1981) so many years ago of two types of communication, where one type is more contextualized, basic interpersonal communication skills (BICS), and the other type is more related to instruction, and therefore, more decontextualized, or cognitive academic language skills (CALP), may still be applicable with a few modifications. The current term for BICS is conversational informal language fluency (CILF), and CALP is referred to as formal academic language fluency (FALF). For more details on these newer concepts, the reader is referred to Paradis, Genesee, and Crago (2011) and Roseberry-McKibbin (2014). Also, keep in mind the comment made ear-

lier that language dominance is a relative term, and bilingualism should be considered "cumulative" rather than "comparative" (Peña, Bedore, & Zlantic-Giunta, 2002).

3. *Type of discourse.* CLD students often experience what Cheng (1994) refers to as "difficult discourse" due to sociological and psychological difficulties that arise when adaption to a different or dual culture and language is necessary. Home tradition may conflict with the rules that govern classroom practices. Although stereotypes should be avoided, having a general knowledge about how various groups adapt to a new linguistic environment is helpful in understanding why some groups may have more difficulty than others. For example, Lao, Khmer, and Hmong families come from more traditional agricultural families where learning English may not be emphasized, whereas families from other cultural and linguistic backgrounds may give formal education a different level of importance.

4. *Home-school differences.* Many CLD students from Hispanic, Asian, indigenous, or other backgrounds may hesitate to participate in class. In some "traditional Hispanic/Latino cultures, children are taught to listen, to obey and not to challenge older persons or persons of authority, such as parents or teachers" (Author).

5. *Nonverbal cues.* Eye gaze, physical contact, and body language influence communication, and cultures differ in ways in which communication is nonverbally transmitted and processed.

6. *Code-switching and language loss.* Code-switching may depend on context and is expected in bilingual communication. Questions about expressive language must take into account the natural loss of a language that is infrequently used.

Several of these factors have been discussed in previous chapters, in particular Chapters 3 and 4 of this guide. Additional information in the areas that have been outlined may be found in other resources such as Langdon (2008), Lynch and Hanson (2011), and Roseberry-McKibbin (2014).

The collaboration with an I/T may be necessary if the parent or a family member does not speak English sufficiently well to be able to understand some of the questions that may arise during the assessment and to interpret in case the child responds to some of the questions in a language other than English. This information can be gathered by sharing information with the parent and/or the child's teacher prior to the assessment session.

ASSESSMENT GUIDELINES PERTINENT TO SLPS AND I/TS

RIOT—A Suggested Guideline for Assessment to Evaluate CLD/Bilingual Children

The review, interview, observe, and test (RIOT) procedure has been found effective in identifying factors that may have prevented students from succeeding in school and other learning environments while ensuring that inappropriate special education referrals and placements are not carried out (Leung, 1995). The steps in the RIOT procedures are as follows:

Review (R) the following pieces of information: school and medical records; reports; teachers' comments; report cards if relevant; students' work and written samples; linguistic, social, and family background; and previous therapy received or testing results.

Interview (I) teachers, peers, family members, and other informants. The interview in Table 5–1 can be helpful in obtaining background information. Often results of a thorough interview assist the team in planning the assessment process. For example, finding out that a student had difficulties learning the first language, is behind in language and communication in L1 (first language) compared to siblings or peers of the same community, or has had a significant medical history assist in determining that the student may be experiencing a language-learning difficulty rather than a language difference. In addition, if the parent reports that the student has had limited exposure to school and literacy, it may indicate that the student needs more time to acquire skills prior to being assessed more formally. Also, finding out the level of literacy that an individual had prior to an accident or traumatic brain injury assists in evaluating the loss of skills resulting from the injury.

The SLP may wish to interview the parents or family to obtain information about play activities, what the child likes to do at home, the student's interaction partners in the home setting, any major event(s) in the student's life that may have compounded the problem, and how the parents and family have reacted to the child's communication skills. These important pieces of information will provide a more complete picture of the child outside the school setting. An interview with the child's teacher assists in gaining his or her perception of the student in a learning environment, his or her progress over time, the child's response to various types of accommodations (if they have been implemented), and a comparison of the child with others who have similar linguistic and scholastic experiences.

Observe (O) the child in multiple contexts if possible while performing various activities with some being more structured than others. Observations of the child's interactions at school and at home assist in gaining a broader picture of his or her overall communication competence, and the I/T may assist in this process. In addition, these observations enable the SLP to define contexts that are conducive to more successful learning. The I/T can assist in providing additional input on the child's behavior and language and can compare the child with peers with similar dual linguistic and environmental backgrounds.

Test (T) school/work and home language competence using multiple sources of information such as informal assessments, language samples, and specific materials (if available in a given language and if norming procedures are taken into account). Having access to a student's work samples enables to understand the student's progress over time.

A comprehensive review by Bedore and Peña (2008) documents some important findings regarding children who were exposed to other languages. Naturally, it is important to consider patterns that arise when children are exposed to two languages. In general, given similar exposure to each language, bilingual children's language patterns in each language are similar to those of children speaking either one of the languages. Their morphosyntax skills reveal the use of particular rules of a given language even when the children mix the two languages. Also, the mixing of the two languages may depend on which language is more dominant. In citing examples from Spanish-English-speaking and Swedish-French bilingual children, the authors indicate that such structures reveal their competence in language rather than signal an error.

The scope of this chapter does not permit us to go into greater detail about the possible patterns that may be noted in assessing children with language impairments who speak other languages than English and/or who are growing up in different L1 and/or bilingual environments. Some highlights of children's profiles who speak another language than English and who have a language impairment include the following:

- In languages such as Dutch, German, or Cantonese, children having language disorders acquire *vocabulary at a lower pace* compared to typically developing peers.
- These children also seem *to have word-finding problems, the number of errors* they make in word use is higher, and they also have *more difficulty using and even* comprehending certain types of end verbs (telic verbs like *build* or *open*) in languages like Cantonese.
- The children's *utterances are shorter and many include errors* that are specific to the particular language structure. For example, some errors in English are in the use of verb tenses, plural, possessive; in Swedish, errors are in the use of verb markings and the omission of indefinite articles, yet their use of definite articles is normal. In French, the use of verb markings is problematic, while in other romance languages, like Spanish and Italian, verb markings are not challenges, but clitic verbs and articles are difficult ("*dámelo*" ["give it to me"]). Overall, children

who have language disorders have difficulties with structures that have less saliency.

Children with possible speech-language disorders who are growing up in a bilingual environment:

- *Seem to have more difficulty* in each language due to less input in each language, and they also may display *more differences* due to cross-linguistic bootstrapping. (In general, bootstrapping refers to procedures in which some built-in or already existing processes or capacities make it possible to advance in operating and building a system.)
- *Will have vocabulary word* deficits in both languages as well as *word-finding difficulties* just like children who are monolingual. The deficits are comparable in both languages.
- *Demonstrate deficits compared to their bilingual peers.* For example, they experience greater L1 loss and use less advanced forms in L2 (Spanish-English).
- *The type of errors made in each language is similar to monolingual children who* have been identified as having a language disorder and who speak either one of the two languages. In Spanish, errors are in use of clitic verbs as well as in use of definite articles, use of appropriate gender for articles (*el/la* or *un/una*), and overgeneralization in use of irregular verbs.

Although there is increasing cross-linguistic research on both monolingual and bilingual children who are experiencing challenges in developing language, it has not been systematic. Therefore, obtaining additional data such as a careful health and development history as well as information on the progress of each language is very important to determine if indeed a child's language patterns reflect a language disorder or a language difference that may be remediated with time.

What to Do When Tests Are Available in the Target Language

As mentioned in previous chapters, the nature of the collaboration with an I/T will be different in a given situation, but a suggested practice is to follow the BID process. Even though there may be norms and procedures to administer tests in the first language (which will be most common in the Spanish language for children living in the United States but might be different in another country, and reference to available materials is listed in McLeod, 2012), there are no provisions on how to factor in the collaboration of an I/T in completing activities. Furthermore, it is important that the SLP or audiologist has confidence in the I/T, and therefore, collaborating with a trained person is essential.

In no case should the I/T be left alone during an assessment without the SLP present.

Briefing: The SLP and the I/T must agree on the procedures they will follow ahead of time. The particular tests with specific item administration and order of presentation should be discussed in testing speech, language, and/or communication skills. Depending on the particular test or test items, the situation, and the I/T's level of training and experience, the I/T may proceed by asking the client to respond to the items without needing the SLP to administer the given item(s) using

English first. The process is facilitated if the SLP refers to the specific test protocols in the child's first language, which will most likely be in Spanish.

As discussed in Chapter 5, there needs to be an agreement between the SLP and the I/T regarding what to do in case the child does not understand directions, if the I/T is unsure of the child's responses, and if the child has behavior issues and/or the task is too difficult or too easy. Also, the SLP and I/T should discuss if the use of recording devices, such as a tape recorder or video camera, would be helpful in the debriefing and evaluation of the process. Depending on the level of training and experience of the I/T, it might be helpful for the I/T to have observed the SLP assessing the same child in English if appropriate to acquaint the I/T with the child.

During the *interaction* phase, the SLP should have a copy of the protocol to gain a general sense of the information being collected. The SLP should record observations about the body language of the child and the I/T or make notations when the I/T appears to use too many words while providing instructions, misuses reinforcement, or seems to give too many or inappropriate hints or clues. The I/T should be prepared for interruptions by the SLP, which may arise, to share his or her observations. Likewise, the I/T should feel at ease and be honest in asking for clarification when unsure of the child's responses and/or behavior. It is recommended that, where appropriate, the I/T briefly communicate with the SLP about the child's overall performance.

If it is important to consider that if the child does not answer in Spanish or the target language, it might be due to a lack of experience with some words or tasks, or simply because of language loss.

Notations should be made to reconsider the item later on for retesting in English. It is best to initiate the assessment using one language at a time, but on certain occasions, shifting to English might be necessary. The SLP might need to ask the question in English just immediately after the conclusion of a certain subtest or after the entire assessment is completed. It is difficult to suggest the best approach to take, and it will be a decision that may need to take place depending on a given situation. If tests such as the PLS-5 in Spanish, the BESA, or the ROWPVT/EOWPVT are used, then the procedure is much easier. Other test items might need to be administered in English at a later date by referring to the English version subtest where an equivalent item might have been included. However, the scoring in Spanish should not be combined with the English because the norms of each version do not allow for this procedure to take place. Table 6–2 includes questions to facilitate recording of the child during testing. The SLP may ask the I/T to watch for some of those behaviors or may ask the I/T to modify some tasks during the session so that these behaviors can be examined.

During the *debriefing* session, the SLP and the I/T should analyze the child's responses to the target testing items, noting which ones were correct and describing the type of errors made by the child. The I/T should try to provide the SLP with relevant cultural and linguistic information that may have influenced the child's performance on specific items such as a possible lack of familiarity with particular situations or words. It is important to discuss deviations from the standard administration, the I/T's impressions, and any difficulties or positive observations that may have surfaced during the process.

What to Do When Tests Are Not Available in the Target Language

During the *briefing* period, the I/T may discuss with the SLP about designing

Table 6–2. *Some Practical Tips in Preparing to Administer a Given Test/Subtest and Recording the Student's Responses*

What are the directions for administering the particular test/subtest?

How do you record the answers?

Do you transcribe the answers and/or circle those that are provided in the protocol?

Are there practice items?

Can you repeat the directions and/or test items?

Where do you begin the test and where you do end? (basals and ceilings)

Are you aware of the pace of reading the items and administering the test?

What do you do if the student does not answer the question or gives an incorrect response?

Discuss what went well and what you need to be aware of the next time.

Discuss how to score the particular test or subtest.

some activities that will not only assess the child's linguistic skills but also evaluate the speed and accuracy of using language. Some suggestions that SLPs and I/Ts can follow are described below and are not listed in any specific order. The SLP may review the availability of one of the tests in several languages listed in McLeod (2012) and McLeod and Verdon (2014). The majority of tests focus primarily on assessment of phonology, with a few focusing on language assessment. Lists of tests in languages such as Arabic (Egyptian, Kuwaiti, Jordanian), Bulgarian, Cantonese, Danish, Dutch, Finnish, French (Canadian and French), German, Gujarati, Polish, Portuguese (Brazilian and European), Somali, Turkish, and Tamil, among several other languages, can be found. If the type of test in a given language is not available or the scope of the tests is not sufficient or appropriate, the child's oral and written skills can be assessed following suggestions described below:

Ask the child's parents if they have any available books or materials in the child's language. If they have books or materials in the target language, the I/T may be requested to comment on whether they would be appropriate for the child's age and experience with the language. If they are, the I/T may plan to read a passage and ask some questions about the content and/or read a passage and ask the child to retell the story. In this case, the I/T may need to tell the SLP about the content of the story, and comprehension questions should be formulated carefully and retranslated into English for the SLP to judge their value in assessing the language skills of the child. All of this material should be written down and prepared ahead of the evaluation time. Depending on the child's age and formal education, the child may be asked to read and write in the target language. Specific activities will need to be planned ahead and require additional time and preparation. For this reason, one of the suggestions made in Chapter 5 in planning for the future is to create curriculum-based activities in various languages that I/Ts and SLPs can utilize when assessing bilingual/CLD children who speak a variety of languages. Additionally, specific activities may be prepared:

Elicit and analyze a language sample. The language sampling and the various language-based activities will depend on the child's chronological and mental ages. A procedure for eliciting and analyzing a language sample is suggested in the next section of this chapter. Gathering a language sample allows the observation of various linguistic and communication features such as phonology, grammar, syntax, pragmatics, and the language formulation abilities of the child.

Have the child name words in various categories in the first language and English, such as foods, animals, body parts, and classroom items to compare and contrast the words used in each language and the ease with which they are elicited.

Use rapid automatic naming tasks such as naming sequences of colors, shapes, and combinations to judge speed and accuracy in word retrieval.

Engaging the child in a card game may be very telling. For example, a card game where pairs need to be assembled or classic games like war may shed light on the child's ability to learn new strategies and/or follow directions. Also, engage the child in board games where turn-taking skills can be observed.

Request the child to draw something and talk about it or complete a simple art activity. This allows the assessment of the child's imagination and creativity as well as his or her ability to follow directions. A conversation may be elicited in this environment.

Prepare a questionnaire as if interviewing the child. Questions may range from learning basic information about the child such as age, birthdate, number of siblings, address, phone number, and so on as well as favorite activities, places to go, games, shows, and music. Depending on a given situation, the child may be asked to respond to questions regarding what is easy or difficult at school; what the child's favorite subjects are; how to play a given game, sport, and so on; and how to retell the plot of a TV show or movie.

Guidelines for Eliciting a Language Sample With the I/T

A language sample can provide useful information about a child's communicative competence, but eliciting and transcribing a representative sample requires special skill, practice, and time. For example, more language is elicited from the child with questions such as "tell me about . . . " or "how do you . . . ?" compared to "where did you . . . " or "do you . . . ?" The first type of question is more open-ended, whereas the second type of question can be answered in a word or short utterance, or even *yes* or *no*.

Many times children may be hesitant to open up even when spoken to in their home language because they may not be used to being addressed by adults they don't know, they may resent speaking in their language for many reasons, or they may be shy, especially at first. Also, some children may not be used to being asked questions where they may be requested to give their opinions or their comments due to lack of experience or practice.

Additionally, those who have language-based learning disorders may not speak much in any language. The SLP and the I/T may need to get used to periods of silence and/or delays between questions/comments and responses from the child. This type of behavior is not unusual because the child may need more time to process what was said and to formulate an answer. The I/T may need to practice more in using various ways of obtaining language samples from different children, beginning with some who speak the language fluently, to experience the process of eliciting language and transcribing what they say more easily. To facilitate the interaction, bringing in a favorite friend to the session is suggested. This author has found that it is helpful to elicit a sample in at least three different contexts to assess the child's linguistic abilities more thoroughly. At first, the process might seem laborious; however, with more practice, it can be completed more quickly. The SLP and I/T should discuss those contexts ahead of time when possible. For example, with *younger children in preschool and up to second grade*, engaging in a conversation while playing with toys or a game might be one context. The second context might be while looking at a pictured book; the I/T may make comments about the ongoing story and solicit responses from the child, such as "what might happen next" or "why do you think . . . " The third context might be elicited while the child draws a picture, completes an art project, or talks about a favorite character in a TV show or DVD as well as provides a narrative using one of the frog stories such as *Frog, Where Are You?* (Mayer, 2003a) or *Frog Goes to Dinner* (Mayer, 2003b). *For older students*, using a conversation to get to know the student's favorite pastimes, sports, and activities, requesting that the student describes the rules of a video game or game, and having the student narrate a story using a wordless book are effective ways to get a more comprehensive language sample. As another method to compare the performance of the student across languages in Spanish and English, the SLP may consider using the Systematic Analysis of Language (SALT) (Miller & Iglesias, 2008). A dilemma is when assessment is completed with an older elementary or upper grade student because comparable samples of students in these ages are not available. Clinicians may find the Structured Photographic Elicitation Test-3 (Spanish version) helpful in encouraging elementary age children to respond in Spanish (Langdon, 2012).

Once the samples are collected, the I/T needs to listen and transcribe what the child/student said verbatim, with no corrections in phonology, grammar, or syntax. It is also recommended to transcribe what the adult said, because more specific interactions can be documented to describe pragmatic skills. Once the samples are transcribed, it is suggested that both the I/T and the SLP review the sample together to analyze the various communicative and linguistic elements included. Specific training of the I/T may be necessary on how to transcribe the sample and what areas need to be considered in the analysis of the sample. The areas are listed below:

Pragmatics: (a) Did the child/student respond to questions and comments appropriately? (b) Did the child/student maintain the topic at hand (if not, could it be due to cultural differences)? (c) Were ideas clearly stated, or it was difficult to follow the child's/student's flow of speech? (d) Could the child/student use language to describe or ask for information (if there were opportunities to do so during the interaction)? (e) Did the child/student seem to use more gestures than needed to get his or her ideas across?

Form and content: (a) Did the child/student use sentences that were grammatically correct, and if they were not, what were some errors noted? (b) What was the nature of the vocabulary used (was it restricted to more general words than expected?) (c) What was the pronunciation like, and if there were errors, what kind were they (examples)? (d) What was the child's/student's overall level of intelligibility?

Manner of language expression: (a) Was there a time delay between the I/T's comments or questions and the child's/student's responses? (b) Were there pauses and hesitations noted, any stuttering or cluttering observed? (c) Was voice quality adequate (any problems with volume, hoarseness, harshness, or breathiness)? (Most likely, the SLP may have observed some challenges in this third area as well while listening to the interaction, but it is important to discuss these observations with the I/T as well.)

Both the SLP and the I/T should keep in mind that the final determination about the child's/student's communication profile and skills is the SLP's charge and responsibility, but the input of the I/T is important to substantiate the SLP's observations. Therefore, the appropriate training of the I/T and trust between the SLP and I/T are crucial.

ASSESSMENT GUIDELINES PERTINENT TO AUDIOLOGISTS AND I/TS

When to ask for assistance from an I/T? The collaboration of an I/T during an assessment may be needed to ensure that the client follows directions accurately. When undertaking an audiological evaluation with a child whose proficiency in English is not fully developed, Dr. McCullough[3] recommends that the I/T gives the client instructions for each test in the test battery, like, "raise your hand whenever you hear a tone, even if it is very low/quiet, as we are trying to find the softest level of sound that you can hear," or, "this is an automatic test that will measure how your eardrum is moving. Please sit still and do not talk while the test is running." Although all audiologists who work with CLD clients may not share these views, they are considered fairly typical.[4]

Most commonly, a child sees an audiologist to evaluate the type and degree of a hearing loss. The procedure includes pure-tone testing and SRT, word recognition, in addition to a tympanogram to assess middle ear function. Dr. McCullough reports that about 80% of her young clients come from homes where Vietnamese, Mandarin, or Spanish is spoken. She is able to communicate through gestures to a child what he or she needs to do when hearing a tone. Under these conditions, the I/T would translate the instructions the audiologist is giving.

Challenges and Solutions

One of the drawbacks of assessing children who speak a different language is the inability to check the results of the pure-tone testing with speech-discrimination testing. It is inappropriate to ask clients to repeat English words because their knowledge of the language may be limited. On the other hand, asking clients to repeat words in their language from a tape does not yield accurate results, because the audiologist who does not speak the client's language cannot evaluate the accuracy of the client's response. The I/T may need to be trained to determine if the child repeated words accurately. However, there is a paucity of phonetically balanced recorded/normed word lists in languages other than Spanish or French. Phonetically balanced lists in languages other than Spanish or French are emerging. McCullough has worked on procedures to develop phonetically balanced lists to include Russian, Mandarin, and Cantonese (Aleksandrovsky, McCullough, & Wilson, 1998; McCullough, Wilson, Birck, & Anderson, 1994). At the present time, an application is being prepared for audiologists to deliver these auditory-visual materials to children and adults who are speakers of these languages. Clearly, a great deal more research in this area is needed to serve patients who are assessed for hearing, not only in the United States but also worldwide. This author could locate other lists for auditory discrimination including Illocano (Sagon, 2006),

---

[3]Personal communication (August 28, 2014).

[4]This author wishes to thank the other audiologists who were interviewed and who offered time in confirming some statements brought about on this topic, namely, Susan Clark, Evelyn Merritt, and Dr. Christine Yoshinaga-Itano.

Jordan Arabic (Abdulhag, 2006), Sesotho (spoken in South Africa) (Khoza-Shangase & Mokoena, 2012), Samoan (Newman, 2010), and Cantonese (Marinova-Todd, Siu, & Jenstadt, 2011). In these publications the authors cite other lists developed in other languages such as Arabic, French Canadian, Mandarin, Russian, and Swedish, among others. However, these lists were tried most often with adults and monolingual speakers.

Assessing SRT and speech recognition may not be conducted unless the client has some familiarity with English. However, speech detection thresholds may be possible to obtain. The instruction might be, "Whenever you hear I am talking in headphones, raise your hand (or push the button), even if my voice is very quiet/low." The child/student does not have to repeat anything; he or she is just indicating whether speech is detected. For individuals without any familiarity with English, word recognition is possible under specific circumstances: (a) The audiologist and the client speak the same language; (b) there are prerecorded words in the patient's language, and someone else who does speak the language (i.e., the I/T) can indicate whether the word was repeated correctly; or (c) the word-pointing or picture-pointing paradigm is used where recorded words are presented in the patient's language, and the client points to the appropriate word or picture on a computer monitor. This way, the audiologist doesn't have to know the language; he or she just has to know whether the client pointed to the correct foil. Most of the time, this is done with a computer, and the computer scores the test using touch-screen technology.[5]

When assessing the client's hearing acuity, for example, it is important that the child understands that he or she needs to respond even when tones are very faint. At times, the procedure may become more difficult because the child has difficulty following the directions of the test. When no I/T is available, some experienced audiologists demonstrate to the child what he or she needs to do using gestures and use a portable audiometer prior to proceeding to the testing booth. Understanding directions and feeling at ease are very important in getting an accurate measure of the client's hearing acuity.

Thus, adequate preparation of the I/T during the briefing is essential to ensure the success of the process. In the case of assessing a younger child, the audiologist may need to train the child to respond through play audiometry. Audiologists typically can condition the children for play audiometry without needing to use any words—the audiologist first demonstrates by presenting tones and throwing a block in a bucket, for example, each time a tone is presented. Then a block is handed to the child, and under most circumstances, he or she understands that it is his or her turn to play by throwing the block in the bucket when the sound comes on. The procedure for auditory brainstem response (ABR) is different—children are usually sleeping, and adults just get instructions to keep very still (for adults, ABR is not performed anymore because magnetic resonance imaging is much cheaper today).[6]

In conducting an audiological evaluation on a bilingual child, the audiologist might not need the services of an I/T to conduct an SRT because the child may be

---

[5]June McCullough, PhD-Aud (personal communication, August 28, 2014).
[6]June McCullough, PhD-Aud (personal communication, August 28, 2014).

familiar with the spondees used to assess this skill, even when the words are administered in English. Pictures for words such as *baseball, bluebird, ice cream, hotdog,* and *toothpaste* may be used. Discrimination testing might also be conducted in English because words are relatively simple such as those used in phonetically balanced lists and include monosyllabic words such as *moon, dad,* and *shoes.* However, if the audiologist administers these words, and the children mispronounce the words, the professional needs to be sure to take dialectal variations into account. For example, a child speaking Spanish might say /da/ for /dad/ because final /d/ is not as common in Spanish, and the word /shoes/ might be pronounced as /tʃous/ because the /ʃ/ does not occur in most Spanish dialects (except for Castilian Spanish).[7]

In case the audiologist wishes to assess the child's speech recognition, it is advised to carry out this task only in cases if the word list has been adapted and recorded in that given language; otherwise, the results may be invalid. Currently, there are a few such lists, and they have been developed only for English, Spanish, and French and are available through Auditec (http://www.auditec .com/). When assessing young clients who speak other languages, it is best not to assess their language if the audiologist is not fluent in that language. A solution is to form a network of audiologists in one's area of service who speak other languages and refer back to those professionals when needed.[8] Translating SRT tests from English into other languages should be

avoided for several reasons: (a) The phonetic repertoire, particular dialect, and the word length are different, and (b) intonation may vary (most evident in those languages that rely on tones to convey different meanings); therefore, a word-by-word translation may be misleading.[9] An audiology faculty member at the University of Puerto Rico, Dr. Mitzarie A. Carlo Colón, reports the following information regarding services in that country.

The only recorded materials for SRT and WRT (word recognition tests) testing in Spanish that I have seen in clinics in PR and Florida (I practiced in FL for some years) is the Spanish Auditec Recordings. My experience has been that if audiologists are native Spanish speakers, they will do MLV (monitored live voice) with the words, and if they are not native Spanish speakers, but feel comfortable enough in scoring the answers, they will use the recorded materials. . . . If the patient is not bilingual, then the audiologist simply does not conduct the WRT/SRT in the evaluation. Of course this is not best practice. These are the cases where the patient brings a family member that translates throughout the test for them but of course cannot translate during WRT/SRT testing. Because WRT and SRT use isolated words, the dialect difference between the audiologist and the patient is not that big of an issue. Just like you may have an African American audiologist from the south testing MLV with a patient from Canada, where there

[7]June McCullough, PhD-Aud (personal communication, August 28, 2014).
[8]Personal communication with Susan Clark, MA-Aud (September 16, 2014).
[9]June McCullough, PhD-Aud (personal communication, August 28, 2014) and Christine Yoshinaga-Itano, PhD-Aud (personal communication, September 8, 2014).

are marked differences. This is exactly why EVERYBODY SHOULD BE USING RECORDED MATERIALS! Of course we know that they aren't.[10]

Another efficient way to assess SRT is to use digit-pairs in individuals who are not proficient in English and may speak other languages, and this has been validated by studies conducted by Ramkissoon, Proctor, Lansing, and Bilger (2002). In his comprehensive article, Shi (2014) provides references to research conducted to obtain SRT measures (Schneider, 1992) and WRT (Comstock & Martin, 1984). Most recently, Calandruccio, Gómez, Buss, and Leibold (2014) report their efforts in developing audiometric tests for bilingual Spanish-English children.[11]

Clearly, more research is needed in developing audiometric tests for bilingual individuals who speak specific languages and who are also bilingual in various language combinations. Nevertheless, every effort should be made to attempt and assess clients as accurately as possible with the collaboration of an I/T whose assistance will be invaluable in taking a careful history and in providing counseling as appropriate to the parent/family and the client.

where there might be normed tests in the child's language (Spanish) as well when there might not be any materials available in his or her language. Some guidelines were suggested about how to supplement the evaluation by administering and scoring a language sample in the child's first language. In reviewing tests that are currently available in Spanish, we highlighted strategies that were developed in getting some normative data for assessing bilingual Spanish-English-speaking children. We emphasized the importance of assessing the two languages and provided some general guidelines.

As far as assessing hearing acuity and auditory processing in bilingual children, methodologies are just emerging, and more research is needed in this area. Nevertheless, it may be necessary for audiologists to train I/Ts to work on collecting an accurate medical history of the client as well as ensure that the client understands the directions of testing, assist in verifying the accuracy of the client in SRT/WRT where appropriate, and very importantly, collaborate in delivering accurate information regarding follow-up and counseling regarding the particular hearing status of the client.

SUMMARY

In this chapter, we have attempted to provide some guidelines about how the SLP might successfully collaborate with a trained I/T in assessing the language and communication skills of a child in cases

DISCUSSION ITEMS AND ACTIVITIES

1. You have to assess the communication skills of a 3-year-old who is primarily Cantonese speaking. He has a vocabulary of only about 40 words. The majority of the words are in Can-

---

[10]E-mail correspondence, September 30, 2014.

[11]The author thanks Dr. Shi, PhD CCC-Aud (Associate Professor at Long Island University, Brooklyn, NY), for some additional references provided in this chapter.

tonese, with about five being in English (*ball*, *TV*, *car*, *juice*, and *book*). All of these five words are pronounced very clearly. How would you assess this child's speech and language? Use the resources mentioned in the chapter as well as other ideas to assess the child's language. What would the I/T's role be? Compare and contrast your notes with another person in your class or group.

2. An audiologist has to assess a 12-year-old student's hearing acuity and word recognition who primarily speaks Spanish. The audiologist does not speak Spanish. What would be the role of the I/T?

3. Practice being an SLP and I/T in eliciting a language sample. As part of your assessment of briefing your interpreter on how to elicit a language sample, select a student who needs a bilingual language assessment. Invite the I/T to observe you working with the student and eliciting as well as analyzing the language sample. This will serve as a model for an I/T when he or she is asked to elicit a language sample in Spanish or another language.

4. Practice being an audiologist and I/T taking a history from a 5-year-old child who is going to be assessed for hearing. He and his family have recently emigrated from Ukraine, and Russian is spoken in the home. The child has never been properly assessed in his home country.

REFERENCES

Abdulhag, N. (2006). *Speech perception test for Jordanian-Arabic speaking children* (Doctoral dissertation). Gainesville, FL: University of Florida.

Aleksandrovsky, I. V., McCullough, J., & Wilson, R. H. (1998). Development of a suprathreshold word recognition test for Russian patients. *Journal of the American Academy of Audiology, 9*, 417–425.

American Speech-Language-Hearing Association. (1988, March). Bilingual speech language pathologists and audiologists definition. *ASHA, 31*, 64.

Bedore, L., & Pena, E. (2008). Assessment of bilingual children for identification of language impairment: Current findings and implications. *International Journal of Bilingual Education and Bilingualism, 11*(1), 1–29.

Bernat, E., & Gvozdenko, I. (2005). Beliefs about language learning: Current knowledge, pedagogical implications, and new research directions. *Teaching English as a Second Language or Foreign Language, 9*(1), 1–21.

Calandruccio, L., Gómez, B., Buss, E., & Leibold, L. (2014). Development and preliminary evaluation of a pediatric Spanish-English perception test. *American Journal of Audiology, 23*(2), 158–172.

Cheng, L.-R. L. (1994). Difficult discourse: An untold Asian story. In D. N. Ripich & N. A. Creaghead (Eds.), *School discourse problems* (2nd ed., pp. 165–170). San Diego, CA: Singular.

Choi, S. (1997). Language-specific input and early semantic development. In D. I. Slobin (Ed.), *The cross-linguistic student of language acquisition* (pp. 41–133). Hillsdale, NJ: Erlbaum.

Comstock, C. L., & Martin, F. N. (1984). A children's Spanish-speaking word discrimination test for non-Spanish-speaking clinicians. *Ear and Hearing, 5*(3), 181–183.

Cummins, J. (1981). The role of primary language development in promoting educational success for language minority students. In Office of Bilingual Bicultural Education, California State Department of Education (Ed.), *School and language minority students: A theoretical framework* (pp. 3–49). Los Angeles: Evaluation, Dissemination, and Assessment Center, California State University.

Cummins, J. (1984). *Bilingualism and special education.* Clevedon, UK: Multilingual Matters.

Dale, P. S., & Penfold, M. (2011). *Adaptations of the MacArthur Bates CDI into non-English Languages.* Retrieved July 14, 2014, from http://mb-cdi.stanford.edu/documents/AdaptationsSurvey7-5-11Web.pdf

Duff, D. A. (2013). Identity, agency, and second language acquisition. In S. M. Gass & A. Mackey (Eds.), *The Routledge handbook of second language acquisition* (pp. 410–426). London, UK: Routledge.

Fenson, L., Dale, P. S., Reznick, J. S., Thal, D., Bates, E., Hartung, J. P., & Reilly, J. S. (1993). *The MacArthur Communicative Development Inventories: User's guide and technical manual.* Baltimore, MD: Paul H. Brookes.

Goldstein, B., & Iglesias, A. (2006). *Contextual Probes of Articulation Competence–Spanish.* (CPAC-S). Greenville, SC: Super Duper Publications.

Hambleton, R. K., Merenda, P. F., & Speilberger, C. D. (Eds.). (2005). *Adapting educational and psychological tests for cross-cultural assessment.* Mahwah, NJ: Lawrence Erlbaum.

Howard, E., Sugarman, J., Perdomo, M., & Adger, C. T. (2005). *The two-way immersion toolkit.* Providence, RI: The Education Alliance for Brown University.

Jackson-Maldonado, D., Thal, D., Fenson, L., Marchman, V. A., Newton, T., & Conboy, B. (2007). *MacArthur Inventarios del Desarrollo de Habilidades Comunicativas (Inventarios) user's guide and technical manual* (2nd ed.). Baltimore, MD: Brookes.

Khoza-Shangase, K., & Mokoena, M. (2012). Speech audiometry in South Africa: In pursuit of resource development of African languages. *Journal of British Communication, I*(2), 1–12.

Kohnert, K. (2013). *Language disorders in bilingual children and adults* (2nd ed.). San Diego, CA: Plural.

Langdon, H. W. (2008). *Assessment and intervention for communication disorders in culturally and linguistically diverse populations.* Clifton Park, NY: Cengage.

Langdon, H. W. (2011, March). *One or two languages? Working with ELL students and their families.* Seminar presented at the annual conference of the California Speech-Language Hearing Association, Los Angeles, CA.

Langdon, H. W. (2012). *Structured Photographic Elicitation Test (SPELT-3)* (Spanish ed.). DeKalb, IL: Janelle.

Langdon, H. W., & Wiig, E. (2009). Multicultural issues in test interpretation. *Seminars in Speech and Language, 30*(4), 261–278.

Leung, B. (1995). Back to basics: Assessment is R.I.O.T. *NASP Communiqué, 22*(3), 1–6.

Lynch, E., & Hanson, M. (2011). *Developing cross-cultural competence: A guide for working with children and their families* (4th ed.). Baltimore, MD: Brookes.

Marinova-Todd, S., Siu, C., & Jenstadt, L. (2011). Speech audiometry with non-native with non-English speakers: The use of digits and Cantonese words as stimuli. *Canadian Journal of Speech-Pathology and Audiology, 35*(3), 220–227.

Martin, N. (2012a). *Expressive One-Word Picture Vocabulary Test (Bilingual) (EOWPVT 4-BE).* Greenville, SC: Super Duper Publications.

Martin, N. (2012b). *Receptive One-Word Picture Vocabulary Test (Bilingual) (ROWPVT 4-BE).* Greenville, SC: Super Duper Publications.

Mattes, L. (1995). *Spanish Articulation Measures (SAM).* Oceanside, CA: Academic Communication Associates.

Mayer, M. (2003a). *Frog, where are you?* (hardcover). New York, NY: Dial Books for Young Children.

Mayer, M. (2003b). *Frog goes to dinner.* (hardcover). New York, NY: Dial Books for Young Children

McCullough, J., Wilson, R. H., Birck, J. D., & Anderson, L. G. (1994). A multimedia approach for estimating speech recognition of multilingual clients. *American Journal of Audiology, 3*(1), 19–24.

McLeod, S. (2007). *The international guide to speech acquisition.* Clifton, NY: Delmar-Cengage Learning.

McLeod, S. (2012). *Multilingual speech assessments.* Bathurst, NSW, Australia: Charles Sturt University. Retrieved December 24, 2014, from http://www.csu.edu.au/research/multilingual-speech/speechassessments

McLeod, S., & Verdon, S. (2014). A review of 30 speech assessments in 19 languages other than English. *American Journal of Speech-Language Pathology, 23*, 708–723.

Miller, J., & Iglesias, A. (2008). *Systematic Analysis of Language Transcripts (SALT)* (English and Spanish, Version 9) [Computer software]. Madison: University of Wisconsin–Madison, Waisman Center, Language Analysis Laboratory.

Newman, J. L. (2010). *Development of psychometrically equivalent speech recognition threshold materials for native speakers of Samoan* (Master's thesis). Brigham Young University, Provo, UT.

Paradis, J., Genesee, F., & Crago, M. (2011). *Dual language development and disorders: A handbook on bilingualism and second language learning* (2nd ed.). Baltimore, MD: Brookes.

Peña, E. D., & Bedore, L. M. (2010, November 1). It takes two: Improvement assessment accuracy in bilingual children. *The ASHA Leader, 16,* 20–22.

Peña, E. D., Bedore, L. M., & Zlatic-Giunta, R. (2002). Category-generation performance of bilingual children: The influence of condition, category, and language. *Journal of Speech, Language, and Hearing Research, 45,* 938–947.

Peña, E., Gutiérrez-Clellen, V., Iglesias, A., Goldstein, B., & Bedore, L. (2014). *Bilingual English-Spanish Assessment (BESA).* San Rafael, CA: A-R Publications.

Ramkissoon, I., Proctor, A., Lansing, C., & Bilger, R. (2002). Digit-speech recognition thresholds for non-native speakers of English. *American Journal of Audiology, 11,* 23–28.

Roseberry-McKibbin, C. (2014). *Multicultural students with special language needs* (4th ed.). Oceanside, CA: Academic Communication Associates.

Sagon, R. (2006). The development of a phonetically balanced word recognition test in the Ilocano language. *Independent Studies and Capstones. Paper 382.* Program in Audiology and Communication Sciences, Washington University School of Medicine. Retrieved from http://digitalcommons.wustl.edu/pacs _capstones/382

Schneider, B. (1992). Effect of dialect on the determination of speech-reception thresholds in Spanish-speaking children. *Language, Speech and Hearing Services in Schools, 23,* 159–162.

Shi, L. F. (2014). Speech audiometry and Spanish-English bilinguals: Challenges in clinical practice. *American Journal of Audiology, 23*(3), 243–259.

Skehan, P. (2013). Language aptitude. In S. M. Gass & A. Mackey (Eds.), *The Routledge handbook of second language acquisition* (pp. 381–395). London, UK: Routledge.

Tardiff, T., Gelman, S., & Xu, F. (1999). Putting the "noun bias" in context: A comparison of English and Mandarin. *Child Development, 70*(3), 620–635.

Ushioda, E., & Dörnyer, Z. (2013). Motivation. In S. M. Gass & A. Mackey (Eds.), *The Routledge handbook of second language acquisition* (pp. 396–407). London, UK: Routledge.

Wiig, E., & Langdon, H. W. (2006). *The Wiig Assessment of Basic Concepts (W-ABC) Spanish version.* Greenville, SC: Super Duper Publications.

Wiig, E., Secord, W., & Semel, E. (2009). *Clinical Evaluations of Language Fundamentals–Preschool Spanish (CELF Preschool-2 Spanish).* San Antonio, TX: Pearson.

Wiig, E. H., Semel, E., & Secord, W. A. (2006). *Clinical Evaluation of Language Fundamentals, Fourth Edition Spanish (CELF-4 Spanish).* San Antonio, TX: Pearson.

Williams, J. N. (2013). Working memory and SLA. In S. M. Gass & A. Mackey (Eds.), *The Routledge handbook of second language acquisition* (pp. 427–441). London, UK: Routledge.

Zimmerman, I. L., Steiner, V. G., & Pond, R. E. (2012). *Preschool Language Scales–Fifth Edition Spanish (PLS-5 Spanish).* San Antonio, TX: Pearson.

Chapter 7

Enhancing Professional Development Programs and the Future of Interpreters

Teresa L. Wolf

- Consider the challenges facing interpreters/translators (I/Ts) working with communication disorders professionals
- Outline a professional development program designed specifically for interpreters working with speech-language pathologists and audiologists
- Provide checklists, which may be duplicated, for speech-language pathologists (SLPs) and audiologists,[1] interpreters (I/Ts), and consumers to use when evaluating their collaboration
- Suggest some activities that may help build the future for interpreters in speech-language pathology and audiology

Inconsistencies in Professional Development Programs

The field of interpreting in allied health, education, or social services has not received the same recognition as international interpreting, court interpreting, medical interpreting, or interpreting for the deaf due to a lack of certification of graduates of professional development programs who are adequately prepared to provide services in those areas.

The success of interpreting programs for specialized fields has been variable due to inconsistency in their scope or duration (Roberts, 1997). University programs often have goals that are focused on the courts or the international arena, which

---

[1]Speech-language pathologists and audiologists as a group are often referred to as communication disorders professionals in this chapter.

are different than goals for community-based interpreters (Carr, 1997). Many university programs focus on international interpreting, which is different from interpreting in contexts such as medical, clinical, or allied health professions (Pochhacker, 1997). Training for the latter purposes has consisted of continuing education programs in large universities. These programs have not been part of a rigorous, established program and have lacked professional status (Gehrke, 1993).

The International Medical Interpreters Association (2014) website (http://www.imiaweb.org/education/training-notices.asp) lists over 300 training programs currently available for medical interpreters. However, these programs do not offer specific training for interpreters who wish to work with communication disorders professionals. Even though these programs may be listed, it does not mean that they are accredited. Most often, individual agencies or school districts have offered training to I/Ts without the participation of special education personnel like speech-language pathologists (SLPs), special educators, or psychologists, resulting in inconsistencies regarding the goals of the program and follow-up training. Table 1–7 lists some examples of institutions in the United States, where conference, medical, and legal interpreters are trained, but none of them specialize in interpreting in specialized fields or allied health professions.

The lack of rigorous professional development programs for interpreters working in allied health professions or community-based organizations has negatively affected efforts to conduct research on the effectiveness of interpreters (Roberts, 1997). Graduates of existing programs often are not given the professional status they deserve. In addition, the limited success of interpreting programs is attributed to the lack of education and involvement of the professionals who use interpreter services (Corsellis, 1997; Nicholson & Martinsen, 1997; Roberts, 1997). In a program designed for speech-language pathology assistants, almost 20 years ago, Manuel-Dupont and Yoakum (1997) concluded that both communication disorders professionals and interpreters need to work together to ensure the success of the process.

Individuals who have been trained as medical interpreters may be best suited to work with SLPs and audiologists. The National Board of Certification for Medical Interpreters provides certification for those who qualify. An oral and written examination is required, and recertification is mandated in order to maintain certification. In 2009, this national board officially launched the process for national certification. Although not currently required for medical interpreters, they are being encouraged to obtain this certification (http://www.certifiedmedicalinterpreters.org/prerequisites).

Inadequate Linguistic Skills of the Interpreter/Translator (I/T)

The process of interpreting has often been of inferior quality because of interpreters' inadequate linguistic skills in one or both languages. Often, personnel seeking this type of job are immigrants themselves and may not have sufficient skills in English or their native language, especially in written language, to fulfill their duties adequately (Benmaman, 1997). Manuel-Dupont and Yoakum (1997) reported that 8 of the 22 candidates for their interpreter education program were unable to complete the program due to lack of proficiency in either their native language or English. Most of the interpreting programs have been available only in English because training in other languages is often very expensive (Roberts, 1997). It is clear that people wishing to become interpreters need to be highly proficient in both languages and be bicultural in order to succeed in the profession (Benmaman, 1997; Mikkelson & Mintz, 1997).

Low Pay and Inconsistent Hours

Another reason for fewer numbers of trained interpreters in the allied health professions is the low salary schedule given the responsibilities and skills needed to perform their duties effectively. Also, many I/Ts work as volunteers and, therefore, do not receive monetary compensation. Organizations that need the services of interpreters and society at large must understand that services provided by interpreters cannot be carried out on low salaries or on a volunteer basis (Fortier, 1997), as the services provided by an interpreter are crucial to appropriate and successful assessment and intervention. Furthermore, the overall low number of full-time positions and the variable or unpredictable hours of employment (services needed on an emergency basis by an agency) make the profession unattractive to skilled workers.

Flores, Martin, and Champlin (1996) surveyed audiologists in the five states with the largest Hispanic populations (New Mexico, California, Texas, Arizona, and Colorado). Only 18% reported they could provide services in Spanish, and 80% provided services with some help. Of those needing help, 50% asked a family member to interpret, and 30% relied on a coworker to interpret. This example illustrates the lack of availability of interpreters and inconsistencies in the training and preparation of interpreters.

Under Title III of the Americans With Disabilities Act (ADA) (1990), health care agencies are required to have an interpreter available if the patient needs one in order to understand the questions and information that are being relayed by the doctor or health care provider. Therefore, SLPs and audiologists working in health care settings should have access to interpreters. Many medical facilities are now using blue phones, which allow access to interpreters in 200 languages 24 hours per day. However, for SLPs and audiologists, using a phone for interpretation can cause problems, such as access to both areas of a sound booth for the audiologist and keeping an active child by the phone during a speech-language evaluation. Therefore, direct access to an I/T is strongly suggested in most cases, especially when clients are younger or have physical or behavioral challenges.

Collaborating with an I/T requires additional time, and is often not factored into the duties of the SLP or audiologist, as well as those of the interpreter. Advocating for this additional time with administrators is important when calculating budgets, since additional time for the process is often not factored into costs, even though the services are required by law. Costs due to inadequate services to patients with limited language proficiency can be great. For example, Quan and Lynch (2011) reported that lawsuits filed by patients who were not proficient in English and who were not provided adequate interpreting services were substantial. In the 35 cases that were analyzed, lack of adequate professional interpreting caused either death or irreparable harm to patients' health. The damages cost the carriers close to 6 million dollars, and several claims were resolved without involving any monetary settlement. Of the 35 cases, 12 included family members or friends who served as interpreters, with 2 being minors. In the case of a public school setting, inadequate interpreting services may not result in death or physical harm unless it involves ingestion of foods causing allergies or swallowing problems, but it may result in emotional stress for students and their families or inaccurate diagnosis or determination for the need of services.

For I/Ts who have gone through a professional training program or may have obtained certification, the responsibilities asked of them when working with SLPs or audiologists may be surprising. Without proper training in the needs of our field, the I/T may be left feeling inadequate and unprepared, questioning if this is really the job for which he or she trained. Therefore, training and open communication between interpreters and communication disorders professionals is essential.

DESIGNING A PROFESSIONAL TRAINING PROGRAM

There is a definite need for SLPs and audiologists to learn to train and work with interpreters. SLPs and audiologists are increasingly different both culturally and linguistically from the clients and patients they serve, and this is mirrored in the special education workforce (Tyler, Yzquierdo, López-Reyna, & Flippin, 2004). Furthermore, the demographic makeup of the American Speech-Language-Hearing Association (ASHA) is not representative of the U.S. population (ASHA, 2008). Carlson, Brauen, Klein, Schroll, and Wil-

lig (2002) found that school-based SLPs reported that, on average, over 25% of their students were from cultural and linguistic backgrounds different from their own and that 9% were English-language learners. However, they did not feel skillful at accommodating the needs of these culturally and linguistically diverse students. Caesar and Kohler (2007) found that only 28% of SLPs agreed that graduate school prepared them to evaluate bilingual students, and only 11% felt that the graduate school practicum with this population was adequate. Yet, the participation of I/Ts is essential in the absence of clinicians who do not speak the same language as their clients (Cooper & Powe, 2004). Baker, Hayes, and Fortier (1998); Flores (2005); and Jacobs, Shepard, Suaya, and Stone (2004) report that onsite interpreters benefit students and clients, and their participation has been found to improve clinical service delivery to people with limited English proficiency. Therefore, it is essential for professionals from both fields to work together.

There are currently few professional development programs available for interpreters and communication disorders professionals to learn their collaborative roles. The hypothetical program proposed here could vary depending on the professional and linguistic background of the individuals who participate and how much time is available for training. This program could be implemented at a university or technical college, in conjunction with a medical interpreter-training course or as an inservice in the schools. SLPs, audiologists, and I/Ts could attend such a program, and specific guidelines regarding recruitment and training of these professionals are described in this section.

Many of the following ideas for an interpreter-training program are based on the implementation of a program for graduate students in speech-language pathology and audiology at the University of Memphis in Tennessee from 2011 to 2014. This program was supported by a U.S. Department of Education Personnel Preparation Grant (H325K100322) to prepare future speech-language pathologists and audiologists to work with non-English–speaking clients by training and working with interpreters.[2]

Criteria for the Program Candidates

Interpreters should be proficient in the two languages in which they perform their duties and should understand the characteristics and variations of the two cultures. People training to be or licensed as speech-language pathology assistants (SLP/A) and nurses' aides, as well as trained medical interpreters, may be especially interested in this program. ASHA specifically indicates that SLP/As may (a) assist the SLP with bilingual translation during screening and assessment activities exclusive of interpretation, (b) serve as an interpreter for patients/clients/students and families who do not speak English, and (c) provide services under SLP supervision in another language for individuals who do not speak English and English-language learners (http://www.asha.org/associates/SLPA-FAQs/). However, those without experience but who possess strong interactive skills and

a desire to learn would also be good candidates. Candidates who work with audiologists may need to receive specific training in working with those specialists.

Establishing Minimum Criteria for Linguistic Proficiency in Both Oral and Written Language Skills

The criteria for the selection of certified I/Ts working with allied health and school professionals may present a challenge for monolingual and even bilingual clinicians when they need to assess clients in a language they do not speak fluently or do not speak at all. It could mirror those required for court and medical interpretation but may need to be adapted to fit schedules and needs. Testing requirements would be waived for those who have proof of completion of an interpreter certification program, as those programs often conduct their own evaluations of participants.

Mikkelson and Mintz (1997) reported that certain states, such as Washington and New Jersey, have implemented rigorous language exams for court interpreters. In California, as of 2013, court interpreter candidates could be certified in the following 14 languages in addition to American Sign Language (ASL): Arabic, Eastern and Western Armenian, Cantonese, Japanese, Korean, Khmer, Mandarin, Portuguese, Punjabi, Russian, Spanish, Tagalog, and Vietnamese (Judicial Council of California, 2013). Examinations consist of multiple-choice questions

---

[2]The contents of the referenced program were developed under a grant from the U.S. Department of Education Office of Special Education and Rehabilitation Services (OSERS), #H325100322, *Working With Interpreters: Preparing Communication Disorders Professionals to Serve Culturally and Linguistically Diverse Children and Families*, November 2010 to October 2014, Linda Jarmulowicz, principal investigator (PI) and Teresa Wolf, co-PI. This report does not necessarily represent the policy of the U.S. Department of Education, nor is it an endorsement by the federal government.

that are related to general vocabulary and word usage, grammar, reading comprehension, and translations of medical and other related vocabulary from English to the second language and vice versa. An oral language proficiency examination is also performed. The examination is tape-recorded and appraised by two examiners. Testing includes consecutive and simultaneous interpreting in addition to sight translation. The candidate's performance is assessed in both interpreting skills and in mastery of language skills. The examination is graded on a pass or fail basis.

The medical interpreting certification is described in a document (National Board for Medical Interpreting Exam, 2014, from the headquarters in Salem, Massachusetts) and consists of both an oral and written examination, just like the exam for court interpreters. The written examination is computerized, is multiple-choice, contains 51 questions, and is in English only. Current languages for which there are oral examinations include Spanish, Russian, Mandarin, Cantonese, Korean, and Vietnamese.

Setting Criteria for the Training Program for Interpreters/Translators

Criteria have already been established for federal court interpreting, medical interpreting, and deaf interpreting, but requirements for different states and agencies may differ. Therefore, inconsistencies in the selection process and training of potential medical interpreters may continue to exist, and consolidation of criteria is therefore necessary. For example, programs should include opportunities to develop short-term memory skills,

note-taking skills, consecutive interpreting with scripts, knowledge of most commonly used phrases and typical sentences, knowledge of terminology specific to the profession, and use of technology in translation (e.g., machine translation and online dictionaries). The National Board for Certification of Medical Interpreters (2009) lists prerequisites for certification, including being at least 18 years old, having a high school diploma, successful completion of a medical interpreter education program (40-hour minimum), and documented oral proficiency in English as well as oral proficiency in the targeted language (http://www.certifiedmedical interpreters.org//sites/default/files/national-board-candidate-handbook.pdf). Once these prerequisites are met, the applicant must complete and pass an oral and written examination. The Commission of Medical Interpreter Education lists the accreditation standards for medical interpreter educational programs. Accredited programs must address cultural competency, interpreting modes, standards of practice, interpreter roles, a code of ethics, and medical terminology. In addition, it is recommended that they include note-taking, simultaneous interpretation, practicum, and the interpretation of research.

An exit examination should be used to validate the proficiency of the candidate (Benmaman, 1997). Michael and Cocchini (1997) have described a program that has been offered to bilingual students at Hunter College in New York. The training has provided students with activities to enhance their interpreting and translating skills following the suggestions given by Benmaman (1997). The training has included a review of a code of ethics, role-playing exercises using videotapes, journal writing to promote reflections, and in-class discussions. The purpose of the program has not been to train students to become professional medical interpreters but for the students to gain a better understanding of interpreting and translating and to strengthen the students' bilingual skills. The existing literature has focused on educating interpreters and translators but not those who collaborate with them.

Some literature describing the requirements for interpreters working with SLPs, audiologists, and educational personnel has been available for quite some time (Fradd, 1993; Langdon, 1994; Toliver-Weddington & Meyerson, 1983). There has been scant information, though, on a description of the actual implementation of a program for such professionals, with the exception of Matsuda and O'Connor (1993) and Manuel-Dupont and Yoakum (1997). Box 7–1 briefly describes these two programs.

MINIMUM QUALIFICATIONS FOR PROGRAM PARTICIPANTS

Knowledge and Skills

Candidates desiring to serve as interpreters with communication disorders professionals should have an interest in learning about communicative disorders and be willing to learn from specific training and on the job as well. They should have excellent interpersonal skills and be willing to engage in teamwork and collaboration. They must be flexible, as each session may be different. Good organizational and time management skills are also valuable. Candidates should be aware that sessions may be emotionally difficult and physically demanding, especially when working with children.

The ideal pool of candidates would be those already trained as medical interpreters. These people already possess the skills required of interpreters but still need to be trained in using their skills in understanding the specific duties performed by SLPs and audiologists. Another group of candidates may be bilingual nurses or nurses' aides who want to specialize in assisting audiologists and otolaryngologists. Finally, bilingual candidates pursuing a career as speech-language pathology assistants are another pool from which to draw. As of March 2013, ASHA reported 25 programs around the country that train speech-language pathology assistants. For a listing of specific training programs around the country, the reader can access http://www.asha.org/associates/SLPA-Technical-Training-Programs, and for additional facts and questions about and responsibilities of these professionals, http://www.asha.org/associates/SLPA-FAQs.htm#e5, based on the Speech-Language Pathology Assistants' Scope of Practice (ASHA, 2013a, 2013b), is a very helpful resource. For example, for those states that have a majority of English-language learner (ELL) students, there are six programs listed for California, three in Arizona, but only one for Texas, and no programs are listed for New York or Florida, where there are large populations of Spanish speakers.

Proficiency in Two Languages

The candidate seeking to become an interpreter working with communication disorders professionals must fulfill a minimum bilingual language requirement, as verified through a formal examination or previous certification from an interpreter-training program. A sample examination

BOX 7–1. DESCRIPTION OF TWO INTERPRETER/TRANSLATOR PROGRAMS

Matsuda and O'Connor, Department of Communicative Disorders, California State University, Los Angeles, CA

Twelve hours of class included a discussion of basics in interpreting, applications to assessment and intervention, and general knowledge of second language development. To qualify for the program, the interpreter passed a language examination that included a written translation and a sight translation of a certain passage in both English and the native language. An oral interview was required for English only.

Manuel-Dupont and Yoakum, Utah State University and Granite School District, Salt Lake City, Utah

Phase 1 included 12 Saturday sessions over a 3-month period. The 20 participants took courses that included normal speech and language acquisition; disorders of speech, language, and hearing; behavior management; materials for intervention; and professional ethics. Participants had little opportunity to implement the knowledge they acquired in the classroom, and many dropped out of the program.

Phase 2 dropped some of the academic requirements to enable the participants to gain more practical experience. This three-weekend program of 21 hours included a brief review of the material covered in Phase 1 and ample time for practice in translation to make participants more aware of their two languages.

In Phase 3, new candidates were recruited because of some difficulties in maintaining interest and commitment from the original participants. The program focused more on practicing the candidate's current language abilities, an aspect that had not been considered before. The program ran for eight Saturdays, with each session lasting 4 to 6 hours, and focused on the translation and interpreting process; child development; case history data-gathering techniques; problems associated with using standardized language tests in assessing culturally and linguistically diverse (CLD) populations; contrasts in normal language development across cultures; techniques in informal assessment, including narratives; and dynamic assessment techniques.

Source: Langdon, H. W., & Cheng, L.-R. L. (2002). *Collaborating with interpreters and translators: A guide for communication disorders professionals* (pp. 135–136). Eau Claire, WI: Thinking Publications.

may proceed in the following manner. Initially, each candidate must pass an oral and written examination in both English and his or her other language to assess his or her linguistic skills. Foreign/modern language specialists may have to be hired to assess the candidate's linguistic skills. Alternatively, if there is a training program for interpreters in the area, it may serve as a site for assessment of language skills. An examination similar to the one proposed by the Foreign Service Institute (FSI), which is based on a scale of 1 to 5 (with 3 being the minimum standard accepted to perform a given professional task), may be used for the oral portion of the examination (Skehan, 1988). Written language skills may be assessed by asking the candidate to write a short essay on a given topic related to education (e.g., writing a letter to a parent announcing a meeting or summarizing the content of an individual education plan [IEP] in both English and the target language). The essay could be scored holistically and using various rubrics to evaluate the ability to convey meaning, sentence formulation, punctuation, and spelling. In addition, each candidate may be asked to translate a portion of a report on a client from English to his or her native language and to translate a letter written by a parent or family member describing his or her child's or relative's communication difficulty into English. Obtaining results from these assessments would assist program leaders in identifying specific areas to emphasize in the translating portion of the program. Assessing the future candidates in both English and their other languages could be based on suggestions to assess their oral and written proficiency in each by using protocols described in Tables 4–4 and 4–5.

CREATING THE PROFESSIONAL DEVELOPMENT PROGRAM

General Components

Ideally, both the interpreters and the communication disorders professionals working with them should attend the professional development program together. This enables both parties to receive the same basic information and to work collaboratively on various assignments. Pairing the I/T with an SLP or audiologist strengthens the quality of the program by ensuring that the interpreter becomes familiar with the policies of a given school, agency, clinic, or hospital. In this manner, the I/T becomes familiar with all procedures that are followed warranting his or her involvement from the beginning to the end of the process.

Interpreters receive a certificate of completion following the fulfillment of all program requirements. SLPs and audiologists receive continuing education units (CEUs) for ASHA or for the American Academy of Audiology (AAA), their state license, or both and may receive graduate credit for advancement on their agency's salary schedule. The following basic areas are addressed:

1. Roles and responsibilities of the I/T and the SLP, including study of a code of ethics, (which were outlined in Chapter 4)
2. Procedures specific to the particular profession and policies followed in the given setting, such as school, clinic, or hospital
3. The process of interpretation and translation (which was outlined in Chapter 5)

4. Locations of necessary materials and references

5. Simulations using various scenarios (e.g., conferences, gathering background information, assessments, and intervention) where SLPs, audiologists, and I/Ts practice using their skills together. Ideally, sessions extend over a 3- to 5-month period. This enables the participants to practice the information presented at each session and promotes discussion and reflection at subsequent sessions about the various issues that emerge during the process of interpreting and translating.

Implementation issues are discussed as part of the training. The interpreter and communication disorders professional should practice following a given assessment procedure together before an actual session. Resources, such as the Internet, research articles, dictionaries, and applications (apps), should be available to all participating professionals. To find out specific information on a given language, a useful resource is the Summary of 250 Cross-Linguistic Studies of Speech Acquisition, which can be found at http://www.csu.edu.au/research/multilingual-speech/speech-acquisition. Phonemic inventories of many different languages can be found on the ASHA website at http://www.asha.org/practice/multicultural/Phono/ or in printed resources such as Campbell and King (2011), Ethnologue (2013), and McLeod (2007). Also, specific tests listed in McLeod and Verdon (2014) may be helpful in assessing the students' speech skills in specific languages. The majority of the tests described by the latter authors focus on speech, but none have been developed to assess receptive and/or expressive skills. However, Table 6–1 lists recommended speech and language tests available in Spanish for bilingual students. The majority have been designed using the participation of bilingual Spanish students from various Hispanic countries living in the United States.

For both trainers and trainees in this type of program, it must be understood that the learning curve for SLPs or audiologists and interpreters working together is steep, especially if the SLPs and audiologists have not had much opportunity to work with culturally and linguistically diverse populations. This learning curve must be taken into account while training together and collaboration through honest discussion is key.

Proposed Syllabus

The ideal professional development program for preparing I/Ts to work with SLPs and audiologists would take place over a 3-month period with meetings occurring for 7 hours twice a month for a total of 42 hours of classroom time. An additional 8 hours would be factored in for various outside assignments, making it a 50-hour course. However, realistically, this type of time commitment may not be possible, and timing may need to be adjusted. Specific topics would be covered in each session. Active participation would be very important in the entire process. Each team (SLP and I/T or audiologist and I/T) would participate and work together in completing and presenting assignments.

Classes are taught by interpreters who have worked in communication disorders fields for at least 2 years and SLPs and audiologists who have collaborated with them. Curriculum and goals would be shared by all instructors. This guidebook and the 5 video clips included in this guide which demonstrate various aspects of the interpreting process prepared by Langdon and Langdon Starr would be used as materials for the program. Participants in the interpreter/translator program would be required to be present at all sessions and complete all assignments. A point system would be used to appraise the quality of the assignments, and participants must receive a certain number of points to obtain the certification. Specific rubrics would be developed for each assignment to maintain objectivity in scoring the participants' performance.

Receiving certification equivalent to that awarded to conference interpreters, interpreters for the deaf, court interpreters, and medical interpreters enables interpreters working with SLPs, audiologists, and other education or health care personnel to gain the professional status

they deserve. In addition, it would serve to inform other communication disorders professionals that the interpreter has already been trained to work with SLPs and audiologists and will require less time training or briefing before a session.

The Process of Interpreting and Translating With Communication Disorders Professionals

Suggested topics and ideas for course activities as well as assignments are included in Tables 7–1 and 7–2. Some topics include brief job descriptions for audiologist, speech-language pathologist, and interpreter; a basic review of the codes of ethics for both professions; and definitions of interpretation and translation. Assignments and activities would include finding research articles to support various

Table 7–1. *Suggested Topics to Address in Covering the Process of Interpreting and Translating*

1. Brief job descriptions for the audiologist, speech-language pathologist, and interpreter.

2. Basic review of codes of ethics for both professions.

3. Definitions of interpretation and translation.

4. Roles and responsibilities of the interpreter.

5. Roles and responsibilities of a speech-language pathologist and audiologist.

6. Review of the briefing, interaction, and debriefing (BID) process.

7. Videotape critique.

8. Simulations and role-plays.

9. Taking notes during sessions.

10. Terminology in the professions of speech-language pathology and audiology.

11. Simultaneous versus consecutive interpretation in different situations.

Table 7–2. Ideas for Course Activities and Assignments

1. Review and critique video recordings of communication professionals working with interpreters. List strengths and weaknesses of sessions.

2. Record yourself doing a session with an interpreter. Critique the session. What was effective? What would you do differently next time? Why?

3. Find research articles to support various dynamic assessment strategies. Discuss the method of the assessment, the age group for which it is appropriate, and how the interpreter and communication disorders professional would work together to implement it.

4. Practice administering a test together. Analyze what you did well and areas that may be difficult. Come up with a list of specific directions for that test.

5. Practice listening to a speaker of a different language and taking notes while he or she speaks. Now practice taking notes while listening to a speaker of a different language with a speech or language disorder. What are some similarities and differences you might note?

dynamic assessment strategies. Students could discuss the method of the assessment, the age group for which it is appropriate, and how the interpreter and communication disorders professional would work together to implement it. Another activity might be to practice administering a test together. Students could analyze what they did well and areas that were difficult and come up with a list of specific directions for that test.

Collaboration With an I/T When Assessing Bilingual/CLD Clients for Speech and Language

Topics to cover are included in Box 7–2. In this section of the training, specific areas would be discussed such as those pertaining to the briefing, interaction, and debriefing (BID) process with an emphasis on the importance of adhering

to test directions, pacing, loudness in item administration, and language adjustment depending on the age and abilities of a given client.

Collaboration With an I/T When Assessing Bilingual Children for Audiology

The same topics as those suggested for SLPs would be discussed (Box 7–3). Although some of the topics are similar, some are very specific to each profession, especially the interaction portions. Therefore, teams might need to be separated into a speech-language pathology group and an audiology group to focus on available tests and modes of administration and evaluation in their respective disciplines. Specific areas for the training of I/Ts who collaborate with audiologists are included in Box 7–3.

BOX 7–2. TOPICS TO COVER IN THE ASSESSMENT PROCESS BETWEEN AN I/T AND SLP

1. Briefing
   a. Plan for the session
   b. Responsibilities
   c. Seating arrangements
   d. Specific instructions

2. Interaction
   a. Introductions and paperwork
   b. Ethnographic interview
   c. Areas of training for testing
      i. Repetitions—allowed or not, number allowed
      ii. Pacing and pausing—fast enough to maintain client's attention, slow enough to give him or her time to process, counting to five before repeating or probing
      iii. Loudness—may need to be adjusted for hard of hearing, may sit on a certain side if hearing is better in one ear; it is important not to increase loudness due to activity in room
      iv. Prosody and expression—small children are engaged with animated prosody and facial expression
      v. Age appropriateness—shorter, more basic language for younger children
      vi. Using verbal and gestural cues—when is it allowed and when not
   d. Standardized speech and language testing
      i. Advantages and disadvantages
      ii. When to use scores
      iii. Issues surrounding translating tests into other languages
   e. Dynamic assessment
      i. An introduction to different types
      ii. Working together to obtain a language sample
   f. Exit interview with parent/family member

3. Debriefing
   a. Sharing notes and scores
   b. Discussing cultural issues and parent/family member conference
   c. Discussing changes for future sessions

BOX 7–3. TOPICS TO COVER IN THE ASSESSMENT PROCESS BETWEEN AN I/T AND AUDIOLOGIST

1. Briefing
   a. Plan for the session
   b. Responsibilities
   c. Seating arrangements
   d. Specific instructions
      i. Taking notes
      ii. Pacing and pausing
      iii. Loudness
      iv. Cues
   e. Areas of training for testing
      i. Pure-tone testing (central auditory processing vs. visual reinforcement audiometry)
      ii. Typanogram-other testing
      iii. SRT/WRT (See Chapter 6 for details)

2. Interaction
   a. Introductions and paperwork
   b. Health and development interview
   c. Following procedure in testing as planned
   d. Parent/family member conference

3. Debriefing
   a. Sharing notes and test results if relevant
   b. Discussing cultural issues and parent/family member conference
   c. Discussing changes for future sessions.

Other Roles for Interpreters When Working With Communication Disorders Professionals

Topics could include the following:

1. Speech-language intervention with culturally and linguistically diverse (CLD) clients
2. Aural rehabilitation with CLD clients
3. Prescription and testing of a hearing aid
4. Case studies

OUTCOMES AND EVALUATION

For this section, suggested topics include the following:

1. Evaluation of each team member's performance
2. Evaluation of team skills
3. Plan for working with administrators to ensure that interpreters are adequately compensated and that there

is adequate time allotted for collaboration and training

4. Course evaluation

On-the-Job Evaluations

It is important that all team members have a way to objectively measure each person's performance and provide meaningful feedback. The checklist in Table 7–3 may be used to evaluate the I/T's performance. Keeping an ongoing record enables the SLP or audiologist and the I/T to focus on specific areas to ensure that the process of interpreting and translating is adequately performed.

Table 7–3. Evaluation of the I/T's Performance

Key: 1 = Always; 2 = Often; 3 = Sometimes; 4 = Rarely; 5 = Never					
General Behaviors					
1. Does the interpreter ask questions to find out what is planned for a given meeting?	1	2	3	4	5
2. Does the interpreter seek clarification when something is ambiguous?	1	2	3	4	5
3. Does the interpreter listen carefully to what is said by all parties?	1	2	3	4	5
4. Does the interpreter share insights about a given culture in a manner that facilitates the process?	1	2	3	4	5
5. Does the interpreter appear to be respectful of both cultures and seem well respected by the community and the families that need the interpreter's services?	1	2	3	4	5
6. Is the interpreter willing to acquire new skills to perform the job more effectively?	1	2	3	4	5
7. Is there evidence that the interpreter maintains neutrality and confidentiality throughout the process?	1	2	3	4	5
8. Does the interpreter accept feedback from parents and other parties involved in the process?	1	2	3	4	5
9. Is the interpreter punctual?	1	2	3	4	5
Specific Interpretations/Translation Skills					
1. Does the interpreter appear to convey a given message clearly?	1	2	3	4	5
2. Does the interpreter retranslate something when it is unclear to any participant?	1	2	3	4	5
3. Does the interpreter use different methods of conveying the same information?	1	2	3	4	5
4. Does the interpreter appropriately use different levels of formality?	1	2	3	4	5
5. Does the translator appropriately use back translation to ensure that a given document has preserved the original meaning?	1	2	3	4	5

Source: Langdon and Cheng (2002).

In addition, a special evaluation form may be used for parents, relatives, and others who have used the services of the interpreter. Box 7–4 is adapted from suggestions by Garber and Mauffette-Leenders (1997). It lists several areas to consider such as general observations of the I/T while performing the job and his or her interpretation/translation skills on a scale of 1 to 5, with 1 being the lowest and 5 the highest score. This assessment would need to be translated into the language used by the consumer who might be the parent, relative, or client, depending on the situation. If clients or family members have difficulty reading the survey, they could be encouraged to complete it at home with the help of a family member or friend.

Interpreters will need to be informed when hired that their performance evaluations will include feedback received from both the professionals working with them and clients (families/consumers). This feedback should be used only as part of the evaluation and is for the purpose of identifying areas of strength and areas targeted for change. It should be emphasized that the changes are meant to benefit the clients served. The survey results should not be the deciding factor in promoting or dismissing an interpreter. The assessment should be completed in a constructive manner and based on several observations or situations. Table 7–4 includes questions for an interpreter to complete to assess the effectiveness of his or her collaboration with an SLP or audiologist. Interpreters can also use this form to evaluate themselves.

BOX 7–4. THE CONSUMER'S FEEDBACK

Dear _____,

Today you participated in a session where the services of an interpreter, Mr./Ms. _____, were used. Your responses and feedback will help us to monitor the quality of services provided by this person. Thank you for your time.

Language: _____
Date: _____

Purpose of Session:

☐ To gather information

☐ To share progress

☐ To share assessment results

☐ To assist with intervention

How many times have you worked with this interpreter?

- ☐ 0
- ☐ 1
- ☐ 2
- ☐ 3
- ☐ 4
- ☐ 5+

How many times have you worked with this specialist?

- ☐ 0
- ☐ 1
- ☐ 2
- ☐ 3
- ☐ 4
- ☐ 5+

On a scale of 0 to 5 please rate the following questions:

(0) = Not applicable; (1) = Very poor; (2) = Poor; (3) = Average; (4) = Good; (5) = Very good

Did the speech-language pathologist, audiologist and interpreter explain their roles to you? _____

How well did you understand this interpreter? _____

What can we do better next time? _____

Please provide any further comments: _____

_____

Source: Obtaining Feedback from Non-English Speakers, by N. Garber and L.A. Mauffette-Leenders, in *The critical link: Interpreters in the community* (pp. 131–143), by S. E. Carr, R. Roberts, A. Dufour, and D. Steyn (Eds.), 1997, Philadelphia: Johns Benjamins. © 1997 by Johns Benjamins.

Originally, adapted with permission in the original version by Langdon, H. W., & Cheng, L.-R. L. (2002). *Collaborating with interpreters and translators: A guide for communication disorders professionals* (pp. 149–150). Eau Claire, WI: Thinking Publications.

Table 7–4. *Interpreter/Translator's Self-Assessment*

Setting:	School	Clinic	Hospital
Date:		Length of conference:	
Conference when the interpreting took place: (Please circle all that apply)			
To gather information	Assessment report	Progress report	To assist with interpretation
How many times have you worked with this SLP/audiologist?			1 2 3 4 5
When do you work with this SLP/audiologist? (Please circle all that apply)			
Interviews for assessments	Reporting results of assessments	Progress reports	Intervention sessions
Which are most frequent?			
What type of interpreting do you typically use when working with this professional? (Please circle all that apply)			
Consecutive		Simultaneous (or whispered)	
Do you have time to brief and debrief with the SLP/audiologist? YES NO			
If yes, how often?			
Almost always	Often	Sometimes	Rarely
If not, please state the reason(s):			
Did you let the SLP or audiologist know if you did not agree with what he or she said after the meeting with the client? YES NO			
Please explain your answer:			
What suggestions do you have to improve service delivery when an interpreter is involved?			
What are some of your personal reactions to the interpreting process when working with an SLP/audiologist?			

Source: Adapted from Langdon and Cheng (2002).

SUMMARY

In this chapter, we have described some of the ongoing challenges experienced by I/Ts who are assigned to work with com- munication disorders professionals and who primarily work with the pediatric population in the schools and educational settings. Difficulty in finding adequately trained interpreters is an important issue to consider. This difficulty stems from the fact that I/Ts and SLPs who work with pediatric populations are sometimes not properly trained, as there are no legal guidelines that direct those individuals and professionals to follow specific protocols. Even when trained medical interpreters may be hired to assist SLPs and audiologists working in the schools or medical settings, they need to be briefed on the particular profession, methods, laws, and regulations. There also is no certification required, and the financial compensation for the job may not be adequate. Suggestions for training those individuals along with SLPs and audiologists were made. It will be helpful if the job provided by I/Ts working in the school/educational setting is recognized as a profession. Creating legislation toward that end can be important and could be attempted by those professionals working in the communication disorders field. By not adhering to specific protocols, we are also running the risk of providing services to CLD populations that are substandard and do not follow the law spelled out by the Individuals with Disabilities Education Act or IDEA. At the same time, more effort could be put toward determining best practices that are evidence based. Specific areas to consider were described in Chapter 5.

DISCUSSION ITEMS AND ACTIVITIES

1. What are two things that could be done to address the challenges that interpreters may face when working with speech-language pathologists and audiologists?

2. What criteria would you use for selecting participants in a training

program for interpreters in communication disorders?

3. Which areas are important to discuss during the BID process from the standpoint of the SLP, audiologist, and the interpreter?

4. Role-play a briefing prior to an evaluation between an interpreter and a speech-language pathologist or audiologist using Box 7–2 or Box 7–3 as a guide.

5. Discuss ways in which you could evaluate your program or sessions. Describe how you might proceed and how the information may be applied to improve sessions for interpreters, communication disorders professionals, families, and clients.

REFERENCES

Americans With Disabilities Act of 1990, 42 U.S.C. §§12181–12189.

American Speech-Language-Hearing Association. (2008). *Highlights and trends: ASHA counts for year end 2008*. Retrieved May 22, 2014, from http://www.asha.org/research/member data/member-counts.htm

American Speech-Language-Hearing Association (ASHA). (2013a). *Technical training programs for speech-language pathology assistants*. Retrieved May 22, 2015, from http://www.asha.org/associates/SLPA-Technical-Training-Programs

American Speech-Language-Hearing Association (ASHA). (2013b). *Frequently asked questions: Speech-language pathology assistants (SLPAs)*. Retrieved May 22, 2014, from http://www.asha.org/associates/SLPA-FAQs.htm#e5

Baker, D. W., Hayes, R., & Fortier, J. P. (1998). Interpreter use and satisfaction with interpersonal aspects of care for Spanish-speaking patients. *Medical Care, 36*(10), 1461–1470.

Benmaman, V. (1997). Legal interpreting by any other name is still legal interpreting. In S. E. Carr, R. P. Roberts, A. Dufour, & D. Steyn (Eds.), *The critical link. Interpreters in the community* (pp. 179–190). Amsterdam, the Netherlands: John Benjamins.

Caesar, L. G., & Kohler, P. D. (2007). The state of school-based bilingual assessment: Actual practice versus recommended guidelines. *Language, Speech, and Hearing Services in Schools, 38*(3), 190–199.

Campbell, G. L., & King, G. (2011). *Concise compendium of the world's languages* (2nd ed.). London, UK: Routledge.

Carlson, E., Brauen, M., Klein, S., Schroll, K., & Willig, S. (2002). *Study of personnel needs in special education: Key findings* [Report submitted to the U.S. Department of Education Office of Special Education Programs]. Retrieved August 27, 2014, from http://ferdig.coe.ufl.edu/spense/Results.html

Carr, S. E. (1997). A three-tiered healthcare interpreter system. In S. E. Carr, R. P. Roberts, A. Dufour, & D. Steyn (Eds.), *The critical link: Interpreters in the community* (pp. 271–276). Amsterdam, the Netherlands: John Benjamins.

Commission of Medical Interpreter Education. (2014). *Accreditation standards.* Retrieved July 11, 2014, from http://www.imiaweb.org/uploads/pages/580.pptx

Cooper, L. A., & Powe, N. R. (2004). Disparities in patient experiences, healthcare processes and outcomes: The role of patient-provider racial, ethnic, and language concordance. *The Commonweath Fund, 753.* Retrieved from http://www.commonwealthfund.org/programs/minority/cooper_raceconcordance_753.pdf

Corsellis, A. (1997). Training needs of public personnel working with interpreters. *Benjamins Translation Library, 19,* 77–92.

Ethnologue. (2013). *Languages of the world.* Retrieved September 15, 2014, from http://www.ethnologue.com

Flores, G. (2005). The impact of medical interpreter services on the quality of health care: A systematic review. *Medical Care Research and Review, 62*(3), 255–299.

Flores, P., Martin, F. N., & Champlin, C. A. (1996). Providing audiological services to Spanish speakers. *American Journal of Audiology, 5*(1), 69–73.

Fortier, J. P. (1997). Interpreting for health in the United States: Government partnership with communities, interpreters, and providers. *Benjamins Translation Library, 19,* 165–178.

Fradd, S. H. (1993). *Creating the team: To assist culturally and linguistically diverse students.* Retrieved September 7, 2014, from https://openlibrary.org/authors/OL610899A/Sandra_H._Fradd

Garber, N., & Maufette-Leenders, L. A. (1997). Obtaining feedback from non-English speakers. In S. E. Carr, R. P. Roberts, A. Dufour, & D. Steyn (Eds.), *The critical link: Interpreters in the community* (pp. 131–143). Amsterdam, the Netherlands: John Benjamins.

Gehrke, M. (1993). Community interpret. In C. Pincken (Ed.), *Translation. The vital link. Proceedings of the XIII World Congress of FIT* (Vol. 1, pp. 417–421). London, UK: Institute of Translating and Interpreting.

International Medical Interpreters Association. (2014). *Training directory.* Retrieved July 11, 2014, from http://www.imiaweb.org/education/trainingnstices.asp

Jacobs, E. A., Shepard, D. S., Suaya, J. A., & Stone, E. (2004). Overcoming language barriers in healthcare: Costs and benefits of interpreter services. *American Journal of Public Health, 94,* 866–869.

Judicial Council of California. (2013). *Fact sheet.* Retrieved May 22, 2014, from http://www.courts.ca.gov/documents/Fact_Sheet-_Court_Interpreters.pdf

Langdon, H. W., & Cheng, L.-R. L. (2002). *Collaborating with interpreters and translators: A guide for communication disorders professionals.* Eau Claire, WI: Thinking Publications.

Langdon, H. W. (with Siegel, V., Halog, L., & Sánchez-Boyce, M.). (1994). *Interpreter/translator process in the educational setting.* Sacramento, CA: Resources in Special Education (RISE).

Manuel-Dupont, S., & Yoakum, S. (1997). Training interpreter paraprofessionals to assist in the language assessment of English language learners in Utah. *Communication Disorders Quarterly, 18*(1), 91–102.

Matsuda, M., & O'Connor, L. C. (1993, April). *Creating an effective partnership: Training bilingual communication aides.* Paper presented at the California Speech, Language, and Hearing Association Conference, Palm Springs, CA.

McLeod, S. (Ed.). (2007). *The international guide to speech acquisition.* Clifton Park, NY: Thomson Delmar Learning.

McLeod, S., & Verdon, S. (2014). A review of 30 speech assessments in 19 languages other than English. *American Journal of Speech-Language Pathology, 23*, 708–723.

Michael, S., & Cocchini, M. (1997). Training college students as community interpreters: An innovative model. In S. E. Carr, R. P. Roberts, A. Dufour, & D. Steyn (Eds.), *The critical link: Interpreters in the community* (pp. 237–248). Amsterdam, the Netherlands: John Benjamins.

Mikkelson, H., & Mintz, H. (1997). Orientation workshops for interpreters of all languages: How to strike a balance between the ideal world and reality. *Benjamins Translation Library, 19*, 55–64.

National Board for Certification of Medical Interpreters. (2009). *National Board prerequisites*. Retrieved June 20, 2014, from http://www.certifiedmedicalinterpreters.org/prerequisites

National Board for Medical Interpreting Exam (2014). Salem, MA. Retrieved from http://www.certifiedmedicalinterpreters.org/contact

Nicholson, N. S., & Martinsen, B. (1997). Court interpretation in Denmark. *Benjamins Translation Library, 19*, 259–270.

Pochhacker, F. (1997). "Is there anybody out there?" Community interpreting in Austria. In S. E. Carr, R. P. Roberts, A. Dufour, & D. Steyn (Eds.), *The critical link: Interpreters in the community* (pp. 215–225). Amsterdam, the Netherlands: John Benjamins.

Quan, H., & Lynch, J. (2011). *The high costs of language barriers in medical malpractice*. Retrieved May 22, 2014, from http://www.pacificinterpreters.com/docs/resources/high-costs-of-language-barriers-in-malpractice_nhelp.pdf

Roberts, R. P. (1997). Community interpreting today and tomorrow. *Benjamins Translation Library, 19*, 7–28.

Skehan, P. (1988). Language testing: Part 1. *Language Teaching, 21*(4), 211–221.

Toliver-Weddington, G., & Meyerson, M. D. (1983). Training paraprofessionals for identification and intervention with communicatively disordered bilinguals. In D. R. Omark & J. Erickson (Eds.), *The bilingual exceptional child* (pp. 379–395). San Diego, CA: College-Hill Press.

Tyler, N., Yzquierdo, Z., López-Reyna, N., & Flippin, S. S. (2004). Cultural and linguistic diversity and the special education workforce: A critical overview. *Journal of Special Education, 38*(1), 22–38.

Part II

A Guide for the Interpreter/Translator

Part II was written specifically for you, the interpreter and translator (I/T), who will be collaborating with the communication disorders professionals (i.e., speech-language pathologist [SLP] or audiologist). It includes three different topics that are important for you to keep in mind as you work specifically with the two professionals mentioned above. Some of the information may be more general, and some may be more specific. However, from my experience, those of you who work closely with SLPs or audiologists, especially in the public school setting, have varying personal and educational backgrounds as well as differing types of preparation and experiences for this important role. The end of this guide includes a glossary, which will hopefully facilitate your learning and use of specific terminology used in the two professions.

Part I was written with my colleague, Terry Irvine Saenz, and is a newly edited and extensively revised version of the same topic previously published in 2002, with a different colleague, Lilly Cheng (*Collaborating With Interpreters and Trans-*

lators: A Guide for Communication Disorders Professionals, 2002). In addition to updating references, we have added chapters on cultural and linguistic issues. Also, five video clips are available illustrating various important points concerning the collaboration of interpreters and the professionals in the fields of speech-language pathology and audiology. Each video clip includes a PowerPoint to reinforce the main concepts and steps to follow.

Part II, which you are reading, is a newer version of a handbook that I originally wrote in 2002 as well, which was for I/Ts' use and was entitled *Interpreters and Translators in Communication Disorders: A Practitioner's Handbook*, addressed specifically to the I/T who will be working with the SLP and/or audiologist.

As you well know, the interpreting and translating process is very complex, and very few people appreciate the knowledge, skills, and responsibilities that are undertaken by those I/Ts who collaborate with SLPs and audiologists. Currently, those I/Ts who work in international conferences, in the medical or judicial fields, or with the deaf can receive specific training to specialize in those areas and are recognized by receiving special certificates.

However, no specific training is offered for those who work in specialized fields such as speech-language pathology, audiology, psychology, and occupational or physical therapy. The information presented in Part II is written for those who will be collaborating with SLPs and audiologists. These individuals work with clients who have hearing, listening, speaking, reading, and writing challenges and are often referred to as the professionals who specialize in communication disorders.

My own experience, as well as that of several colleagues who need to work with an interpreter and/or translator, has demonstrated that those individuals do not receive specific training, and their skills are often taken somewhat for granted. There are no guidelines for either the professional (SLP or audiologist) or you (I/T) on how to best collaborate in order to meet the language needs of those clients and their families who do not speak the majority language (in this case, English in the United States). Often, individuals who are not familiar about the process of interpreting or translating assume that knowing two languages is sufficient to do the job. We know that it is much more complex, and it requires training and practice. Part I provides information on various aspects of the process; it includes a summary on the current demographics of the second-language-speaking population in the United States, cultural and linguistic variables that need to be considered in working with this multilingual and multicultural population, a procedure to follow in order to provide professional interviews

and conferences for family members as well as fair speech and language and audiological assessments for clients, the roles and responsibilities of both parties (SLPs or audiologists and I/Ts), and suggestions for the setup of training for both the communication professional and the interpreter/translator.

Part II includes three chapters covering the following topics: (a) the interpreting and translating process, (b) the interpreter/SLP or audiologist collaboration process, and (c) evaluation and outcomes of the process. At the end of the guide, there is a glossary of terms that I thought would help you with your work. Each chapter begins with a listing of the main points discussed in that chapter and includes a varying number of tables and boxes. Each of the three chapters included in Part II ends with some activities for practice and what I refer to as "self-assessment items" in order to prepare yourself for the various facets of your job.

You may be familiar with the content included here to varying degrees, depending on your individual formal training and/or your experiences. It is recommended that you refer to the specific chapters of Part I to supplement your prior knowledge or a given skill. I will make reference to specific pages where I feel it will be necessary to review prior information. However, if you wish, you may want to read the information as needed. The guide addresses issues that pertain to the young population (infant to age 21), but the content may be applied to the older population as well.[1]

---

[1]*Client, child,* or *student* will be used interchangeably.

Chapter 8

The Interpreting and Translating Process

Henriette W. Langdon

This chapter includes the following:

- What you should know about speech-language pathologists (SLPs) and audiologists
- Interpretation and translation terminology
- Expectations of interpreters and translators who collaborate with SLPs and audiologists
- A proposed code of ethics for interpreters and translators who work with professionals involved in the field of communication disorders
- How to facilitate the interpreting and translating process and a description of some common errors
- Activities to practice your interpreting and translating skills
- Self-assessment items[1]

Your role as an interpreter or translator (I/T) is essential to the success of SLPs and audiologists working with clients who are culturally and linguistically diverse (CLD). In this chapter, you will learn about the essentials of the professional charges of SLPs and audiologists and what to expect when working with professionals in this field. You will also learn about your role as an I/T and the skills you need to have to perform your important function in working primarily in the educational setting such as a special clinic or public school. Ethical practices are important for you and for professionals who work in the field of communication disorders. Some proposed guidelines in the form of a code of ethics are proposed. You will also have the opportunity to practice translating orally and in writing some common statements used with a variety of clients in the two fields as well as practice some interpreting with subject matter that is specific to the two professions.

[1]You will find much of the content illustrated in video clips 1, 2, and 3.

WHAT YOU SHOULD
KNOW ABOUT SPEECH-
LANGUAGE PATHOLOGISTS

Job Responsibilities of Speech-Language Pathologists

The job responsibilities of an SLP that most directly affect your interpretation or translation work include the following:

- Identify and assess clients of various ages (this content is directed to the infant or birth to 12th-grade population but may apply to older clients as well) who have challenges in communicating adequately (e.g., difficulties in articulating sounds); problems with language (using correct grammar, syntax, expressing ideas); fluency challenges (stuttering); difficulties using adequate voice pitch, stress, or loudness; and challenges in performing adequately in tasks requiring reading and writing. Once these clients are diagnosed, the SLP is responsible for drafting intervention plans and treating these clients.
- Conduct interviews and conferences with family members and clients, if appropriate, to obtain additional information to facilitate the assessment or intervention plan or to report results of an assessment.
- Collaborate with other professionals to enhance the success of the intervention plan. In the school setting, other professionals may include the general and/ or speech education teacher, the

psychologist, the counselor or other mental health professional, the occupational or physical therapist, and adaptive physical educator (APE). In a clinic or hospital, it may be a physician, a therapist, or a social worker.

Interviews and Conferences

An interview or a conference follows a certain format. Specific topics are covered in each situation. Most typically, information about a client's challenges and general communication skills as well as development in general is collected during an interview. Results of an assessment or intervention are discussed during a conference for an IFSP (individual family service plan) for the birth/infant to 3 years of age population or when an IEP (individual education plan) is developed for the school-age child 3 to 21 years of age.

The use of specific vocabulary is needed when conducting an interview or a conference. For example, during an interview, the SLP might bring up medical issues that relate to information about birth and early infancy history as well as motor and speech developmental milestones. The child may also have some other medical issues, such having heart or breathing problems, ear infections, some craniofacial anomalies like a cleft palate, syndromes like Down syndrome, some metabolic anomalies, motor difficulties due to cerebral palsy, and/or swallowing issues, for example. Other questions may be related to the child's favorite games and activities as well as a description of a typical day. During a conference, the SLP reports the results of an assessment and/ or goals for intervention, and other terms might be used related to the profession. For a typical interview, you may want to refer to Table 5–1 in Chapter 5, page 111.

Assessment and Intervention

Various types of tests exist (e.g., normed, criterion referenced, and inventories). SLPs select tests based on their purpose and their usefulness with various age groups or suspected disabilities. Each type of test has limitations on its usefulness, so that the SLP may use a variety of instruments to develop a fuller picture of the client's strengths and challenges. You may be requested to converse with the child, to play with the younger child, and/or to read/look at a book together to collect a language sample from the student, and the SLP will need to train you on how to best obtain this sample. And, you will need to analyze it together to find out how the child produces sounds, words, and sentences and how the child understands and expresses him or herself. Reading Chapter 2 would be helpful for you to gain more insight into this matter. In some cases, the SLP may seek your opinion about the child's general speech and language skills. Therefore, he or she is expecting you to provide some guidance in deciding whether or not you feel there is a problem. However, the SLP will need to use his or her own expertise and clinical judgment based on this information and what he or she hears from the child and your input to make an ultimate decision. In addition, the SLP will work with you to teach you what you need to know regarding various methods of assessment. Computerized materials such those included in an iPad may be utilized, especially in therapy, and augmentative communica-

tion materials may be used such as cards and/or a variety of computerized devices, in addition to various toys, games, and books. Again, the SLP will work with you to help you learn the language needed for the setting, and be sure to ask for help if you need direct help or clarification.

Paperwork Procedures

The process of interpreting and translating is enhanced if you are familiar with the admission and dismissal procedures and the paperwork involved in a school setting. Understanding the referral, assessment, and conference protocol related to the development of an IEP or IFSP will enhance the efficiency of your job performance. Your SLP will be responsible for teaching you the specific information you will need to be successful in each setting.

WHAT YOU SHOULD KNOW ABOUT AUDIOLOGISTS

Job Responsibilities of an Audiologist

The job responsibilities of an audiologist that directly affect your interpretation or translation work may include the following:

- Assess a client who has difficulty with hearing and/or processing auditory information by following the directions provided by the professional.
- Conduct conferences with parents to obtain a clinical history about the client with a focus on hearing

as well as counsel them regarding the use of hearing aids and devices, in addition to suggesting specific educational programs for hearing-impaired clients as well as those who may have received cochlear implants.

- Collaborate with other professionals such as general and special education teachers as well as SLPs and possibly ear, nose and throat specialists (otolaryngologists) to enhance the success of assessment and intervention.

Interviews and Conferences

Specific issues are addressed in each type of context. For example, during an interview, the audiologist asks questions about the extent of the hearing problem and its possible origin, asks about the situations where the client feels most uncomfortable, and collects pertinent background medical history. If hearing aids are prescribed, the audiologist holds a conference with the parents and the client, if appropriate, to discuss recommendations regarding the use of the hearing aids and the best learning and communication environment for the client.

The audiologist uses specific professional terms related to this specialty. Your understanding of these terms is important in facilitating the interpreting or translating process. Refer to the Glossary to begin learning specific terms.

Assessment and Intervention

Many types of tests are used (e.g., pure-tone, air and bone conduction, auditory brainstem response [ABR], speech dis-

crimination, speech reception, tympanogram, and acoustic impedance). Test results may be recorded on an audiogram or other report formats. The kinds of hearing losses that are identified may involve deafness, conductive hearing loss due to otitis media, or sensorineural hearing loss. The various tests are described in video clip 3.

Intervention may involve a session to fit a hearing aid and to explain its use and care, followed by one or more return visits to check on its effectiveness. In schools, the audiologist may participate in an annual IEP meeting to update information on the student's needs and progress and make recommendations for the following year.

Paperwork Procedures

The success of the interpreting or translating process is enhanced if you are familiar with the admission and dismissal procedures and paperwork involved in a school setting or a clinic, just as when you collaborate with an SLP. Understanding the referral, assessment, and conference process related to the development of an IFSP for an infant/birth to 3-year-old or an IEP for a 3- to 21-year-old enhances the efficiency of your job performance.

INTERPRETING AND TRANSLATING TERMINOLOGY

Interpreting involves orally transmitting the same message from the first language (L1) to the second language (L2). *Translating* involves transmitting the same written message from L1 to L2.

Interpreting is considered more demanding than translating because the interpreter needs to continually shift from L1 to L2 and vice versa. Interpretation takes place during interviews, conferences, assessments, and intervention. Interpreters must have knowledge and use of specific vocabulary, good auditory memory, and the ability to respond quickly while under pressure. There are two types of interpreting:

- **Consecutive interpreting** involves transmitting segments of a speaker's message while the speaker pauses for the interpreting to be carried out. The segments that are conveyed should be neither too long nor too short to be well understood. In consecutive interpreting, there is lag time between what is said by each speaker. This is the most frequent type of interpreting used in the setting (public school or clinic) that you will be using.
- **Simultaneous interpreting** involves interpreting the message from one language to the other without lag time. This method is used primarily in the international relations field. An interpreter may want to use this method in a clinical setting to keep the meeting flowing without interruption.

Using either type of interpretation, the interpreter may whisper the interpretation to the parents or family members as the meeting is proceeding if it can be carried out without disrupting communication.

Translation is used to transmit information from letters and documents such as the IFSP or IEP or from informal tests. Knowledge of specific vocabulary is necessary for translation. Translation speed is important in some cases (e.g., when the

translator is asked to translate a written document orally). There are two types of translation:

- **Prepared translation** involves preparing a written version of any type of document, such as a letter or a report, in advance. This is the most common type of translating in the field of communication disorders.
- **Sight translation** involves providing a spoken translation while reading a written document. Fewer formal terms and structures are used in sight translation than in prepared translation.

EXPECTATIONS OF INTERPRETERS AND TRANSLATORS WHO COLLABORATE WITH SLPS AND AUDIOLOGISTS

In this segment, we review the *linguistic* and *procedural* skills that you need to have and know to perform successfully as an interpreter and translator when you collaborate with an SLP or an audiologist. We also focus on your specific *roles* and *responsibilities* during this process. Tips on facilitating the interpreting and translating process are also offered.

Linguistic Skills

Six linguistic skills are needed to ensure that you can successfully bridge the communication between two parties who do not share the same language:

1. **Oral and written proficiency with two languages.** You must understand and

speak both languages fluently and at a normal rate. You must also have accurate written language skills, including grammar and spelling, for both languages. A condition to be hired will be that you fulfill some important requirements, which were listed in Table 4–4 on page 93 in the guide for the oral examination. The oral examination proposed is similar to that of the Foreign Service Institute (FSI), which is based on a scale of 1 to 5, with 3 being the minimum standard accepted to perform a given professional task. Ideally, native speakers of both English and the target language will need to interview you. The oral interview may take place in the group session or different sessions for each language. The topics will vary from general and conversational to those more specifically related to the job. For example, how are you able to respond to a parent who tells you she missed her appointment because she did not have transportation, or how would you respond if a parent did not understand she could not stay the entire time during her child's assessment? According to the FSI criteria for level 3, you must be intelligible in most instances, although you may make some occasional grammar and pronunciation errors that are not severe enough to interfere with communication.

For the written portion, you will be asked to translate a letter to a parent into your language or a fragment of a report from English, and you will need to achieve a score of 3, which will follow a certain rubric judging if you have conveyed the meaning and your use of grammar, spelling, and punctuation. As I mentioned earlier,

familiarity with expectations of language skills of children proficient in the language in which you are interpreting will be helpful to the SLP to guide her in her diagnosis of a possible speech and/or language problem. However, the ultimate decision will rest on the SLP's clinical judgment and professional expertise. More on oral and written requirements will be discussed in Chapter 10.

2. **Knowledge of two cultures and non-verbal communication.** You must be sensitive to social and cultural variations, including dialectal variations, pronunciation differences, and paralinguistic messages (e.g., intonation, use of gestures, and facial expressions). You must also be sensitive to differences that are tied to a given cultural background and that may affect the client's understanding of procedures, interpretation of assessment results, or acceptance of medical and educational labels. Common cultural differences fall in the areas of child-rearing practices, beliefs about possible medical conditions, illnesses, communication and educational performance, and understanding of the role of parents and families in carrying out communication disorders professionals' suggestions and recommendations. For example, the word *enfermito* in Spanish is used to mean "a little child who is sick" as well as "a little child who is experiencing anywhere from moderate to severe developmental and/or learning problems." Humorous statements are often difficult to interpret because of their use of idioms and multiple-meaning words. You may need to clarify intended meanings of ambiguous statements to avoid miscommunication. Reading

Chapter 3 of this guide may be very helpful to you to gain a broader perspective on considerations related to various aspects of culture.

3. **Ability to convey the same meaning in two languages.** As you know, variations across languages are reflected at the sound, word, and sentence levels. Some languages use sounds that do not exist in other languages. Words with the same meaning but spoken in two different ways may be quite different in their length and speech sounds. Some passages require many more syllables or words to use in one language compared to another. In addition, words are located in different positions within a sentence depending on the language. For example, adjectives may be placed before or after a noun. Pronouns may have formal and informal forms that indicate the relationship between the speakers, or this distinction may not be marked at all in some languages. Rather than interpret word by word, the interpreter must understand the message from the first language and restate it accurately in the second language. Thus, when interpreting or translating, you must convey messages without changing the meaning. A word-by-word translation or interpretation cannot convey the same meaning because grammar and word use are different in each language. For example, translation of a Spanish statement that means "Would you please sign this assessment plan?" would become "Do me the favor of signing this plan of assessment" ("*Hágame favor de firmar este plan de evaluación*") following a word-by-word translation.

4. **Knowledge of professional terminology.** You should be familiar with specific terminology and procedures used in speech-language pathology and audiology to perform with greater speed and accuracy. If you are not sure of the meaning of a certain word in the target language, it is permissible to use a dictionary even when a meeting is being held. If a word in English does not exist in a given target language, a definition for a given term or concept may be necessary. But first, you need to be sure that the definition is accurate by double-checking with the professional. In those instances, you need to interpret all that is happening.

5. **Familiarity with dialectal differences.** Dialects are regional variations within a language. These variations may result in vocabulary differences (e.g., the same word may indicate different meanings, or different words may be used for the same meaning). Many pronunciation differences occur between regional dialects. None of these differences should be judged as less correct than another. Interpreters must be aware of usages that are correct in a particular dialect in order to transmit messages accurately and to assist the SLP or the audiologist in distinguishing between language differences and disorders. Therefore, you must be aware of potential dialectal variations in a language. Vocabulary differences may lead to confusion of word meanings. Differences in grammar or speech sounds may be misinterpreted as errors. You can find more useful information by reading Chapter 2 in the guide.

6. **Ability to adapt to the speech and language of people with communication disorders.** You need to use careful listening skills when working with

people who have communication disorders. A client may present varying degrees of challenge in comprehending and expressing information. This is especially important during the assessment process. Quite often, a younger child or an older one with more severe language difficulties will be difficult to understand because he or she may misarticulate or omit sounds (or do both), and this will interfere with his or her intelligibility. During assessments, pay close attention and transcribe what the client says verbatim (sound by sound, word by word) and do not edit what is said or do not change sounds. (Note: You will need to explain to the SLP what is said versus what should have been said.) Two important linguistic phenomena should be considered:

a. *Code-switching:* Code-switching is the use of two different languages in the same response or responding to a question using an alternate language. This phenomenon is common in competent bilingual individuals and may be noted in interpreted or translated contexts. You may need to code-switch when there is no equivalent word or concept in the other language. In doing so, it may also be necessary to give an explanation of the concept, since it is likely that the recipient of the message will not know the foreign term. Ask the SLP or the audiologist to provide that explanation. Code-switching by the client should not be considered a sign of a disability without diagnostic information collected by the SLP.

b. *Language loss:* Language loss is a regression of skills in an individual's first language. It may occur for many reasons, such as the person's lack of practice, use of the language only in certain situations, or social or political reasons that may discourage the use of the language. Language loss by the client should not be considered a sign of a disability without other diagnostic information collected by the SLP. Your observations as an interpreter will assist the professional to document the extent of the language loss and possibly the reasons for the loss as well.

Procedural Skills

1. **Familiarity with specific procedures followed in each job setting.** You must be familiar with procedures followed by the specialties of speech-language pathology and audiology. Procedures may differ according to where the child or student may receive services. For example, even within a public school, a child may receive special education services in a pullout situation (small room), within the classroom setting or both, or in a resource room. A younger child or infant may receive services in a center, at home, or both.

2. **Understanding of your function and role.** You must remain neutral and accurate in your communication. Your responsibilities may be redefined as your relationship with the SLP or audiologist develops. Remember to function within the guidelines of the code of ethics, which is spelled out in Table 4–6 on page 98.

3. **Flexibility.** You must be able to work with a variety of people with all sorts of ages, personalities, and levels of education. In all cases, you should be patient and respectful. Flexibility is also required when called on to provide services with short notice or no advance preparation time.

Roles and Responsibilities of Interpreters and Translators

The interpreter or translator's responsibility is to bridge communication in various contexts between parties who do not share the same language. Consider the following list of roles and responsibilities:

1. **Maintain neutrality.** Remain neutral about the behaviors and statements conveyed by all parties involved in the interpreting process. No value judgments should be made about a person's beliefs, practices, or skills. Maintaining neutrality also means not becoming actively involved in a situation. You may be tempted to take on an advocacy role or provide advice to a client or a family member. However, your role is to represent the other speaker's meaning, not to interject your own ideas.

    The role of an interpreter is difficult because you are the only one in the meeting who understands the interaction of two languages and cultures. When I mean *neutral*, it does not indicate that you should not care about the topics being discussed; it means that you need to convey the information from either party as faithfully as possible. However, your role may change, but not during the interaction between two parties that do

share the same language. Nevertheless, this alternative role needs to be discussed with the professional you are working with ahead of time. For example, you may also act as a *cultural broker*, which implies that you may offer some suggestions to the professional you are working with before or after the meeting. Specifically, if you suspect that a particular family is likely to have difficulty accepting the fact that their child may have certain challenges, it is important to discuss this fact prior to a meeting so that you and the professional can have some strategies about how to respond to the parents' concerns. Also, if you feel that a child or student may not respond well to interacting with a stranger, you may need to plan to meet prior to the assessment or interaction to acquaint that child with you and the SLP or the audiologist. The SLP or audiologist may ask you to administer some tests or interact with the client directly during parts of an assessment or ask your opinion about the child's general expressive language skills, for example, whether or not you understand the child in his or her language and/or if the child uses sentences that are comparable to those used by other children who speak the same language. However, if you feel an assignment may be too challenging, do admit it. Perhaps with extra practice or assistance, you might be able to do it well. You may want to review the section on the interpreter as *cultural broker* described on pages 92 to 97 in Chapter 4.

2. **Interpret faithfully.** Serve as a bridge between two or more parties and interpret everything that is said, including offensive and negative remarks. You

must interpret all that the professional says or expresses, including both verbal and nonverbal messages, as accurately as possible in order to convey the underlying meaning. If something is unclear, it is fine to interrupt the interaction to ask for clarification from the SLP or audiologist, the parent, or any other person present at a meeting.

3. **Respect confidentiality.** All information shared during a session must remain behind when you leave. Information learned during interpretation or translation should not be used or shared with others outside the professional setting.

4. **Participate in ongoing learning and remain flexible.** Respond positively to constructive criticism to increase success on the job. Continue to update your knowledge about procedures to follow in a given work setting, and follow up on suggestions made by the professionals you work with. Identify areas where you need more training, and ask for assistance in locating sources of information or training.

Facilitating the Interpreting and Translating Process

As you engage in interpreting or translating for interviews, conferences, assessment, or intervention, you must remember your role in facilitating the communication process. Keep the following strategies in mind:

1. **Maintain a continual dialogue during all phases of the process.** Request that the SLP or audiologist provide ongoing supportive feedback to you and stress the importance of his or participation in the process. For example you may use Table 7–3 and Table 7–4 as guides on pages 177 and 180. Encourage the SLP and/or audiologist to support your development as a well-informed member of the team. Resist the occasional desire to provide advice or advocacy for a client of family member when not appropriate. Instead, discuss any needs the family may have, so that assistance can be provided through appropriate channels.

2. **Remind the professionals you are collaborating with about:**
   a. *Keeping grammatical constructions as simple as possible.* Remind them that the quality of an interpretation depends on the clarity of the original message. Thus, the professional should attempt to convey ideas clearly, one idea at a time, checking regularly to make sure the message has been understood. The speech rate should be neither too slow nor too fast.
   b. *Avoiding idiomatic expressions.* Idioms use one or more words that have a figurative meaning (e.g., *pull one's hair out* or *talk one's ear off*). The intended meaning is often lost in a literal translation, and it is difficult for nonnative speakers to memorize and quickly recall meanings of idioms.
   c. *Defining professional terms.* Professional terms such as *auditory processing skills, visual motor integration,* or *percentile* may not have equivalent words in other languages. To be clear, the term should be followed by a definition and a concrete example applicable to the home or work context.

d. *Watching for indicators of translation difficulty.* All professionals, including you, should watch for indicators of comprehension difficulty such as a puzzled look from a parent or family member, even when the message appears to have been interpreted faithfully.

e. *Remaining as clear as possible.* Make a note of something that was said, which was too long or too complex, or a response that does not coincide with the original question or statement. Avoid assuming the meaning of nonverbal communication, which may vary widely due to cultural and individual differences. For example, a smile may indicate embarrassment, friendliness, or a warning of tension. When in doubt, it is the SLP's or audiologist's responsibility to ensure that what is said is clear and understandable to all parties involved.

f. *Addressing the client directly.* Position yourself so that the SLP or audiologist can face the client and his or her family, and address all comments directly to them. Maintaining eye contact facilitates more direct communication and helps the professional establish rapport with the client and/or family.

g. *Maintaining linguistic skills.* Constantly refine the skills cited previously that are necessary for you to successfully bridge the communication between two parties who do not share the same language: (a) oral and written proficiency with two languages, (b) knowledge of two cultures and nonverbal communication, (c) ability to convey the same meaning in two languages, (d) knowledge of professional terminology, (e) familiarity with dialectal differences, and (f) ability to adapt to the speech and language of individuals with speech and language communication challenges.

COMMON INTERPRETATION AND TRANSLATION ERRORS

Errors in interpretation and translation cannot be avoided. However, they may be minimized through more practice working with the SLP or the audiologist. There are five frequent errors in the process of interpreting:

1. **Omissions.** You leave something out, whether a word, a phrase, or an entire sentence. This could happen because you do not think the extra words are important (e.g., instead of saying "rather difficult," you might say "difficult"). In some cases, however, even a single word can make a difference, as in *mildly* versus *moderately* delayed. Omissions can also occur because you are unable to keep up with the speaker's rate of speech. As an interpreter, you can request repetition and/or slowing down of the speech rate to assist your accuracy.

2. **Additions.** You add words, phrases, or sentences that were not said or written. This may happen because you elaborate or editorialize by adding your own thoughts. This should be avoided. At other times, you may need to add a word when a concept does not translate directly into the

other language. This second type of addition is not considered an error as long as the same meaning is conveyed.

3. **Substitutions.** You use other words, phrases, or entire sentences in place of the actual words. Substitutions can occur because you do not remember the specific word, phrase, or grammatical construction. In other instances, you may confuse words that sound almost the same (e.g., *entendre* [hear] vs. *attendre* [wait] in French, or *sold* vs. *cold* in English). Lack of understanding or ability to keep up with the speaker may cause incorrect usage of pronouns.

4. **Transformations.** You change the word order of the original statement. It may result in an error if the meaning is altered, as in saying, "Peter was hit by Paul," instead of "Paul was hit by Peter." However, if the sentence were delivered as "Paul hit Peter," the meaning would not be altered, even though a transformation occurred. This change would not be considered an error during a conference or an interview but may have implications during an assessment of language skills that is examining a client's understanding or use of the specific grammatical construction.

5. **Misinterpretations of nonverbal communication.** You omit information that was conveyed nonverbally or may misinterpret the nonverbal information conveyed by a person from another cultural background. For example, nodding may be interpreted as agreeing with what you said, instead of meaning that the person is just listening. In addition to paying attention to nonverbal communication, you and the SLP or audiologist should pay attention to stress on words and intonation in sentences. For example, there is a difference in saying, "Your child performs much better on tasks that require visual attention," compared to, "Your child performs *much* better on tasks that require visual attention."

CODE OF ETHICS

The SLP or audiologist needs to abide by the Code of Ethics (2010) drafted by the American Speech-Language-Hearing Association (ASHA). You may want to review it by going directly to the website (http://www.asha.org/policy). In Chapter 4, Terry Irvine Saenz, the second writer of this guide, reviews portions of the current ASHA Code of Ethics that apply directly to working with and supervising support personnel like you. You may want to read that portion of the chapter to familiarize yourself with the contents of pages 82 to 83. However, no code of ethics for interpreters and translators working with SLPs and audiologists has been written except for an outline, which I wrote in the 2002 handbook. In the same Chapter 4, Terry Irvine Saenz discusses some rules from "A National Code of Ethics for Interpreters in Health Care," by the National Council on Interpreting in Health Care, 2004, retrieved from http://www.ncihc.org/, which she included in Table 4–6 on page 98 of Chapter 4. The document highlights some important roles and responsibilities, such as confidentiality, maintaining impartiality, adhering to your professional boundaries, expanding your awareness of your own culture and that of others, and treating everyone with respect. It also states situations where it is recommended you act as an advocate and encourages you to continue your professional growth and act in a professional and ethical manner.

I have created the activities below to offer you opportunities to practice your interpreting and translating skills. The first set of activities includes common sentences that are used during interviews, conferences, and assessments so that you can practice translating them orally and in writing. The second set of activities includes scenarios and/or case studies to practice interpreting, sight, or written translation skills.

Practice Exercises for Translation

This first set includes common sentences used by SLPs or audiologists during either interviews or conferences with parents about their child or during assessments.

Conferences and Interviews

- When did you first notice that your child had a speech/language/hearing problem?
- Do you think your child has difficulty understanding oral directions? For example, if you ask him or her something, does he or she stare at you or not do it instead?
- Did your child babble, or in other words, say a string of sounds that do not really make too much sense, such as /bababa/ or /mamama/ or /babagee/?

- Is your child saying any true words? Can you give me an example, please?
- Does your child use sentences that are complete? For example, "I want some bananas" instead of "I want banana," or "Take me to the park" instead of "Take park"?
- Can you understand your child when he or she speaks? What about other people who do not know him or her?
- Children may have problems with language comprehension (understanding) and expression or just in expressing themselves, meaning speaking clearly. Your child has difficulty saying sounds in words, and this is why he is so difficult to understand.
- An individual education plan (IEP) can be implemented only after the parent has given written consent for the content of the plan and the placement for specific services.
- A student needs to receive special education in the least restrictive program possible.
- Your child can understand what he or she hears well, but his or her major difficulty is using complete sentences and saying some sounds consistently. This is why it is hard to understand him or her.
- Your child hesitates when he or she speaks. He or she repeats the first syllable in words, and he or she seems aware of his or her speech problem. I think I will need to work with him or her, and I will give you some ideas on how to help him or her at home as well.
- Does your child require that the TV be set at a higher volume? Do you have to call his or her name

many times before he or she responds to you?

• This audiogram shows that your child has a conductive hearing loss in the left ear in the low frequencies. You need to see the ear, nose, and throat specialist to seek medical management. He or she might need to put tubes in to drain the fluid. It is a common procedure but requires some anesthesia. We have seen a lot of improvement afterward, and it will help with his or her language development.

• Whenever you speak with your child, you should be careful that he or she can see you, and there is not too much noise in the environment.

During Assessment

• I am not going to hurt you; I just need you to put these headphones on your ears.

• Put a block in the bucket when you hear a beep even if it is very soft/quiet/soft (like this).

• Raise your hand when you hear a beep even if it is very soft/quiet/faint (like this).

• Tell me if these two words sound the same or different.

• I am going to show a book that has only pictures. After you look at them, I want you to tell me a story.

• I am going to say some sentences, and I want you to say them back to me. Don't change anything; just say what I say. Here we are going to try: "I will go to the park." Now you say the whole thing (the child repeats the sentence). "Good."

• I want you to name these colors and figures/shapes as fast as you can. Go.

• Point to the picture that goes with what I say.

• I want you tell me all the names of animals you know as fast as you can. For example, cow, hen, dog. . . . When you are ready, let me know.

Practice Exercises for Interpreting

Box 8–1 and Box 8–2 are scripts from interactions that I have transcribed for you to practice your interpreting skills. They are written as role-play activities. Box 8–3 is written for you to practice your sight translation skills.

Conferences

1. Select Box 8–1 or 8–2 to use with your team.
2. Make sure each item includes the members identified in the script plus one or two observers. The observers will fill out the observation sheet in Table 8–1.
3. Decide if you will use consecutive or simultaneous interpreting during the role-play.
4. Request that role players and observers discuss the effectiveness of the interpretation. Discuss how role players decide when to stop to enable the interpreter to communicate in the other language with consecutive interpreting.
5. Discuss the advantages and disadvantages of each method.

Some self-assessment items are listed at the end of this chapter to enable you to review the information presented.

BOX 8–1. MEETING TO REVIEW PROGRESS (IEP)

Team Members: Parent, SLP, Interpreter

SLP: We have been working on helping John understand and remember directions. Do you recall when we talked about how he had trouble following along in class?

PARENT: Yes, I am glad you are working on this skill, because I have noticed he tends to remember things better lately.

SLP: I am glad to hear this. With the cooperation of all his subject teachers (English, math, science, social studies), we have been having John use a tape recorder at the end of each class to hear the directions for homework. When we have therapy in my room, I check how he has been transcribing his homework into his daily planner, and this has helped him keep things organized.

PARENT: I have seen him use his daily planner much more now. I am also making him talk to me about the homework and how he is going to work on it.

SLP: That is excellent. Eventually, I would like him to improve in his ability to record his homework directly into his planner. We are practicing taking notes, and we are starting by going over previous recordings and learning how to write down the main ideas. We have also been listening to the teachers' lectures and practicing the same skill. He has been very conscientious about coming to therapy. I am going to rewrite this goal and focus more on subject content. Another thing is for John to pay more attention in class and learn to recognize when he does not understand something.

BOX 8–2. RESULTS OF AN AUDIOLOGICAL EVALUATION

Team Members: Parent, Audiologist, Interpreter

PARENT: I am so glad I came here; I am very concerned about Billy's hearing. I have to raise my voice with him. You know he had multiple ear infections when he was an infant. We were at the doctor's at least once a month at that time. We had those little tubes, you know, when he was 2 years old, and then they came out. His hearing has been good, but lately, with this terrible spring, I think he has allergies as well.

Audiologist: What we found today is that he has fluid in his ears once again, and no wonder he has been complaining about earaches, especially in his right ear. What I am going to do is ask you to go to the ear, nose, and throat specialist. It is possible he might recommend another procedure to put tubes in. Please let me know what he decides by calling Lilly, our interpreter here, and she will let me know.

PARENT: But I can't make the appointment because I don't feel good about my English. Maybe Lilly can help me do this.

Audiologist: Yes, she will call your doctor and set up an appointment as soon as possible.

PARENT: Oh, thank you so much, but what can I do in the meantime?

Audiologist: Be sure he does not get a fever. If he does, take him to your pediatrician right away. He might need antibiotics. And then please make sure you come back for a follow-up. Thank you for seeing me today.

BOX 8–3. SIGHT TRANSLATION

Tom was referred for special education because the school team has attempted to provide him extra assistance with reading using a program recommended for children who are referred for problems in that area. Other children with similar difficulties have been able to catch up, but this was not the case for Tom. Although he tries very hard, he still has a great deal of trouble. He does understand what he listens to very well and he pays attention.

Several different formal and informal tests were administered to see how well he knows his alphabet, sound-letter correspondences (for example, that the sound /s/ is for the letter *s* or *c*), ability to recognize sounds within words (for example, to tell which one is the first sound in /pet/) and blends (if we say sounds in isolation and ask him to put them together like /f/-/a/-/ t/), and recognize number of syllables (for example, that /pet/ is one syllable in English or /calendar/ has three syllables). Tom knows his alphabet, but when he says it, he sings it instead of saying each individual letter. He recognizes a few upper- and lowercase letters. He needs a lot of repetition even though he tries very hard. We will work with him on a one-on-one basis, and we will give you some ideas of how you can help him at home. You mentioned you want to hire a tutor.

Table 8–1. Observation of Interactions During Interviews and Conferences

The SLP and interpreter reviewed the purpose of the interview or conference prior to the meeting?	Yes	No
The critical pieces of the information to be presented were reviewed?	Yes	No
Seating arrangement was appropriate for the interaction?	Yes	No
The SLP/audiologist introduced the participants?	Yes	No
The SLP/audiologist stated the purpose of the meeting?	Yes	No
The I/T used the "I" form instead of "Mr./Mrs. X says . . ."	Yes	No
The I/T appeared to convey all that was said by all parties without editing?	Yes	No
The I/T appeared to interpret all clearly and precisely?	Yes	No
The I/T asked clarification questions when needed?	Yes	No
The parent seemed to comprehend what she or he was told?	Yes	No
The environment seemed comfortable?	Yes	No
The I/T and the SLP/audiologist met following the meeting to discuss what went well and what to emphasize at a future meeting?	Yes	No
Comments:		

Source: Adapted from Langdon, H. W. (2002). *Interpreters and translators in communication disorders: A practitioner's handbook* (pp. 26–27). Eau Claire, WI: Thinking Publications.

SELF-ASSESSMENT ITEMS

After studying the information in this chapter, review the following items by yourself or with another person who is receiving the same training as you.

1. Compare and contrast interpreting and translating. Which required skills are your strengths and which do you need more practice in?

2. Refer to the code of ethics proposed for interpreters and translators in Table 4–6 on page 98. Select one item and identify potential negative effects of not following the code.

3. Describe the way in which you would expand your knowledge of professional terminology.

4. The SLP and audiologist know how and why to avoid idiomatic expressions, but a family member may not. What will you say to the person if he or she were to use an idiomatic expression?

5. Identify at least three pieces of information you would want to learn about before beginning an interpreting session with an SLP and/or an audiologist and your reasons for needing to have that information beforehand.

6. Based on your knowledge of an audiologist's responsibilities, do you believe

interpreting services should be used more during assessment or during interview and conferences? Why?

7. After practicing the translation and interpretation activities, what seemed easier or more difficult? State your reasons.

8. What would you do if a client approached you with a question that you felt you could answer regarding some of the content of a conference during which you interpreted a few days before?

Chapter 9

The Interpreter/SLP or Audiologist Collaboration Process

Henriette W. Langdon

This chapter includes the following:

- A discussion of three steps that should be considered when planning an interview, a conference, or an assessment in which an interpreter/translator (I/T) is part of the team, that is, in briefing, interaction, and debriefing (BID)
- Desired strategies to ensure an interview or a conference yields positive outcomes with the assistance of the I/T for audiological and speech-language assessments
- Preparation and interaction in an assessment or treatment session where the I/T is involved

This chapter provides guidance for situations or scenarios most commonly needing the services of an I/T in the field of communication disorders: interviews, conferences, and assessment of a client's communication performance.

Here I should pause for a moment and say that I have tried to use the word *collaboration* with an I/T instead of the common word that one hears, which is *use*. You often hear well-meaning people say, "We need to use an interpreter." For me, *use* refers to an object, and you are a person. Therefore, I try to say and write phrases such as "collaborate with an interpreter" or "use the services of an interpreter." You never hear anyone say, "I will use a speech-language pathologist" or "I will use a surgeon," rather "I will use the services of . . . ," "I will work with . . . ," "I will seek . . . ," and so on. So, all together, I would like to avoid *use* by itself. However, this term is commonly heard and read in the literature all over the world.

Anyway, I hope that the procedures recommended here will help make your interactions with speech-language pathologists (SLPs) and audiologists as productive as possible. Procedures include the briefing, interaction, and debriefing (BID) process, which will be your guide for preparing in advance for collaborating with the SLP or the audiologist during interaction with a client. In other words, to secure a more seamless process, it is recommended that you meet with the SLP or the audiologist prior to any interaction with the family member(s) or the client to review the main points that will be discussed in an interview, in gathering some background information about the client, in participating in a conference to discuss the results of an assessment and draft an intervention plan, or simply, in discussing the progress made by the client during a certain period of time. When an assessment is considered, you need to prepare to know the purpose of the interaction, the tests and materials that will be used, and your role in this instance. In either case, this first phase is referred as the **briefing**, like a legal case, where some preliminary preparation takes place prior to the actual trial. The actual interview, conference, or assessment is referred as the **interaction**. Once the latter is concluded, it is strongly recommended that you meet with the SLP or the audiologist to discuss the outcomes of the interaction and what is planned for a follow-up. This portion is referred as the **debriefing**, hence the acronym, **BID**.

It is important for all participants to be reminded that any interaction where an interpreter/translator will be involved will be at least one and a half times longer than any other interaction, even if the method of interpreting ends up being simultaneous or even if not all of the information needs to be interpreted because the parent has ascertained that it was understood in English.

THE INTERVIEW OR CONFERENCE ENVIRONMENT

Briefing

For either scenario and for purposes of briefing, it is important to meet prior to

the interaction to discuss the following points. A meeting can take place to either interview a parent and/or a client, or it may take the form of a conference to share results of an assessment. To make it easier I have put an (I) for interview and/or a (C) if it applies to conference. Many of these points are illustrated in video clip 2.

1. **Review the purpose of the meeting** and the critical pieces of information that will be discussed = [I] and [C]. This will be a good moment to prepare together about what you might need to do in case a parent is reluctant to answer questions because of embarrassment or how you may want to convey information about the results of an assessment where the parent might have difficulty accepting a given diagnosis or following up with a decision.
2. **Limit the number of participants**, if possible, to decrease the stress on the family or the client to make your interpreting task more manageable = [C].
3. **Find out which other disciplines will be represented** at the meeting and if there is specialized terminology you will need to interpret = [I] and [C].
4. **Make the setting as comfortable and nonthreatening as possible** = [I] and [C].
5. **Seat all people so that they are able to make eye contact with each other**. We discussed this issue in the previous section. However, consider that in some cultures, direct eye contact is avoided as a sign of respect = [I] and [C].
6. **Immediately before the meeting begins, politely** = [I] and [C].
   a. Ask participants to refrain from side conversations so you are able to interpret everything that is said during the meeting.

b. State that your responsibility is to interpret all that is said, both what may appear "good" as well as "bad." Indicate that you may not edit or change any of the information conveyed by any of the participants.

c. It is helpful to request everyone to speak using a slower rate of speech and shorter sentences so that you may complete your job with greater ease.

7. **Avoid being a direct participant in the interaction.** All those involved should direct their gaze directly at the family member or client when called for = [I] and [C].

8. **Remember to use the *I* form when interpreting.** For example, instead of saying Mr. X or Mrs. X says, use the pronoun *I* = [I] and [C].

You may wish to refer to Table 8–1, on page 204, to ensure that all of these areas are covered as you prepare for an interview or a conference.

Interaction

Interviews

During an interview, the SLP and/or audiologist will need to review two critical pieces of information: (a) legal rights and (b) gathering background information about the client by asking specific health and developmental questions, including his or her performance at home and school. Also, during that time, there should be an opportunity for the parent(s) to ask questions and voice concerns.

Legal Rights. Parents and/or clients who are over 18 years of age must be given all information regarding their legal rights. It is necessary that the SLP or the audiologist explain these rights, even though the laws may have been translated into the target language and provided in written form. This includes rights when undergoing an assess-ment or developing an individual family service plan (IFSP) or an individual education plan (IEP). In reality, many of these documents include legal language that is often difficult to understand even for the native English speaker. Receiving rights about possible special education may be particularly difficult for those individuals who are unfamiliar with such a protocol. In many countries of the world, general education is often not accessible to everyone, let alone special education services like speech and language and hearing. Families have often asked me if they will need to pay out of pocket for these services, and they are relieved to know that they are free of charge. It is your duty to interpret documents containing these laws and rights using language that is understood by the family member or client. However, the SLP or audiologist will facilitate the process by providing important highlights of the documents, and you need to interpret that information. On some IFSP or IEP forms, the person signing the papers is asked to check if he or she has received his or her rights. Asking the parent to retell what he or she understood in his or her comfortable language is a practical way to ensure that the content was clear to him or her. It is also recommended that a note be written that the meeting was conducted in the parent's preferred language and that you acted as an interpreter.

From the start, parents must know that they are full participants in their child's education, both general and special education. The Individuals with

Disabilities Education Act reauthorization act (IDEA) of 2004 requires that parents actively participate in the process of assessment, program planning, and placement in a program for children with special education needs. Therefore, the SLP or audiologist needs to ask parents directly for their opinions and seek their feedback. In many instances, parents and other family members may not be comfortable giving their opinions for various reasons, including unfamiliarity with the process followed in the U.S. school system or feeling intimidated due to their own limited formal education. They may also have unquestioning trust in the expertise of professionals. In any event, the parent needs to ensure that he or she will be heard. The process may take time, but it ultimately helps protect and assist the client.

Gathering Background Information. The SLP or audiologist will have a set of questions to ask or may need to check information with the parent and/or the client prior to an assessment. It is important that you have the majority or types of questions ahead of time to prepare yourself adequately. I have developed a questionnaire, which you can find in Table 5–1 on page 111. To expedite the meeting, it would be helpful to have the major questions translated into the target language ahead of time. If a given language occurs frequently in a given district, equivalent questionnaires can be developed in several languages. While the I/T asks the questions directly, the SLP or audiologist can follow along with the English version of the questionnaire, making sure that the interpreter cues the professional about the particular question and interprets all of the parent's responses for the professional while writing the responses on the questionnaire.

It is important that you are familiar with the specific terminology as it relates to birth and development, as there might also be some medically related terms for which you may need to know the equivalents in the target language you are interpreting and translating, like *jargon language, articulation, hearing acuity,* and so on. All these terms appear at the end of the guide in the Glossary, but if you are faced with a term for which you don't know the translation, you will need a regular or computerized dictionary. As previously stated, in reviewing the questions prior to the meeting, you can also alert the professional that a parent may be reluctant to answer some of them, as they are considered too personal. This will enable both of you to plan how you may ask the questions and/or what you may do in case the parent is reluctant or too embarrassed to answer.

Conferences

For conferences where results of an assessment and plans for intervention are entered on the IFSP or IEP form, it is a good idea to have the information that will be shared ahead of time to prepare adequately in using the necessary terminology, whether the presentation is oral, or if the IFSP or IEP will have to be translated orally (sight translation).

In this chapter, I discuss some tips that will facilitate the interaction and follow-up of a conference. The first set is related to the interaction regarding information presented, and the second set is related to what to do if the parent seeks your advice because you share the same language and culture and, therefore, feels comfortable communicating with you. The third set concerns issues of follow-up and your role in this type of situation.

To ease the interaction and your job, it will be helpful if the SLP or audiologist uses some concrete examples, pictures, or diagrams to make a point. These may include a normal curve diagram to help explain test scores (if the SLP decides that these measures are fair in the case of a given client), a picture of the vocal cords to demonstrate the location of nodules, or an illustration of the hearing mechanism to indicate where the hearing difficulty might originate. It is important to invite the parent to ask about or comment on any of the information shared, and here you may want to indicate to everyone present that this is the case by reading the parent's nonverbal communication signals, which may be missed by others. At the end of the meeting, the professional may make suggestions to the parent on how he or she might be able to help the client at home. It is a good idea for everyone to ensure that the parent is comfortable with the follow-up suggested.

Important reminder: Typically, a parent or family member may feel comfortable sharing personal information with you before, during, or after a meeting. You should listen but be honest and remind the individual that you may need to share this confidential information with another professional who can assist or solve the concern or dilemma. You should not provide advice, give counseling, or discuss very personal matters. On the other hand, you may assist a client by contacting a person at a given agency on behalf of the client or contacting the parent's place of employment indicating that the parent was absent for some time that day because of an important meeting in regard to his or her child. Always keep the SLP or audiologist you are collaborating with informed about your activities, and seek his or her guidance when uncertain whether to assist an individual.

Another important component of a meeting is the follow-up. A follow-up telephone call will allow the family time to reflect on the meeting so that they may voice their questions or concerns. The call allows you to confirm that the parent understood the content of the interview or the conference. In turn, the parent can indicate whether he or she agrees with the assessment, the recommendation, or whether he or she has further questions for the SLP or the audiologist to clarify something. You should not respond to any questions before consulting back with the professional you have been collaborating with. The best practice is to place the follow-up call only if you have participated in the previous meetings and only with the approval and guidance of the professional.

Debriefing

It is highly recommended that the I/T and the professional take time to debrief at the conclusion of an interview or a conference to discuss whether the meeting was productive and why, to determine which areas went well, such as whether the professional obtained the information desired and the manner in which the interview or conference was conducted, or what other strategies might be used to make it run smoother. Also, decide on the type of follow-up and what your role might be.

ASSESSMENTS

Many of the concepts that are discussed in this section are illustrated in video clips 4 and 5. Assessing someone in a language other than English to find out if he or she might have a hearing, speech, and/or language challenge in his or her own language is quite a challenge. This first segment will provide you with some background knowledge that will be helpful to understand why this process is so difficult even for the seasoned SLP or audiologist. It will also offer specific strategies to follow the BID process for audiological and speech-language assessments.

In the United States, federal and state laws stipulate that individuals who are referred for an assessment because they may have possible challenges in hearing, speech, language, or learning *need to be evaluated using their stronger language.* As stated in Chapter 8, this is not the case with many parts of the world, where not all students have access to even general education. However, despite our laws and efforts, the likelihood that we may find bilingual audiologists or bilingual SLPs may be minimal. There are many bilingual specialists in those fields, but the majority speaks Spanish. Yet, there may be numerous languages that are represented in one single school district; therefore, an interpreter/translator like you will be needed to work side-by-side with the audiologist or the SLP to assist him or her in the evaluation. Furthermore, tests in languages other than English are still limited in number, and different tests normed on bilingual individuals who speak specific languages are almost nonexistent. This dilemma applies to the entire globe.

Often, the terms *testing, assessment,* and *evaluation* are used interchangeably. *Testing* means to give someone a task to do once to measure his or her performance on a given skill, and typically, the items administered are very specific with specific responses required. *Assessment* means administering several types of tasks over time, and this includes tests but also a language sample, observing how he or she responds when given more time or more trial items, as well as considering his or her overall performance over time with and without assistance in the classroom and/or at home. *Evaluation* means taking into consideration all the data on a given individual, that is, tests as well as assessment results that include also feedback from persons who know the client well like parents and teachers. It also includes deciding whether or not this individual does have or does not have a significant problem in hearing, speech, and language requiring special education intervention.

THE BID PROCESS IN AUDIOLOGICAL ASSESSMENTS

Important Information to Keep in Mind

Many of these concepts are illustrated in video clip 3. The following information will help you prepare for and successfully participate in audiological assessments. You should be aware of the general procedures and common terminology used by audiologists. The audiologist will orient you to the specific information needed.

Audiologists typically work in a clinic, private practice, or hospital. Educational audiologists provide services in schools. Audiologists use more instrumentation than SLPs. The two most common tasks audiologists perform are (a) measuring hearing sensitivity and (b) hearing aid assessment and fitting. Today, audiologists also calibrate and measure cochlear implants, which are becoming almost routine for many individuals who qualify and/or desire to have them.

Testing rather than assessment is a more appropriate term to use in audiological examinations because the audiologist conducts objective measures of the hearing sensitivity of the client. Testing can occur at any age. In fact, with the increased use of infant hearing screening, which is required in most states today, you are likely to assist families with newborns. Tests typically performed by an audiologist include the following:

- **Pure-tone thresholds:** air and bone conduction audiometry measure hearing sensitivity. Frequencies (tones) are tested at varying decibel (loudness) levels. Headphones deliver air conduction signals to identify air conduction loss. A behind-the-ear vibrator delivers bone conduction signals to identify sensorineural loss. Results are recorded on an audiogram. The type of audiogram obtained will determine the type of hearing loss.
- **Speech reception threshold (SRT):** measures the intensity (loudness) needed for the client to repeat 50% or more of spondaic test words (two-syllable words that have equal stress, for example, in English *cowboy*, *sunset*, and *baseball*). One of the major challenges is that lists of words of this type have been developed in other languages but may not have been calibrated. Several audiologists hesitate using the original words in other languages, as many have not have been calibrated. The audiologist who does not share the language with the client is often hesitant to administer it because he or she may not be able to judge if the repetition is accurate. Therefore,

he or she does not request the interpreter to either administer the list as he or she cannot verify if the words are repeated accurately. For more discussion on this topic, you may want to read the section on audiological assessments available in Chapter 6 of the guide.
- **Word recognition test (WRT):** measures the intensity (loudness) needed for the client to repeat words accurately. This measure may also be problematic to administer for the reasons stated above.
- **Typanometry:** measures movement of the tympanic membrane (ear drum) and corresponding middle ear function. It is administered with a tympanometer. Results are charted on a tympanogram. You may want to refer to this website retrieved on April 18, 2015: http://www.utmb.edu/pedi_ed/ AOM-Otitis/tympanometry/ tympanometry.htm
- **Otoacoustic emissions (OAE):** measures cochlear function, using sounds naturally emitted by the inner ear.
- **Auditory brainstem response (ABR):** measures the brain response to sound. It identifies newborns' hearing losses or the site of a lesion along the auditory nerve. Results are recorded on a graph.

After performing one or more of these tests depending on the client's needs, the audiologist will evaluate the results. Most typical findings are that the client may have the following:

- **Conductive hearing loss** caused by damage to the outer or middle ear. Causes include accumulation of earwax (e.g., cerumen or fluid) in the middle ear (i.e., otitis media if the fluid is infected), tumors, physical discharge, or otosclerosis in older patients (fixation of the small bones of the middle ear).

- **Sensorineural hearing loss** caused by damage to the inner ear or the auditory nerve (VII cranial nerve).
- **Mixed hearing loss**, a combination of both conductive and sensorineural loss.

The following website retrieved on April 18, 2015, may be helpful in reviewing audiograms illustrating the various types of hearing loss described just above: http://www.audiologyawareness.com/hearinfo_agramdem.asp

BID During Audiological Assessments

Briefing

Preparation might include discussion of the following:

- You and the audiologist meet to review the client's medical history or chart and plan the testing process. Questions related to the onset or progress of a hearing loss, past use of a hearing or amplification device, or other medically related questions are discussed.
- The audiologist explains the level of participation needed for a given client. In many cases when an interpreter is not available, the audiologist can explain the procedure directly to the client through demonstration using a combination of verbal and nonverbal directions. In Chapter 6 of this guide, I discuss this point as well. But you may be of assistance using the client's preferred language by explaining that the client must raise his or her hand when hearing a given signal, even if it appears to be very faint. As mentioned in Chapter 6, the word *faint* may have several translations in various languages, so you will have to be careful which word(s) you will use to describe or even mimic various levels of quiet/faint sounds. With younger clients, you may need to assist in training the child to throw a peg or block into a box or basket when hearing a sound. Obtaining a tympanogram typically will not require your help because the reading is done automatically without the client's direct participation.
- When assessing speech discrimination or reception, the audiologist will need to decide to address this issue and will have to discuss how he or she needs you to assist. You may be asked to present the words or to record the accuracy of a client's responses. Study any word lists ahead of time, and make the audiologist aware of any words that might be problematic for the client because of dialectal differences or because the word may be too difficult for a child of a given age.
- You need to make a plan in case the client does not understand his or her role or when testing cannot be appropriately conducted because the client is uncooperative.

- You should prepare to answer the questions of the client's parent in case there have been concerns about the procedures or the outcome of testing.

Interaction

The following are tasks that you may need to engage in when face-to-face with the client.

- During an interview or conference, remember to interpret every participant's questions, comments, and responses that are heard.
- Ensure the client understands his or role during testing, such as raising his or her hand or throwing a peg in a box to signal that a tone is heard.
- Assist the audiologist when the client appears to be confused about directions or does not seem to respond to what is asked, using the audiologist's guidance to fix any misunderstanding on the part of the client.
- Present and/or record the word list according to the directions of the audiologist made during the briefing portion of the testing session.
- After completing the testing, you and the audiologist should take a few minutes to discuss the results and plan how to share them with the family member or the client.
- During the conference, the audiogram, the tympanogram, and other testing results are explained. The audiologist indicates if the client's hearing loss is conductive, sensorineural, or mixed because the course of intervention is different in each case. The audiologist

explains the effects of the hearing loss on the client's performance on communication as well as performance in school and/or home.

If the fitting of a hearing aid is indicated, the audiologist will typically follow six steps, and it is important for you to be familiar with them. However, for each case, make sure that you and the audiologist have a few minutes to discuss the highlights of the conference. You may want to take notes to feel more at ease, no matter how much experience you may have had.

1. **Evaluation:** You may be asked to assist the audiologist in explaining test procedures or administering test items. The results of the testing will help the audiologist determine the degree and type of hearing loss and if the client is a candidate for a hearing aid or possible cochlear implants, which are electronic devises that are surgically implanted in the inner ear. An audiologist may explain this option to the young adult client or the parent of a minor.

2. **Treatment planning:** The client's hearing needs in daily life activities are assessed. For example, what are the most common environments in which the individual will be working and interacting with others? Will it be a noisy place, and if so, what type of noise? You may be asked to interview the client or the parent to collect this information, which will help determine the type of amplification needed.

3. **Selection of the hearing aid:** The audiologist will make the selection depending on the degree of hearing

loss and the hearing demands that occur in the daily activities of the client. As background information, you may want to know that the size of hearing aids and devices has changed dramatically in the past 30 years. Initially, body hearing aids were always used, and they were much larger than today's models. The miniaturization of electronic circuits and batteries has allowed increasingly smaller hearing aids to be produced. Significant hearing losses typically need a larger style of hearing aid for more power and louder amplification; milder losses can be adequately served by smaller hearing aid styles. These smaller styles are referred to as *behind the ear* (BTE) and *in the ear* (ITE). Recent advances in miniaturization have resulted in ITE models known as *in the canal* (ITC), which fill the outer part of the ear canal and *completely in the canal* (CIC), which fit farther inside the ear and are barely visible.

4. **Verification:** The audiologist verifies that the hearing aid includes basic electroacoustics, cosmetic appearance, comfortable fit, and electroacoustic performance.

5. **Orientation:** You may be asked to interpret while the audiologist counsels the parent or client on the use and care of the hearing aids. The audiologist may be able to demonstrate some of this information nonverbally. This is the stage where the audiologist also describes realistic expectations that the client should have for the performance of the hearing aid.

6. **Validation:** In a follow-up session, the audiologist verifies that the hearing aid is appropriate given the client's hearing loss and daily communication needs. Your assistance may

be needed in receiving feedback from the client or the parent/child on hearing and performance.

Debriefing

Recall that the BID process is not complete without taking a few minutes to discuss how the interview, assessment, or conference unfolded with the audiologist. During this time, the debriefing, you and the audiologist should review what was successfully accomplished and identify areas that need more attention in the future. You may also want to discuss if the family understood the results of the tests and the follow-up that may need to take place, such as referral to an ear, nose, and throat specialist (otolaryngologist) because of necessary medical intervention as well as recommendations for the home and classroom environments, or the need for a phone call.

> ## THE BID PROCESS IN SPEECH AND LANGUAGE ASSESSMENTS

Some Preliminary Considerations

Your role will change during this interaction section of a speech-language assessment: In an interview or conference scenarios, your role will be to interpret or translate information from one language to the other. During an assessment, which means asking a client to respond to various activities to determine how well he or she understands and uses his or her native/first language, **YOU** will be the one directly interacting with the client. It is a much more natural process than having the SLP administer a test item, or interact directly with the client, instead of having you interpret the same information for him or her. Therefore, in this context, adequate and intensive preparation needs to take place between you and the SLP. In this case, you are the one who provides the information to the client, and the professional will observe what and how you work with the client, in essence, your take on that professional's role; you are the representative of that professional in using the target language instead of English. You can now appreciate why your role *is very important and cannot be taken lightly.* In the next paragraphs, I talk about testing and assessment in speech-language pathology and some properties of tests in general, including their content and construction. In subsequent segments, I talk about scenarios on how to best collaborate with a professional and execute your job when there are tests in the target language and what to do when there are no tests in the language, which is the most frequent case. I also discuss helpful strategies to obtain a language sample and assist the SLP in analyzing it. These concepts and strategies are illustrated in video clip 4 and video clip 5.

When there are tests in a given language: If you are asked to assist in the assessment of a child in Spanish, there are several tests that have been adapted and normed through standardization for children of various ages. Many of the tests are also described in Table 6–1 on page 143, and you are encouraged to go over those and study them. However, you will need to be specifically trained to use each one of them.

The existing tests were developed to evaluate several different areas of language such as articulation, grammar, syntax, sentence construction, and vocabulary. The various tests include sections, which assess the child's understanding or reception of language, and his or her ability to put together sentences of different types. You will need to take time and practice each one under the supervision of a Spanish-speaking SLP who will coach you on how to administer a given test and how to record responses. There are several tests, which include many sections, so you will need to practice those as well.

Standardized tests assist in comparing individuals to a normed population. The scores used for these comparisons are called *norms.* The tests include specific items that need to be administered following consistent directions for use. Only a limited number of tests have been developed using norms from a group of individuals whose primary language is other than English, and most of these have been developed, as I mentioned earlier, for Spanish-speaking groups. A few other tests exist in a few languages, but there are not that many. Your SLP might have some that he or she may have obtained from a particular reference, or you may locate the following website (http://www.csu.edu.au/research/multilingual-speech/speech-assessments, retrieved on December 24, 2014) and/or retrieve a list included in the article by McLeod and Verdon (2014).

Standardized tests are helpful in determining how well a client performs in a particular area compared to other clients of the same age or grade level. In designing test items, the authors have a specific purpose in mind that is based on a theoretical or empirical framework. To develop norms, these test items are administered to be statistically representative but often have a relatively small (often no more than 200 per age or grade level) sample of subjects. Groups differing in social or cultural backgrounds may be included in the sample, but the SLP should consider the results of the client's performance by taking into account the specific characteristics of the client and the normed population. That is, a client whose background is different from that of the normed group may score lower on the test despite having adequate speech-language or hearing abilities, just because the client has not had the same cultural experiences.

Standardized tests must be valid and reliable to draw useful conclusions from their results. *Validity* means the test truly measures what it purports to measure (e.g., language comprehension or memory). *Reliability* means that the results will be consistent when administered in the same way to the same type of people.

Even when tests are normed on a particular bilingual population, their validity and reliability are compromised because each bilingual speaker's language proficiency varies a great deal based on individual experience and differs from the sample population used in the norming of the test. Furthermore, more discrepancies can be found when an interpreter is involved in the testing process because no standardized tests have been normed using the assistance of an interpreter. Nevertheless, there is value in administering the items, because one can draw a general idea of the individual's performance on specific tasks, such as his or her ability to comprehend sentences, follow directions, respond to various types of sentences from a story, and use expressive vocabulary or specific grammatical structures. You may also obtain information on how well a client can read (but prior experience in reading in that language is important). And, it is recommended that the final determination of a diagnosis and eligibility for services be based on additional factors other than results on standardized tests.

A synopsis of what you should know about tests: It is important to keep in mind the following when using any tests:

- *Test limitations:* Most standardized tests do not provide norms when an interpreter or translator is involved in administering the test. This is one reason why the results of interpreted tests need to be deciphered with caution.
- *Subtests:* A comprehensive test is generally composed of several subtests. If the test is normed, the manual may have specific rules on what item should be used to begin (*basal*) and where to end the test (*ceiling*). Directions may change from subtest to subtest. These details are included in the test manual, and some tests may include these directions on the individual administration form also referred to as a protocol. The SLP is responsible for making certain you know where to begin and end any given subtest.
- *Demonstration items:* Most tests and subtests have demonstration items to ensure that the client understands the directions. For example, "I am going to say something and I want you to repeat/say it back to me exactly the way I said it; don't change anything." Or, "I will tell you a story, and when I am done, I am going to ask you some questions about what I told you. So listen carefully." Administer these items exactly according to the directions in the manual. The SLP can show

you where to find the directions and can answer any questions you might have.

- *Repetitions and wait-times:* The directions for the test specify whether repetitions are allowed and how long to wait for the client to respond before going on with the administration of the next item. When in doubt, consult with the SLP (who should be present at all times during this process, regardless of how many times you have worked together or how well prepared and competent you are). There are three reasons for this: (a) It is important for the SLP to observe the responses provided by the client, observe how you respond to the client, and make his or her own observations about the process to compare notes with you; (b) it is necessary that the SLP answer any questions or clarify any information you may need because no two cases are the same, even though they may appear to be so from the surface; and (c) ultimately, the SLP is responsible for the assessment, the evaluation as well as the diagnosis, and the outcome of the evaluation as well as the implementation of the treatment plan. We live in a very litigious society, and in the event that the family is not satisfied with the process or results or disagrees with what went on in the process, the SLP or the audiologist will be the one responsible and liable. And, you should remember that, when in doubt, you should ask for clarification and guidance from the SLP or the audiologist without compromising the client's performance. You should not be embarrassed to ask questions, because ultimately it will benefit the client you are trying to assess.

- *Cuing:* The manual may indicate how to cue the client to provide other responses if the response is inaccurate. For example, a phrase such as "Tell me more," or "Can you think of another word" might be used. Only the particular cues that are spelled out in the test directions should be used. Again, when in doubt, consult with the SLP.

- *Observing client behaviors:* Observe the client's responses to the test items to gather a more comprehensive impression about his or her ease or difficulty in responding to various tasks, including a longer time to respond or a lack of attention/distractibility. Discuss your observations with the SLP during the assessment (if appropriate) or after, as part of the debriefing.

- *Deviations from directions:* Be certain to inform the SLP about instances when you vary from the directions provided by the manual, and discuss how they may have affected the client's responses. Expect to be asked for a rationale as to why you deviated from the instructions. Ideally, make the SLP aware of the alteration at the time it is occurring. If this is not feasible, discuss the deviations during the debriefing part of the assessment process.

- *Item readministration:* Once the administration of a given subtest is completed, the SLP may ask you to readminister some of the items under modified conditions.

Modified conditions may include repeating the instructions, repeating the target items, providing more examples, giving the client more time to respond, or providing a second chance to respond. This will have value in determining if the client can perform with greater success a second time and predict the client's progress. For example, if the client responds to questions after hearing a short story when the information is read a second time and/or at a slower pace, it may mean that simply repeating the information may be helpful in facilitating recall. Thus, the general education teacher may help the client in the classroom by repeating directions for the client and perhaps others who may miss them the first time. Readministering a test item in the original form or with modifications like extra time to respond or providing some cues to facilitate correct responses is called *dynamic assessment.* You want to find out if the student can succeed and under which conditions. Here, the SLP will guide you, and it would be easier if you plan it as you go along.

- *New scores:* New scores may have been obtained through readministration but should not be considered as comparisons with the performance of the normed population if they are part of a normed/standardized test.
- *Raw scores:* A raw score is obtained when the total number of correct items is computed. The new score is converted by the SLP to one or more statistical measures to compare the client's performance

with a normed population. These scoring systems often are based on numerical scales called *standard scores* or *percentiles.* Each scale has reference points that indicate an average range and where the individual's performance falls within or outside that average range. Again, you will likely be called on to explain raw score and numerical scales to clients and/ or family members during the conference that follows assessment. Thus, you will need to make certain you have a complete understanding of the scoring system(s) for the subtests/tests you have administered. Table 6–2 on page 151 might assist you in preparing you for administration of tests that have been normed in Spanish and other languages.

When there are no tests in a given language: When there are no tests in a given language, the SLP may ask you to assist him or her in creating and adapting some materials in the language. The information provided in the body of the guide in Chapter 6 is duplicated here to ease your reading. The strategies are illustrated in video clip 5.

- *Ask the child's parents if they have any available books or materials in the child's language.* If they have books or materials in the target language, the I/T may be requested to comment on whether they would be appropriate for the child's age and experience with the language. If they are, the I/T may plan to read a passage and ask some questions about the content and/or read a passage and ask the child to retell the story. In this case, the I/T may need to tell the SLP about the content of the story, and comprehension questions should be formulated carefully and retranslated or back translated into English for the SLP to judge their value in assessing the language skills of the child. All of this material should be written down and prepared ahead of the evaluation time. Depending on the child's age and formal education, the child may be asked to read and write in the target language. Specific activities will need to be planned ahead and require additional time and preparation. For this reason, one of the suggestions made in Chapter 5 in planning for the future is to create curriculum-based activities in various languages that I/Ts and SLPs can utilize when assessing culturally and linguistically diverse (CLD)/bilingual children who speak one or two other languages in addition to English.

However, you and the SLP should keep in mind that language differences are especially critical in tests of speech and language skills. When words are translated, they may be shorter or longer than the original version, which may make the task easier or harder. Tests of grammatical usage may vary in difficulty depending on how a grammatical feature (e.g., verb tense, like present or past [*go, went*]; feminine article [*el* or *la* in Spanish or *le* and *la* in French], or noun-verb agreement as in *he goes* and *they go*) occurs in the other language and if it occurs at all. Even tests of vocabulary can be very different when translated because some

words or concepts are less common in another culture or may have multiple meanings that do not occur in the other language. Therefore, it is highly recommended that you **DO NOT TRANSLATE ANY ITEMS OF ANY TESTS.** There is a high likelihood that the translated version, although correct in that language, may have a completely different meaning from the original version. Therefore, instead of translating or adapting test items, it is suggested that specific activities be prepared such as:

- *Elicit and analyze a language sample.* The language sampling and the various language-based activities will depend on the child's chronological and mental ages. A procedure for eliciting and analyzing a language sample is suggested in a subsequent segment of this section. Gathering a language sample allows for the observation of various linguistic and communication features such as articulation/phonology, grammar, syntax, pragmatics, and the language formulation abilities of the child.
- *Have the child name words in various categories* in the first language and English, such as foods, animals, body parts, and classroom items to compare and contrast the words used in each language and the ease with which they are elicited.
- *Use rapid automatic naming tasks* such as naming sequences of colors, shapes, and combinations to judge speed and accuracy in word retrieval.
- *Engaging the child in a card game may be very telling.* For example, a card game where pairs need to be

assembled or classic games like War may shed light on the child's ability to learn new strategies and/or follow directions. Also, engage the child in board games where you can observe how the client follows directions during an informal activity.

- *Request the child to draw something and talk about it or complete a simple art activity.* This allows the assessment of the child's imagination and creativity as well as his or her ability to follow directions. A conversation may be elicited in this environment.

- *Prepare a questionnaire as if interviewing the child.* Questions may range from learning basic information about the child such as age, birthdate, number of siblings, address, phone number, and so on, as well as favorite activities, places to go, games, shows, and music. Depending on a given situation, the child may be asked to respond to questions regarding what is easy or difficult at school, what the child's favorite subjects are, how to play a given game or sport, and so forth, and may be requested to retell the plot of a TV show or movie.

Eliciting a language sample: A language sample is a collection of the client's consecutive utterances (words, phrases, or sentences) during an interaction. The interaction should be structured to elicit a sample that is as close to the client's typical conversation as possible. Alternatively, the SLP may have to collect a narrative sample (e.g., "tell me a story" or "tell me the story you just heard" as suggested in the section above) in addition to

or instead of a sample collected during a conversation.

A language sample can provide useful information about a client's communication skills, but eliciting and transcribing a representative sample requires skill, practice, and time. For example, more language is elicited from the clients with questions like "tell me about . . . " or "how do you . . . " or "do you . . . ?" The first two types of question are open-ended and usually require full/longer sentences to provide a complete answer. The third type of question can be answered with one word or a simple "yes" or "no."

You may be asked to collect a language sample during an interaction in the client's first language. You will need to practice language sampling prior to performing this task with a client. A client may be shy or reluctant to speak at first. Clients may also not cooperate or may have very poor expressive language skills. Use a variety of comments and activities to encourage the client to verbalize. A period of silence may follow your own comments or questions before the client responds, and you need to be quiet and patient to enable the client to respond when ready.

Ask the SLP to provide you with one or more practice opportunities in collecting and transcribing a language sample. The SLP should observe your techniques and instruct you in how to transcribe the sample accurately. You should analyze the transcript together to identify techniques that were effective or ineffective in eliciting a valid language sample.

To obtain a representative sample, vary the context of the conversation to obtain a comprehensive sample. Discuss possible topics of conversation with the SLP ahead of time. You should provide feedback to the SLP on topics that might be sensitive or difficult to discuss because of cultural differences.

For a preschool-aged client, consider topics and settings related to play with favorite toys and games, describing a favorite TV program, or discussing a hypothetical situation (e.g., what to do when the client cannot find a favorite toy or has a hard time falling asleep). For the school-aged client, include topics related to school or activities with friends and TV shows, including rules for favorite games/videogames.

To collect a narrative sample from a preschool or elementary school client, use a wordless book where the client has to make up the story to go along with the pictures. For the adolescent or young adult client, use topics such as favorite hobbies or how to resolve a difficult situation, such as convincing parents to borrow their parent's car to go to a party or join a group on a trip to another country. Make certain that the sample is audiotaped or videotaped. (Remember that most computers can be used for recoding samples now if the microphone is close enough for the client to pick up the sound.)

Once the sample is completed, listen to the recording and write down what the client said word for word. This process is referred to as *sample transcription*. Include notes about speech sound and grammatical errors that you noticed in the first language.

- *Analyzing a language sample:* Remind the SLP that cultural differences must be respected when evaluating narratives. For example, a narrative is the organization used when telling a story, but narratives

may vary between cultures. In addition, recounts (talking about what happened) and eventcasts (talking about what will happen) may not be as frequent among certain cultural groups. Keeping in mind these cultural differences, provide input to the SLP when assessing the areas summarized in the next section. It is important to keep in mind that there may have been a lack of opportunity for the client to express some of the language features described in the next paragraphs. For example, he or she may not have had an opportunity to use questions or to convey language to inform about something.

- *Pragmatic skills:* This section is related to how language is used. Be prepared to comment on the following questions: (a) Did the client respond to questions or make comments appropriately? (b) Did the client maintain the topic at hand or switch often? (c) Were ideas sequenced logically so as not to interfere with communication? (d) Could the client use language to describe, ask for information, explain something, retell, and inform? and (e) Did the client appear to use more gestures than needed (i.e., did the client use gestures instead of using specific words)?

- *Form and content:* This section has to do with using sentences that are complete and correct. Questions to consider are as follows: (a) Did the client use sentences that were grammatically correct? Be prepared to explain incorrect grammatical

features you noted, such as a lack of use of gender articles in Spanish (*el* vs. *la*), or an incorrect verb form to denote the past tense, or incomplete sentences where there were no articles (like "I went to store").
(b) Did the client use appropriate vocabulary words or did he or she have a tendency to use fillers such as *like a* . . . or closely related words, such as *fork* instead of *knife*, or simply *thing* instead of the word?
(c) Did the client pronounce words correctly (if not, what errors were noted, and provide examples)? and (d) Could you understand the client at least 90% to 95% of the time, and why?

* *The Manner of language expression:* Finally, be prepared to answer these questions: (a) Was there a time delay between the interpreter's questions and comments and the client's responses? (b) Were there pauses and hesitations when the client seemed to search for words? (c) Was voice quality adequate (i.e., did the voice call attention to itself because of hoarseness, harshness, or breathiness)? and (d) Were there any signs of stuttering? If yes, how often did they occur?

Below I describe some steps that should help you plan and execute a speech and language assessment where you will be acting as a "very direct bridge" in the process. Box 9–1 will help you follow the process.

Briefing

Determine an agreeable time and location for the assessment. To ensure that the process runs smoothly, you and the SLP should work together as much as needed prior to the scheduled assessment session. The SLP should meet with you to discuss the client's background information and brief you on the tests and procedures that will be used if you are going to test in Spanish or any language where there are norms available. You can refer to Table 6–1 on page 143. The information you are seeking includes the reason for referral, the results of other testing, and pertinent medical, developmental, social, and educational background data. It is possible you may already know the client and his or her family if you interpreted for the SLP during an initial interview.

You should take notes, ask questions, and review the background information presented by the SLP and the parent(s) when applicable.

Next, the SLP should explain the test items that you will readminister, including their purpose, procedures, and manner of recording responses. You must become familiar with the test items to be certain that procedures are clear. Ask for clarification prior to and even during the assessment process when necessary. Keep a list of the tests with notes about administration handy during the session.

You and the SLP should discuss strategies to follow in case the client does not cooperate or performs below or above expectations. More stretch breaks, shifting the test items, or postponing the session may be necessary. Also talk about the use of recording devices, such as a tape recorder or video camera, which may aid in the debriefing process.

When there are no tests or materials in a language, you will have to prepare those ahead of time as well. Ideas were provided on pages 220 to 224 of this chapter.

BOX 9–1. COLLABORATION WITH AN INTERPRETER DURING A SPEECH AND LANGUAGE ASSESSMENT: A CHECKLIST

Briefing

- Purpose of the assessment or intervention is explained
- Procedures to be followed are reviewed
- Use of gestures, voice patterns, and other body language that might cue the client is discussed
- The interpreter is reminded to write down relevant information and keep notes
- The SLP has test protocols to follow during the assessment

Comments: _____

Interaction

- The SLP is present
- The interpreter asks questions immediately as needed
- The SLP takes notes

Observing Relevant Client Behaviors

- Perseveration, short attention span, distractibility
- Needs repetition and cuing
- Uses more gestures than words to express ideas
- Has difficulty with expressive language (pauses, hesitations, delays in responding, reauditorization, short answers)
- Benefits from various strategies such as repetition, modeling, or breaking down information

Comments on other behaviors observed: _____

_____

Noting Relevant Interpreter Behaviors

- Uses appropriate nonverbal communication
- Gives clear instructions
- Provides adequate amount of reinforcement
- Cues or prompts for the client were appropriate

- Takes notes
- Asks for information from the SLP when needed

Comments: _____

Debriefing

- Client's responses are reviewed
- Interpreter relates what the client should or should not have said in response to specific questions
- Any difficulties in the process are reviewed
- Language sample is documented, annotated, and reviewed

Comments: _____

Source: Langdon and Cheng (2002).

It is highly recommended that a language sample be taken in one or two different contexts as suggested previously. In either case, it is important for you and the SLP to develop a sequenced list of the various tests and activities that you will be using as a guide in the testing.

Interaction

During testing, the SLP should follow along on another copy of the test protocol to gain a general sense of the information being collected if it is in a language that he or she might read. If not, an assessment plan, which lists a sequenced list of various tests and activities, should be helpful in following your lead. The SLP may write down observations about the body language of the client and your reaction to the client or make notations when you may have appeared to use too many

words while providing instructions, to misuse reinforcement, or give too many or inappropriate hints or clues. For example, the SLP may have heard you repeat the instructions when you were not supposed to. These notes help the SLP understand the client's performance more fully and will help him or her provide valuable feedback to you.

You should record all responses, take notes, and immediately ask for clarification when questions arise. Be honest and observant when unsure of what to do next. For example, ask the SLP what to do when the client gives you an answer that might be acceptable but is not included in the list of possible responses.

You may interrupt the testing process from time to time to inform the SLP about the client's progress. Make interruptions at appropriate times to minimize disrupting the client's concentration. These interruptions help the SLP stay informed about the entire procedure. When interrupting, make sure the client understands what is happening.

You and the SLP must keep in mind that a client may not respond in the first language because of language loss or lack of experience with the particular task or vocabulary when hearing it in the first language. Therefore, when in doubt, read-minister the items in English. Here is the advantage of using tests that adhere to the idea of conceptual scoring, where you can take into account responses in two languages. This is only possible for Spanish and English thus far, as reviewed for specific tests listed in Chapter 6. Please read on pages 141 to 142 of Chapter 6, which states the following information: Four recently published tests that are norm-referenced—the Expressive One-Word Picture Vocabulary Test (Bilingual) (Martin, 2012a) and the Receptive One-Word Picture Vocabulary Test (Bilingual) (Martin, 2012b), the Preschool Language Scales Fifth Edition Spanish (PLS-5 Spanish) (Zimmerman, Steiner, & Pond, 2012), and the Bilingual English-Spanish Assessment (BESA) (Peña, Gutiérrez-Clellen, Iglesias, Goldstein, & Bedore, 2014)—are scored using the principle of *conceptual scoring*. Specifically, the child's total score compiles performance in the two languages. It includes all items in both Spanish and English. For example, on the PLS-5 Spanish version, the child is allowed to complete the items that were not answered in Spanish using English, thus yielding a more accurate score of the child's general language competence. On the BESA, scores in each language may be compared on the various subtests to determine which ones were performed better and in which language. If the SLP wishes to have normative data on language samples in English and Span-

ish, he or she may administer the English version and then request the I/T to administer the Spanish-available version.

Also, it is not unusual for a bilingual client to *code-switch* (i.e., to use two languages in the same response or to respond to a question using the alternate language), as I noted previously in Chapter 2, pages 43 to 44. This type of response should be documented and analyzed at the end of the assessment by the SLP with your assistance. It may not signal that the client has a language disability. Generally, a bilingual assessment is completed best if each language is tested first during different segments of one session or during two different sessions. If the client does not respond in the first language, readminister the item in the other language once the session is completed. Observations about the client's behavioral responses may be recorded using Table 9–1.

Debriefing

You and the SLP should compare the client's responses to the target responses suggested in the protocol or manual, noting which were correct and what types of errors the client made. If necessary, provide the SLP with relevant cultural and linguistic information that may have influenced the client's performance on specific items, such as lack of appropriate terms in the target language or possible unfamiliarity with particular objects or activities. Discuss deviations from the standard administration, your impressions, and any difficulties related to the interpreting process.

If you administered materials that you prepared, review the responses and their accuracy. Determine with the help of the

Table 9–1. *Observation of the Client During Testing*

Can the client follow oral and written directions as expected?
Is the client easily distracted by noise or visual stimuli? How sustained is the client's attention?
Does the client perform with greater ease when the input is shorter, repeated, or rephrased?
Does the client need more time to respond?
Does the client perform better when visual cues or pictures are provided?
Does auditory cuing aid in expression or recall of information (for example, saying the first sound or syllable of a word, as in "na" for "narrow")?
Does the client's performance improve with more practice?
Can the client respond with greater ease when examples are provided?
Can the client retain newly acquired information (for example, provide an answer to a question at the beginning of the session and probe to determine if the client can recall it in the middle or the end of the session)?

Source: Langdon (2002).

SLP the type of errors that were made, and in all cases discuss the behaviors that you observed. After transcribing the language sample, review all of the different areas as described on pages 223 to 224 in this chapter.

The SLP makes the final determination about the client's communication profile, but your input is important to substantiate the SLP's observations. For example, you may indicate that the client used many sentences that were ungrammatical or that he or she was also difficult to understand because of many articulation difficulties. However, you may indicate that, overall, your impression was that the client's comprehension skills were adequate. But, it is up to the SLP to decide the impact and importance of this aspect in judging the client's overall communication skills.

ACTIVITIES TO PRACTICE ASSESSMENT PROCEDURES

Standardized Test

In this segment, you are going to practice using the Listening to Paragraphs subtest of the Clinical Evaluation of Language Fundamentals (CELF-4) (Wiig, Semel, & Secord, 2006) to respond to the questions written in Table 6–2, on page 151.

1. Assign team members to role-play an assessment session. You will need an interpreter, a client, and an SLP. One or more may be assigned as observers/evaluators of the process. To assist in conducting the observation, use items from Table 9–1.

2. Role players prepare and practice your interactions, referring to the manual instructions, the test's individual administration form, and the items listed in Box 9–1.
3. Review the questions in Table 9–1 while you become familiar with the subtest.
4. Team members role-play BID procedures while observers/evaluators use the checklist to note the performance of the role players. Follow the items to consider in Box 9–1.
5. Role players and observers/educators discuss how well the BID procedures matched the checklist and how well the test administration procedures were followed.

IEP for Ana

This activity can be divided into two segments. The first segment will provide practice sharing the results of a written report on a bilingual speech and language assessment (Spanish and English) of a 10-year-old girl; the second segment will serve as practice in developing goals for her.

Sharing Information About an Assessment (Conference)

Assign a specific role for an SLP, a Spanish-speaking parent, and a bilingual Spanish-English-speaking interpreter. One or more individuals can be assigned as observers/evaluators. Use Ana's case (see Box 9–2) to practice this activity. Follow the protocol proposed in Table 8–1, page 204.

Developing Goals and Objectives

At the end of the report on Ana, there is a section for the team to develop goals and objectives. This is a good opportunity for the SLP to plan some of these goals and objectives prior to meeting with the interpreter and then the parent. The SLP will develop some of these goals and objectives ahead of time, and as required by law, they will have to be discussed and modified during the parent meeting/IEP conference. This is a good opportunity for everyone in training to create the elements of the conference. Again, you may want to use Table 8–1 to ensure that all steps are followed during the meeting.

Sharing Results About the Results of an Audiological Test

Use Box 9–3 where YYY is a 20-year-old individual who is primarily a speaker of ZZZ attending junior college with a hearing complaint, and role-play a conference in which an audiologist will share his or her results with YYY using the services of an interpreter. Select a language where the audiologist may have a list of words to determine SRT and WRT. Use the protocol proposed in Table 8–1. Two additional cases, both conducted with an interpreter, Ali (Speech and Language Assessment Report Conducted With the Assistance of an Interpreter), and Samantha (Audiological Assessment Report Conducted With the Assistance of an Interpreter), can be found in Boxes 5–1 on page 121 and 5–2 on page 126 for your further practice.

BOX 9–2. ANA: SPEECH AND LANGUAGE REPORT

Background Information

Ana is a 10-year-old (9:9) bilingual Spanish-English speaking child who lives with her parents and two younger siblings, aged 5 and 3. Her family is originally from Michoacán, a state neighboring Mexico City. She was raised by her maternal grandparents beginning at the age of 6 months; after 5 years, she was reunited with her parents in the United States.

Ana attended kindergarten in Arizona but moved in the middle of that year when her parents found better jobs in California. She is in the fourth grade in a school where her mother works in the school cafeteria. Ana has learned English quite well, but she is behind in reading. All of her schooling has been in English. Ana has always attended the same school. Her teachers voiced no concerns until this year because she was able to complete her work and because previous teachers attributed some of her difficulties only to her bilingualism.

Ana speaks Spanish to her parents and some relatives who live nearby, but she talks to her siblings in both English and Spanish. Her parents insist that only Spanish should be spoken at home.

Mrs. S., Ana's mother, reported that she herself attended only elementary school in Mexico and could not continue her studies because she had to work to help her family. She is taking classes to improve her English and plans to go back to school to eventually receive a high school equivalency diploma. Mr. S. completed high school in Mexico and is attending a community college to be trained as a mechanic. He is working in an auto shop. Both parents are eager to see their children achieve in school.

Ana's parents read newspapers, magazines, and some books in Spanish. They visit the library every week and encourage their children to take out books in both Spanish and English as well as tapes and movies. The family watches TV together and goes to different places on the weekends—places such as the flea market, amusement parks, and restaurants.

No health or developmental difficulties were reported. Ana's parents indicated that even though they had not seen her for a long time, she had had no ear problems or infections that they were aware of. Since she has lived with them, she has had no health issues. The last school vision and hearing screening was unremarkable.

Assessment Procedure

Ms. HWL, a bilingual Spanish-English speech-language pathologist, evaluated Ana. In addition to administering tests in Spanish, Mrs. HWL supplemented the school SLP's English evaluation to obtain results in equivalent language areas.

The assessment began in Spanish and ended in English, as one language was assessed at a time. However, if Ana responded in the other language, her responses were acknowledged. The following materials were used to assess Ana's speech, language, and communication in Spanish and English.

1. Bilingual Syntax Measure (BSM-I)
2. Bilingual Receptive One-Word Picture Vocabulary Test (ROWPVT)
3. Bilingual Expressive One-Word Picture Vocabulary Test (EOWPVT)
4. Clinical Evaluation of Language Fundamentals (CELF-4) (Spanish and English versions) (selected subtests)
5. A language sample taken during informal conversation. In addition, Ana was asked to make up a story in each language using a wordless book: Mayer's (1975) *One Frog Too Many*
6. Brigance (Spanish and English): Reading Decoding and Reading of Paragraphs
7. Informal writing tasks

Classroom Observation

Ana was briefly observed in her classroom. The students were asked to answer questions from their social studies book. Ana worked with an assigned peer. The classroom teacher worked with the pair to ensure that they understood the assignment. Ana copied her friend's answers using very neat but labored handwriting.

During the Assessment

During the one-on-one interaction, Ana did not have difficulty transitioning from task to task or language to language. Initially, she did not say very much, as it took her some time to feel at ease in interacting with the clinician. Overall, she seemed to enjoy the individual attention; this was noted by her smiling. She seemed to try her best, and often she asked if she was doing well.

It was easier for Ana when questions were paired with pictures and when she did not have to elaborate on her answers. For example, she formulated responses on the BSM and the Formulated Sentences subtests (CELF-4) much faster. More hesitations and repetitions of words or phrases were noted when she had to narrate a story using the wordless book. These hesitations were more prevalent in English. This is not unusual for a second-language learner. However, persons working with Ana need to continue using visual aids and allow her to take time to respond.

Results and Discussion

Ana's performance in each language must be interpreted by taking into account the fact that her exposure to each language has been varied and contextually different. Specifically, her formal exposure to English began in kindergarten. She communicates in Spanish with her family and in both languages with peers and siblings. The reader must also remember that her performance in Spanish may not be as strong in some areas due to language loss. For example, it was difficult to elicit the conditional tense from her in Spanish. This is one of the last grammatical forms that appear in a child's speech and the first one to be lost once the language is not used as often.

Results of the CELF-4 in each language need to be interpreted with care as well. The English version was standardized on monolingual English-speaking students; the Spanish was standardized on bilingual Spanish/English-speaking children in the United States.

TEST/TASK	Spanish	English
BSM-1	RS: 15/18 Level 5-Proficient	RS: 16/18 Level 5-Proficient
ROWPVT Bilingual	RS: 63 SS: 74 34th percentile	
EOWPVT Bilingual	RS: 64 SS: 101 53rd percentile	
CELF-4	Spanish	English
Recalling Sentences	RS: 62 SS: 9 37th percentile	RS: 42 SS: 6 9th percentile
Paragraph Comprehension	RS: 6 SS: 8 25th percentile	RS: 8 SS: 7 16th percentile
Formulated Sentences	RS: 32 SS: 10 50th percentile	RS: 37 SS: 9 37th percentile
Word Associations	RS: 28 Met criterion.	RS: 24 Did not meet criterion.
Rapid Automatic Naming	Could not be completed because Ana could not recall the names of the figures in either language. Training did not help her recall the names of the figures. She could perform the color sequences in both languages, but at a lower speed in each language.	
Phonological Awareness	RS: 35 Does not meet criteria. Difficulty is indicated for this area.	RS: 50 Does not meet criteria. Difficulty is indicated for this area.
SAMPLE Wordless Book: *One Frog Too Many*	Total: 24 sentences Nine compound sentences joined with mostly *y*, *porque*, and *que*	Total: 24 sentences Eight compound sentences joined with mostly *and*, *after*, and *because*.
Brigance Reading	About primer level—less fluent Read 7/10 words at primer.	About primer level—more fluent Read 8/10 words at primer.

Ana maintained the same language of interaction as the clinician and communicated in both languages with almost equal ease. She appeared more confident telling a story (narrative) in English (even though more hesitations and repetitions of words and phrases were noted) than in Spanish. She has definitely reached the Basic Interpersonal Communication Skills level in English (BICS) and is beginning to acquire more academic language in English (CALP)—but at a much slower pace as compared with her peers.

Language Comprehension and Processing

Ana had no difficulty comprehending information presented during a conversation in Spanish or English. However, she had more difficulty remembering information when asked questions in Spanish about orally presented short paragraphs (CELF-4—Paragraph Comprehension subtest); there was less difficulty when the same task was administered in English. Ana missed several vocabulary words on the ROWPVT. She was unfamiliar with words such as *reflection, eruption, protection,* and *injury* (in both languages). These words are generally learned through academic experience and reading.

Short-term memory/processing difficulties were noted when Ana was asked to repeat sentences of various length and complexity in either Spanish or English. However, she had somewhat less difficulty in Spanish, but her overall performance was weak.

In summary, Ana's comprehension skills in both languages are adequate during conversation. She has more difficulty when she needs to respond to more abstract information or novel information, where she cannot depend on contextual clues.

Language Expression

At first Ana was somewhat reluctant to converse with the clinician. As she began to feel more comfortable, she was willing to share personal information and continue the clinician's conversation. Comments provided below pertain to both languages.

Pragmatics. Ana was able to maintain the topic of conversation. She was also comfortable initiating and expanding on topics presented during the evaluation. For example, she described how her family took a trip to the beach in Acapulco (she spoke Spanish). She switched from one language to the other with no hesitation. She could use the two languages for various purposes, for example, to denote cause and effect as in: Spanish, *"Ya después el niño estuvo contento porque la rana regresó"* ("And then the boy was happy because the frog came back"), or in English ("The boy was sad because he couldn't find his frog").

Grammar/Syntax. Ana used sentences that varied in length and complexity in each language depending on the context. Some typical sentences in Spanish included: "*Y ya después el niño llegó a su casa y se fue subiendo a su cuarto*" ("And then the boy arrived at his home and he went upstairs to his room"), and "*El otro con el que se iba a casar lo abandonó porque se iba a morir*" ("The other one, the one whom she was going to marry, she left him because he was going to die"). While Ana's grammar and syntax was more correct (not surprisingly—in Spanish), she made occasional errors in English such as using the incorrect form of the past ("They fall down" and "The boy tooked"). These errors are usual for early second-language learners but should not be present in the language of students who have had as much exposure to English as Ana has.

Vocabulary/Content. In Spanish, Ana used words like *abandonó* (abandoned) while describing a fragment of a TV show. She could label items and concepts such as *statue* and *footsteps* and identify the map of the United States. When she did not know the label, she would define the use of the item to some extent. For example, when naming a telescope, she said, "to see things." She was unable to remember the word for *shield* and called it *knight*, saying, "*We have those here in school.*" Ana's vocabulary appeared more restricted and she hesitated more while expressing detailed ideas in English. Thus, she repeated words or phrases while searching for terms to express her ideas.

Ana's voice appeared hoarse. She denied having a cold or abusing her voice. The clinician did not have a chance to ask her mother if her voice has the same quality. It is advised that she be checked again. In case of doubt, a referral to an ENT is indicated.

Academic Skills

Ana could not say the alphabet in order in Spanish, but she could in English. She knows most of the days of the week in both languages. She can answer questions about which day was *yesterday, tomorrow, before yesterday, and after tomorrow* in both languages. She does not know the months of the year. She seemed very confused when asked to detect sounds in various positions of words in either language—except for initial-position sounds. She had difficulty blending and segmenting words. It was very difficult to explain to her the meaning behind the concept of rhyming. The RAN (Rapid Automatic Naming) could not be completed because she could not recall all of the shapes in either language despite being trained by the clinician. On this test, the client is timed as she is asked to name a sequence of colored circles, followed by a sequence of colored shapes, and finally, a sequence of combinations of different colors and shapes like "blue circle, green triangle, etc." Assessing this skill provides information on speed and accuracy that relates to reading where different symbols in the form of sequences letters representing words need to be recognized accurately and at a certain speed.

Ana is currently reading at about the primer level in both languages. She feels more confident reading in English. When she reads, she can remember the words she has not been able to identify previously, and she is also reading with comprehension. She does not guess a word but tries to decipher it so that it makes sense in relation to the rest of what she reads.

She is also more willing to write and spell words in English than in Spanish. She can write words like *pizza, book, brown, stop,* and *baby.* She misspelled words like *shoe* (sho) and *grass* (gras).

Summary

Ana is an almost 10-year-old bilingual Spanish/English-speaking student who was referred by her teacher in fourth grade because of concerns about her progress with academic subjects (primarily reading). She has received some tutoring, but very limited progress has been noted. All of her instruction has been in English.

Ana cooperated and attended well during the one-on-one interaction with this clinician. She appeared to try her best and seemed to enjoy the one-on-one interaction. Results of this assessment indicate that Ana's Basic Communication Skills (BICS) are fairly intact in both languages but that she has occasional difficulty in using grammar in English. However, she has underlying difficulties with working memory and processing that are evident in both languages. These difficulties are more pronounced in English than in Spanish. Ana experiences challenges with recall of auditory information, phonemic awareness, and comprehension of information when she has to rely on auditory processing, which is weak. She performs much better when visual support is provided (Formulating Sentences). Even though she can express herself fairly well, the vocabulary words sampled on a test like the ROWPVT revealed limited vocabulary in both languages. The gap is most likely due to lack of exposure to and experience in reading to learn new material.

Ana was able to talk about different topics, and her grammar usage in Spanish was adequate, but errors were noted in English. Her BICS skills are adequate, but not her CALP, due to difficulty with processing auditory information and lack of phonological awareness skills. These challenges have impacted her ability to acquire reading fluency skills. Her challenges do not reflect a second-language acquisition problem but signal a language-learning disability that is apparent in Spanish and more so in English. The prognosis for her progress is good (if she obtains adequate instruction) because she has been able to maintain some of her skills in Spanish, even though she uses the language only at home and only for certain purposes.

Developing Goals and Objectives

1. Ana needs to have some goals written for speech and language intervention. Write two goals with two objectives and support your goals with your prior knowledge.
2. What other educational services does she need?
3. What suggestions do you have for her teacher?
4. What suggestions do you have for her family?

BOX 9–3. YYY, A 20-YEAR-OLD PRIMARILY SPEAKING XXX LANGUAGE WITH A HEARING COMPLAINT

YYY is a 20-year-old primarily XXX speaker who is attending junior college. He only came to the United States six month ago and he/she still prefers interacting in his/her home language for topics that are medically related. YYY has always had a hearing difficulty that prevented him/her from hearing easily, but he/she was able to get by without any hearing aids. There is no history of hearing loss or impairment in his/her family. As a child, he/she never had any ear infections. He/she expresses him/herself clearly in XXX, but sibilants are slightly distorted, and there is a somewhat monotonous rhythm and loudness quality to his speech.

Audiological data indicated a mild to moderate hearing loss in both ears with SRT levels of 45 dB (right ear) and 40 dB (left ear). WRT was at 86% in the right ear and 62% in the left ear. Tympanograms were normal.

The diagnosis was a sensorineural hearing loss, probably cochlear of unknown etiology. The audiologist counseled him/her to consider a hearing aid fitting and tried to point out the advantages for his/her use of hearing aids. The patient was advised to consult with a physician to verify the audiologist's findings. The possibility of an FM system was suggested as well.

Source: Adapted from Langdon, H. W. (2002). *Interpreters and translators in communication disorders: A practitioner's handbook* (p. 76). Eau Claire, WI: Thinking Publications.

SELF-ASSESSMENT ITEMS

After studying the information presented in this chapter, review the following items by yourself or with another person who is receiving the same training as you.

1. Why is it important to have the SLP or the audiologist present during an interview? Imagine you have done many of them in another field, and you feel very secure about the process.
2. You have a couple of people who are talking with each other in Eng-

lish while you are interpreting. How would you handle the situation?

3. Imagine you are called to a school where the SLP has never worked with an interpreter, and you have a conference in 5 minutes. How would you handle it?

4. Explain using your own words the reason for not translating tests from English to the language you would be interpreting.

5. Describe how you would use Box 9–1.

6. What would you do if the SLP does not make the test manual available to you prior to your administration of a test? How would you explain your actions to the SLP?

7. What would you do if you began talking to a client in his or her first language, which is reportedly his or her preferred language, and he or she speaks to you in English instead? How would you interact with the SLP about this?

8. There are no tests in your language, and your SLP is recommending that you use some activities that will be difficult for the child because he or she has never been to school. How would you approach the SLP about this issue?

9. Describe three strategies you would use to learn and practice skills for eliciting a valid language sample.

10. You explained to the client he or she is supposed to listen to very faint/quiet sounds, and he or she raises his hand inappropriately. Do you have any ideas of what you would recommend to the audiologist?

REFERENCES

Individuals with Disabilities Improvement Act. (2004). *Act of 2004.* Publ .L.No.108-446.

Langdon, H. W. (2002). *Interpreters and translators in communication disorders: A practitioner's handbook.* Eau Claire, WI: Thinking Publications.

Langdon, H. W., & Cheng, L.-R. L. (2002). *Collaborating with interpreters and translators: A guide for communication disorders professionals.* Eau Claire, WI: Thinking Publications.

Martin, N. (2012a). *Expressive One-Word Picture Vocabulary Test (Bilingual) (EOWPVT 4-BE).* Greenville, SC: Super Duper Publications.

Martin, N. (2012b). *Receptive One-Word Picture Vocabulary Test (Bilingual) (ROWPVT 4-BE).* Greenville, SC: Super Duper Publications.

McLeod, S., & Verdon, S. (2014). A review of 30 speech assessments in 19 languages other than English. *American Journal of Speech-Language Pathology, 23,* 708–723.

Peña, E., Gutiérrez-Clellen, V., Iglesias, A., Goldstein, B., & Bedore, L. (2014). *Bilingual English-Spanish Assessment (BESA).* San Rafael, CA: A-R Publications.

Wiig, E. H., Semel, E., & Secord, W. A. (2006). *Clinical Evaluation of Language Fundamentals, Fourth Edition Spanish (CELF-4 Spanish).* San Antonio, TX: Pearson.

Zimmerman, I. L., Steiner, V. G., & Pond, R. E. (2012). *Preschool Language Scales–Fifth Edition Spanish (PLS-5 Spanish).* San Antonio, TX: Pearson.

Chapter 10

Evaluation and Outcome of the Process

Henriette W. Langdon

This chapter includes the following:

- Techniques for you and the speech-language pathologist (SLP) or the audiologist to provide feedback to each other regarding your collaboration
- Ways to gain feedback from the client or a family member regarding the interpreting and translating process during his or her interaction with you and the SLP or the audiologist
- A method for self-evaluating your performance following an interpreting or translating session

The information presented in Part II and training provided by an agency of the SLP or audiologist are just the first step in your continuing education. This final short chapter provides tools you can use to help identify ways to improve the collaboration process with other professionals and areas in which you need further study or practice.

You may use the assessment of oral and written language to develop prac-tice activities or to anticipate questions that may be presented at an interview for an interpreter or translator position, or use some of the questions suggested in the guide for the SLP or audiologist for practice. It does not mean that you will be asked these same questions but similar ones. Recall that I mentioned on page 93 in Chapter 4 that one of the conditions to be hired is for you to receive a score of 3 suggested by the Foreign Service Institute (FSI) over time. I have also provided suggestions on how to score translations, and you may use those with any of the cases that are presented in the guide. Because I did not include the criteria for scoring translations, I will mention them in one of the sections below.

The evaluation of a collaborator's skills provides a vehicle for the SLP or audiologist to give you feedback on performance during an individual session or over a period of time, and you can provide similar feedback on the effectiveness of the communication disorders professional in his or her collaboration with you. A form can be handed to clients or family members to provide you as a team written feedback on the interpreting services they receive. You can perform your own self-assessment with another copy of the form.

ASSESSMENT OF YOUR ORAL AND WRITTEN PROFICIENCY IN TWO LANGUAGES

As I have mentioned in this guide, the selection and hiring of interpreter and translator candidates should be based on the candidate's oral and written language proficiency in English and the target second language. Some or all of the following components may be used for candidate assessments.

Oral Language Skills

The oral examination is similar to that of the FSI and is based on a scale of 1 to 5, with 3 being the minimum standard accepted to perform a given professional task. Ideally, native speakers of both English and the candidate's target language will interview the candidate. This oral interview may take place in one group session or different sessions for each language. A collection of topics appears in Table 4–4 on page 93.

Translation Skills

You may practice your translation skills by practicing the different sentences suggested under Activities at the end of Chapter 8, page 199. The rubric for scoring translation skills that I propose can be found in Table 4–5 on page 96, along with other activities you may want to use as practice.

EVALUATION OF COLLABORATORS' SKILLS

The collaboration process can improve if key members are evaluated periodically, that is, you and the SLP or audiologist as well. Table 7–3 on page 177 and Table 10–1 are suggested to ensure success in the process.

Evaluation by the Consumer

You may want to request feedback from family members and/or clients, where appropriate, to identify areas needing improvement or topics to pursue for your continuing education. Box 7–4 on page 178 provides a format for clients to use to provide feedback. The SLP or audiologist may want to use this form to collect information regarding each interpreter that has been asked to provide services for the purpose of program improvement.

Self-Assessment

It is important to evaluate yourself to improve your growth. Table 7–4 on page 180 may be helpful to you.

Table 10–1. Evaluation of the SLP/Audiologist's Performance

Key: 1 = Always; 2 = Often; 3 = Sometimes; 4 = Rarely; 5 = Never					
General Behaviors					
1. Does the SLP/audiologist provide sufficient information to prepare the I/T before a job?	1	2	3	4	5
If not sufficient, please indicate what could be improved:					
2. Does the SLP/audiologist debrief with you following a meeting and/or assessment session?	1	2	3	4	5
If not sufficient, please indicate what could be improved:					
3. Does the SLP/audiologist use language forms that are not too difficult to interpret?	1	2	3	4	5
4. Does the SLP/audiologist listen to parents/clients even though he or she may not understand their language?	1	2	3	4	5
5. Does the SLP/audiologist seek your insights about a given culture as a way to facilitate the process to serve the client more fairly?	1	2	3	4	5
6. Is the SLP/audiologist willing to use the suggestions you provide?	1	2	3	4	5
7. Does the SLP/audiologist provide you with the feedback you need to perform your job satisfactorily?	1	2	3	4	5
If not sufficient, please indicate what could be improved:					
8. Does the SLP/audiologist provide you with sufficient resources to perform your job satisfactorily?	1	2	3	4	5
Comments:					

Source: Adapted from Langdon (2002).

CONCLUSION

I hope that the content of Part II will assist you in your interview and on-the-job work. I welcome your comments and suggestions all the time at Henriette.Langdon@sjsu.edu.

REFERENCE

Langdon, H. W. (2002). *Interpreters and translators in communication disorders: A practitioner's handbook.* Eau Claire, WI: Thinking Publications.

Epilogue

Communication is a human right. Human beings use the various languages they have created to communicate among themselves. These languages have evolved over a long time, and they are purposeful as well as meaningful among the users of those languages. But, when wanting to communicate, the same codes must be used to decode and encode the messages that are being conveyed.

Currently, more than 6,000 languages have been identified in the world. Some are different from each other in every way, while others share some similarities such as Italian and Spanish or Polish and Russian. The diversity in using different languages in one single encounter is a common phenomenon occurring not only in the United States but also throughout the entire globe. The challenges we face in working with children and adults from all over the world are enormous. When teachers work with new English-language learners, they are often unable to communicate with the family and the students because they do not share the same language. Communication is broken or sometimes nonexistent. The need for proper interpretation and translation is absolutely paramount.

Our nation is a nation of diversity. Americans come from all over the world. In the past 50 years, we have seen an increase of linguistically and culturally diverse populations in our nation. The influx of Spanish-speaking individuals from south of the border has never stopped. In the mid-1970s, the refugees from Southeast Asia came over to the United States in large numbers (the so-called boat people). Unrest in the Middle East brought to us refugees and immigrants who speak Farsi, Arabic, Dari, and other unfamiliar languages. Most recently, internal unrest and civil wars brought many people from Sudan, the horn of Africa, and other parts of Africa. Immigrants and refugees from the former Soviet Union and current-day Russia have continued since the 1990s. The list goes on and on. Practitioners in speech-language pathology and audiology are on the front line when it comes to assessment of speech, language, and hearing. They need to engage the services of translators and interpreters to facilitate communication with the students, clients, and their families.

The purpose of this guide is to provide some direction for speech-language pathologists (SLPs) and audiologists to train interpreters/translators (I/Ts) in order to solve this problem. The coauthors of this guide, Henriette W. Langdon and Terry Irvine Saenz, both have significant experience in dealing with children and adults from linguistically and culturally diverse families. In this guide, they attempt to answer the following questions and dilemmas: How can we serve the children and their families when we do not know the language they speak? What can we do to improve the quality of communication between the professionals and the families? How can we ensure that communication is effective?

Although many clinicians (both monolingual and bilingual) are bilingual personnel who could perform as I/Ts, they do not have appropriate training on how to work effectively with SLPs or audiologists, and potential interpreters are often not trained to work in our professions. The responsibility often rests on the SLP or audiologist to provide this training. Therefore, having access to the content of this book will provide important current best practices in working effectively with interpreters and translators in the communication disorders field.

In this guide, the authors have laid out the ingredients for a successful process, adding their collective insight known among interpreters/translators in the phrase "lost in translation." Clearly, it is very difficult to translate and/or interpret the meaning of a speaker or a writer from one language to the other. The authors tried to include all the elements that need to be considered when working with an interpreter face-to-face. They stress the importance of evidence-based practice and look for substantive documentation and validation in this dynamic process. They draw upon their many years of research and practice to present the content of this book. They also updated the many research papers in the literature pro-

viding a wealth of information for readers. In addition to presenting the proper process of using an I/T in the assessment of linguistic competence, they are also very cognizant of the significance of discourse analysis. They understand the notion of difficult discourse in human communication. They reviewed the concepts of basic interpersonal communication skills (BICS) and cognitive academic language proficiency (CALP) also referred to as Conversational Informal Language Fluency (CILF) and Formal Academic Language Fluency (FALF).

Overall, the authors manage to present a fair and current picture of the state of the art of interpretation/translation. Many years ago, a few colleagues and I got together, and we proposed a model of assessment, namely, the RIOT approach. This concept includes the process of to review, to interview, to observe, and to test. The RIOT concept was mentioned in this book in detail and indeed represents a best practice model for practitioners.

It gives me great pleasure to have a chance to review this guide, and I had a great time reading the manuscript. I am honored to be able to write this epilogue for the authors, both of whom I have known for many decades, and I admire their work and resilience. Indeed, this is an important contribution to the speech and hearing field. This guide fills the gap of knowledge between working with monolingual English speakers and multilingual families. Happy reading!

—Li-Rong Lilly Cheng, PhD,
   H-CCC-SLP
   Managing Director of Confucius
      Institute, SDSU
   Professor Emerita, School of
      Speech Language and Hearing
      Sciences, SDSU

Glossary

With today's availability of the Internet, definitions can be easily found for many terms. However, I feel definitions of some basic terms in our profession might be helpful to begin with.

Accent. Phonetic traits of an individual's speech.

Acoustic gain. A ratio of the output power or input power (gain = output – input).

Acoustic impedance. Measurable contraction of the tympanic membrane in response to a tone.

Adaptive behavior. Effectiveness of the individual in adjusting to the natural and social demands of his or her environment.

Affective. Related to the emotions and feelings of a person.

Air conduction. Transmission of sounds to the inner ear through the external auditory canal and the structure of the middle ear.

American Sign Language (ASL). The language of the deaf community in the United States. ASL has its own system in all areas of language form, content, and use.

Aptitude test. A test that measures capacity, abilities, or talent for learning something.

Articulation. The way in which sounds are produced during speech.

Audiogram. A chart that shows an individual's hearing capacity. Sensitivity to sound conducted in the air and by the ear bones can be shown on this chart.

Audiologist. A specialist who identifies and measures hearing loss and also helps in the rehabilitation of those with hearing disabilities by recommending specific hearing aids or devices.

Audiometric evaluation. An evaluation of an individual's hearing sensitivity and acuity.

Auditory brainstem response (ABR). A test that helps determine the site of a lesion to the cochlea, the brainstem, or the auditory nerve (VIII cranial nerve).

Auditory cuing. Any strategy, such as stress, pitch, or intonation, that may assist in enhancing communication.

Auditory memory. The ability to recall information that is presented auditorily.

Auditory processing. The ability to make full use of what is heard and includes the ability to discriminate, analyze, and associate what is heard.

Augmentative and alternative communication (AAC). Any approach to support, enhance, or supplement the communication of individuals who are not independent verbal communicators. It may use approaches such as picture boards and computer-assisted devices.

Autism. Abnormality in interpersonal relationships exhibited in early childhood. The effect on language development is variable. Reactions include resistance to change and possible peculiar interest in or attachment to animate or inanimate objects.

Back translation. Translation of a document from a second language into the original language. For example, French to English and English back to French to check accuracy of the translation.

Basal. In testing, the lowest level at which testing is initiated on a given set of items.

Basic interpersonal communication skills (BICS). Term introduced by Cummins (1981, 1984) defining the level of an individual's language ability as it is related to communicating in daily situations or situations that are highly contextualized, meaning that he or she can understand them because they are immediate, within his or her experiences.

Behavior modification. A process based on the belief that every behavior is learned and, consequently, must be unlearned. One must decide specifically which behaviors should be changed and how to make the changes in a definite way.

Behind the ear (BTE). A certain type of hearing aid that is worn behind the ear.

Body language. Nonverbal features of communication, including gestures, facial expressions, and body language.

Bone conduction. Transmission of sound to the inner ear through vibration applied to the bones of the skull. It

allows determination of the cochlea's hearing sensitivity while bypassing any middle ear abnormalities.

Ceiling. In testing, the highest level at which an individual gives a response.

Central auditory processing disorder (CAPD). Difficulty in discriminating speech resulting in an inability to process the information, even when there is no loss of hearing sensitivity.

Cerumen. Earwax.

Cleft lip or palate. A space or opening that may occur in the lip and/or hard palate. It is a congenital condition.

Cochlea. The coiled tube in the inner ear that contains the sensory cells for hearing.

Cochlear implant. An electronic device that is implanted in the cochlea to stimulate hearing.

Code-switching. Alternating use of two languages at the word, phrase, or sentence level with a complete break between languages in phonology.

Cognitive ability. The act of the process of knowing. It is the ability to think in a logical and analytical form (used interchangeably with *intelligence*).

Cognitive academic language proficiency (CALP). Term introduced by Cummins (1981, 1984) differentiating the level of an individual's language ability as it relates to performing tasks that are academic in nature.

Completely in the canal (CIC). A certain type of hearing aid that fits inside the ear and is barely visible.

Conductive hearing loss. A loss of hearing sensitivity caused by damage to the outer and/or middle ear.

Congenital. A disorder that occurs at birth or early in the developmental period.

Conversational Informal Language Fluency (CILF). Type of language used in conversations and environments that are contextually based.

Craniofacial anomalies. Malformation of the cranium (skull) and facial areas.

Criterion-reference test. A test that assesses the ability to perform a certain skill. For example, such a test could include the ability to read paragraphs of certain length and complexity, the ability to comprehend directions, or the ability to write definitions of specific words.

Cuing. Any strategy that will enhance a correct response (visual or auditory or gesture).

Decibel. Measurement of the intensity of a sound, abbreviated as dB.

Dialectal variation. Variation in the pronunciation, word usage, and even grammar and syntax within a given language.

Disfluency. Interruptions of the flow of speech sounds marked by repetitions, prolongations, or hesitations.

Distractibility. Difficulty paying attention.

Dominance. The language that is predominantly used or is more easily used by an individual exposed to two languages. Attention needs to be given to a particular area of language. Sometimes a bilingual individual may be more dominant in speaking in one language but in reading and writing in another.

Dynamic assessment. Assessment of an individual's skills using various methods to enhance his or her performance through repetition of information presented, demonstration of examples, or simplification of the information.

Dysarthria. A motor speech disorder due to impairment originating in the central or peripheral nervous system.

Dysphagia. Difficulty swallowing, which may include inflammation, compression, paralysis, weakness, or hypertonicity of the esophagus.

Endoscopy. Refers to the examination of the interior of a canal or hollow space.

Ear mold. A fitting usually made of plastic and fitting in the auricle of the ear. Designed to conduct amplified sound waves from the receiver of a hearing aid.

Eventcast. Refers to the use of language to describe events or information.

Expressive language. Communication through the use of oral or written words.

Fine motor coordination. The ability to use minor muscular groups, such as for writing or cutting.

Fluency. Absence of hesitations or repetition during speech.

FM system. One of several possible assistive listening devices to increase reception of information presented auditorily.

Formal Academic Language Fluency (FALF). Language that is used in more academically related contexts, generally of more abstract nature.

Free appropriate public education (FAPE). The right of all children in the United States by federal law to receive free general and special education services.

Frequency. Number of repetitions of compressions and rarefactions of a sound wave that occur at the same rate over a period of time. Expressed in hertz (Hz). For example, a vibration of 125 Hz consists of 125 cycles per second.

Grammar. Principles or rules for speaking or writing according to the form and usage of a language.

Gross motor coordination. The ability to use major muscular groups, such as for jumping or running.

Hearing aid. An electronic amplifying device to bring sound more effectively into the listener's ear. Consists of a microphone, amplifier, and receiver.

Idiom. An utterance that has a hidden meaning (e.g., *out to lunch*).

Idiomatic expression. A part of speech that includes an idiom.

Individual education program (IEP). An individual education plan written to meet the special education needs of students 3 to 21 years of age.

Individual family service plan (IFSP). An individual education plan written to meet the developmental needs of a child aged birth to 3 years.

Individuals With Disabilities Education Act (IDEA). Federal law passed in 1997 to ensure educational access and fair assessment and intervention for students experiencing a variety of learning difficulties.

Intelligence. Aggregate capacity to act purposefully, think rationally, and deal effectively with the environment, especially in relation to the extent of perceived effectiveness in meeting challenges. Used interchangeably with cognitive ability.

Intelligibility. Ability to be comprehensible while communicating with someone orally.

Interpreting. Transmitting a message from one language to another orally.

In the canal (ITC). A specific type of hearing aid that fills the outer part of the ear canal.

In the ear (ITE). A specific type of hearing aid that is worn in the ear.

Jargon language. Verbal behavior of children beginning at about 9 months and ceasing at about 18 months. It includes a variety of syllables that are inflected that approximate meaningful connected speech in advanced stages; some true words may be heard.

Language. Any accepted structured symbolic system for interpersonal communication composed of sounds arranged in ordered sequence to form words. Includes rules for combining words into sequences that express thoughts, intentions, expression, and feelings. Composed of phonological, morphological, syntactical, and semantic components.

Language loss. A regression of skills in an individual's first language as a result of a lack of opportunity to use the language or forgetting some of it. It is frequent in individuals who use more than one language at a time. A loss that is very rapid may indicate a language disorder.

Language sampling. A manually gathered or taped sample of an individual's consecutive utterances during an interaction (e.g., telling a story) or a conversation on various topics.

Learning disability. A significant difficulty with the acquisition and use of one or more of the following abilities: listening, speaking, reading, writing, mathematical computation, or mathematical problem solving.

Lexicon. Vocabulary of a language.

Marriage and family therapist (MFT). Diagnoses and treats mental and emotional disorders, whether cognitive, affective, or behavioral, within the context of marriage and family systems. Applies psychotherapeutic and family systems theories and techniques in the delivery of services to individuals, couples, and families for the purpose of treating such diagnosed nervous and mental disorders.

Mixed hearing loss. A combined conductive and sensorineural hearing loss.

Modality. The way to acquire or receive sensations. Sight, sound, touch, smell, and taste are the common senses.

Morphology. The study of the smallest speech unit that has a differential function: for example, *-s* for plural and *-ed* for past in English.

Multiple meaning word. A word that can have more than one meaning (e.g., *orange*, or *glasses*).

Neurologic examination. Tests to determine if an illness exists or there is damage to the nervous system.

Nodules. Caused by inflammation to the vocal folds, resulting in a generally benign callous-like growth. The nodules are generally paired and located in the midpoint of the vocal folds.

Nonverbal communication. See *paralinguistic*.

Norm. A set standard or pattern derived from a representative sampling of median achievement of a large group (meaning how many are higher or lower within an average). It offers a range of values against which individual comparisons can be made.

Normal curve. A graph (curve) that represents the distribution of performance of a sample that has been normed.

Observations. Recording of behavior or performance.

Occupational therapist. A specialist who helps patients/clients develop useful physical and mental attitudes toward all the areas of daily life.

Oral manometer. An instrument that measures the air blown into a tube to measure the amount of oral pressure that is exerted during respiration.

Oral peripheral examination. A speech-language pathologist examines the structures (and their functions) responsible in the production of speech, such as the lips, tongue, and so on.

Organic disorder. Disorder with a known physical cause.

Other health impairment. Having limited strength, vitality, or alertness, including a heightened alertness to environmental stimuli, that results in limited alertness with respect to the educational environment, that (a) is due to chronic or acute health problems such as asthma, attention-deficit disorder or attention-deficit hyperactivity disorder, diabetes, epilepsy, a heart condition, hemophilia, lead poisoning, leukemia, nephritis, rheumatic fever, sickle cell anemia, and Tourette syndrome and (b) adversely affects a child's educational performance.

Otitis media. Infection of the fluid in the middle ear.

Otoacoustic emissions. Sounds generated within the normal cochlea.

Paralingustic. Includes all nonverbal features used in communication. For example, gestures, facial expression, body posture, speech volume, and intonation (synonymous to *nonverbal communication*).

Percentile. Converted score compared to a ranking based on a normed population. For example, 90th percentile means that only 10% of the population sampled scored higher.

Perception. The process of interpreting sensory information. It consists of the mental association of present stimuli with memories from past experiences.

Performance score. What a person can do without needing to speak or verbalize.

Perseveration. Continuing to behave or to answer in a certain way when it is not appropriate. It is the difficulty in changing from one action, thought pattern, or assignment to another.

Phonology. The study of the sound system of a language, including pauses and stress.

Physical therapist. A specialist who helps clients in the treatment of disorders of bones, joints, muscles, and nerves by means of heat, light, massage, and exercise.

Pitch. Acuteness or gravity of a sound, dependent on the frequency of the vibrations producing it and its intensity.

Polyp. Bulging growth generally appearing on one of the vocal folds and located in the front middle portion of the vocal fold.

Pragmatics. The study of speaker-listener intentions and relations and all elements in the environment surrounding the message.

Proficiency. Referring to the degree to which an individual is fluent in a given language.

Prosthesis. Artificial device, which substitutes for a missing body part.

Protocol. In testing, the sheet that is used to record an individual's responses.

Psychologist. A specialist who studies individuals' thinking and behavior processes. Overall, he or she helps to assess thinking, feeling, and behavior in individuals and also can administer learning, cognitive, behavior, and academic tests.

Psychomotor. Refers to the traction of the muscles, including development of the small muscles (e.g., cutting something) and the large muscles (e.g., walking and jumping).

Radiographic study. An X-ray of a given body part, like the chest, neck, or skull.

Raw score. In testing, the score that is obtained by subtracting total missed items from the ceiling.

Receptive language. Ability to understand spoken (oral) or written communication.

Recount. Retelling a story or event.

Reinforcement. A procedure where a certain stimulus is offered to elicit a response. For example, a student is given verbal or tangible praise when responding to a question or request.

Reliability. Means consistency. It refers to the consistency of scores obtained by the same people when retested with the identical test or with an equivalent form of the test. Should include interscorer/interexaminer and internal consistency measures.

Resonance disorders. Abnormalities in the use of the nasal cavity when speaking. Resonance can be hypernasal (excessive nasality) or denasal (insufficient nasality).

Reverberation. Persistence of a sound in a closed space that results from multiple reflections after the sound has ceased.

Sample transcription. Writing down exactly what the individual says (verbatim).

Scaffolding. Any strategy used to facilitate an individual's comprehension and/or response to a task.

School counselor. School counselors help students develop social skills and succeed in school. They also assist them in making a career decision, by helping them choose a career or educational program.

Self-concept. The idea that a person has about himself or herself.

Self-help skills. Refers to actions such as dressing oneself, eating, and other activities for functioning in the family, in the school, or in the community.

Semantics. Study of the meaning of language, which includes the relationships between language, thought, and behavior.

Sensorineural hearing loss. A hearing loss that stems from damage to any part of the inner ear and/or auditory system.

Social maturity. The ability to take on the social and personal responsibilities that are expected for people of a similar age.

Social worker. Helps people solve and cope with problems in their everyday lives. One group of social workers, clinical social workers, also diagnose and treat mental, behavioral, and emotional issues.

Special education. Special instruction for children who have learning difficulties. These children must have an IFSP or IEP.

Specific language impairment (SLI). Characterized by difficulty with language that is not caused by any known neurological, sensory, intellectual, or emotional deficit. Several areas may be affected such as vocabulary, grammar, morphology, syntax, and receptive and expressive language skills in general.

Specific learning disability. (Federal Definition). (a) General. The term means a disorder in one or more of the basic psychological processes involved in understanding or in using language, spoken or written, that may manifest itself in an imperfect ability to listen, think, speak, read, write, spell, or do mathematical calculations, including conditions such as perceptual disabilities, brain injury, minimal brain dysfunction, dyslexia, and developmental aphasia. (b) Disorders not included. The term does not include learning problems that are primarily the result of visual, hearing, or motor disabilities; of mental retardation; of emotional disturbance; or of environmental, cultural, or economic disadvantage.

Speech. Medium of oral communication that uses a linguistic code (language).

Speech discrimination. Ability to compare sounds with other sounds, nonsense syllables, and monosyllables or multisyllabic words.

Speech reading or lip reading. Using visual cues to determine what is being said.

Speech-language pathologist (SLP). A specialist who works with children and adults in assessment and intervention for speech and/or language problems.

Speech reception threshold (SRT). The level at which a client can repeat correctly 50% of two-syllable words referred to as spondees, like *baseball, doormat, birthday,* or *cowboy.*

Standard score. Derived score obtained by comparing a score to that of a normed population.

Standardized test. A test consisting of specific items that must be administered and scored using a consistent method to compare the results to a normed population. The test must have data on reliability and validity.

Stroboscopy. A method by which an instrument enables one to examine the vibration of the vocal folds.

Stuttering. Disruption in the normal fluency and time patterning of speech.

Syntax. Order of words forming a sentence. The order varies across languages.

Threshold. The lowest intensity necessary to produce an awareness of a stimulus. In the context of audiology, it means the perception of a signal, tone, or word.

Total communication. The use of any method, including finger spelling, singing, speech, or speech reading, to enhance face-to-face communication.

Translating. Transmitting a message from one language to another in writing.

Traumatic brain injury (TBI). An acquired injury to the brain caused by an external force resulting in total or partial functional disability and/or psychosocial impairment that adversely affects an individual's performance. Impairments can be in one or more areas, such as cognition, language speech, memory, attention, reasoning, abstract thinking, judgment, problem solving, physical functioning, and information processing.

Tympanic membrane. The thin concave membrane that separates the external and the middle ear.

Tympanogram. A graph obtained from tympanometry indicating the function of the middle ear.

Tympanometry. Measure of the resistance of the tympanic membrane to various pressure changes.

Validity. Verifies that a test measures what it claims it does and how well it does it.

Verbal performance. The ability to solve problems through the use of language.

Videoendoscopy. The results of an endoscopy that are recorded on video.

Vocal cords or folds. Membranous cords located in the larynx composed of folds. The vocal folds vibrate when air is pushed through the larynx.

Vocal stress. Difficulty in using voice at a normal pitch/loudness.

Voice quality. A description of the voice that is produced by the vibrations of the vocal folds. Quality may be described as hoarse, breathy, or harsh.

Word attack skills. The ability to analyze words, recognizing word endings, prefixes, and root words.

Word recognition test (WRT). A test to determine the intensity at which a given word may be heard.

REFERENCES

Cummins, J. (1981). The role of primary language development in promoting educational success for 140 language minority students. In Office of Bilingual Bicultural Education, California State Department of Education (Ed.), *School and language minority students: A theoretical framework* (pp. 3–49). Los Angeles, CA: Evaluation, Dissemination, and Assessment Center, California State University.

Cummins, J. (1984). *Bilingualism and special education.* Clevedon, UK: Multilingual Matters.

Index

Note: Page numbers in **bold** reference non-text material.